Clinical Gastroenterology

Series Editor

George Y. Wu, University of Connecticut Health Center, Farmington, CT, USA

More information about this series at http://www.springer.com/series/7672

John R. Romanelli · David J. Desilets
David B. Earle
Editors

NOTES and Endoluminal Surgery

Humana Press

Editors
John R. Romanelli
Department of Surgery
University of Massachusetts/Baystate Medical Center
Springfield, MA
USA

David B. Earle
Lowell Surgical Associates
North Chelmsford, MA
USA

David J. Desilets
Division of Gastroenterology
University of Massachusetts/Baystate Medical Center
Springfield, MA
USA

ISSN 2197-7399 ISSN 2197-7704 (electronic)
Clinical Gastroenterology
ISBN 978-3-319-50608-1 ISBN 978-3-319-50610-4 (eBook)
DOI 10.1007/978-3-319-50610-4

Library of Congress Control Number: 2016961663

Printed on acid-free paper

This Springer imprint is published by Springer Nature
The registered company is Springer International Publishing AG
The registered company address is: Gewerbestrasse 11, 6330 Cham, Switzerland

Foreword

In 2004, Dr. Anthony Kalloo and his colleagues introduced a disruptive concept involving passing an endoscope through the wall of the stomach and into the peritoneal cavity in order to perform a gastrojejunostomy. Shortly following this, Drs. Rao and Reddy demonstrated a transgastric appendectomy performed via an endoscope through a patient's mouth. These creative innovations ignited a firestorm of discussion and research in endoscopic surgery.

A group of surgeons and gastroenterologists came together to form the Natural Orifice Surgery Consortium for Assessment and Research (NOSCAR). This group intended that this new concept be introduced with attention to patient safety and careful outcomes assessment.

Industry responded admirably to the needs of the researchers and developed a host of new technologies to facilitate these endeavors. In the research laboratory, new procedures were developed by essentially every surgical specialty and through every natural orifice.

Practical application of the methods was begun under careful institutional review board supervision. Initially, however, results demonstrated the procedures to be somewhat difficult to perform, labor-intensive, and costly. Many were ready to abandon the concept.

Yet, throughout the world, others continued to study and perfect the procedures, gaining great success and acceptance. Additionally, concepts gained from the study of NOTES were adapted to new areas, and single-port surgery and intramural procedures such as per-oral endoscopic myotomy (POEM) emerged.

Today, it seems clear that NOTES is quite alive. New and improved concepts and technology continue to enhance the procedures and expand the applications.

This monograph will serve as an important milestone in documenting the progress and growth of natural orifice surgery and crediting those who have made great contributions to the field.

Jeffrey L. Ponsky, M.D.
Professor of Surgery
Cleveland Clinic Lerner College of Medicine
Case Western Reserve University
Cleveland, OH
USA

Acknowledgements

I would like to thank my wife Kirsten and my children Julia, Justin, and Daniel, for affording me the time to complete this project.

I would like to thank my early surgical mentors, Dr. John K. Edoga and Dr. Demetrius E. M. Litwin, both of whom taught me the value of innovation in the search for better and less invasive therapies to treat disease.

I would like to thank my surgical leaders, Dr. Richard B. Wait and Dr. Neal E. Seymour, for supporting our NOTES research and encouraging us to keep forging ahead.

I would like to thank my co-editors and research partners, Dr. David J. Desilets and Dr. David B. Earle, for their spirit of adventure and for teaching and reinforcing the concept of teamwork.

Lastly, I would like to thank all the authors of this book, without whom there is no project. Good will can only be thanked with true gratitude.

John R. Romanelli

I would like to thank my wife Carla, for putting up with my frequent absences from the family during this project. Without your support, I can do none of the things that I do.

I would like to thank interventional endoscopy mentor, Doug Howell, who taught me the value of persistence, risk-taking, and ignoring naysayers who tell us "it will never work."

I would like to thank my co-editors and research partners, Dr. John Romanelli and Dr. David Earle, for their faith in me and my skills, for their can-do attitude, and for pushing me in directions I did not know I would love.

I would also like to thank the authors of this book, who gave freely of their precious time and effort, and without whom the textbook would not exist. Thank you colleagues. You are the best!

David J. Desilets

I would like to thank my wife Noreen and three daughters, Emily, Lindsey, and Allison, for supporting me to read and write about my life's passion—surgery. I would also like to acknowledge my mentor, Felicien Steichen, M.D., a true surgical innovator, and whose surgical stapling techniques are used worldwide on a daily basis. Dr. Steichen started the Institute of Minimally Invasive Surgery in the mid-1990s, to foster an innovative spirit that thrives today. During the final year of his life, he expressed interest and concern about going through a normal organ to get to a diseased one, yet never tried to stifle the innovation. I would also like to acknowledge John Bookwalter, M.D., another surgeon innovator who also has a daily impact on the global practice of surgery. John has given me much encouragement to help complete this book. And without Richard Wait, M.D., Ph.D., believing in me during and after my training, I would never have had the opportunity to start and run a minimally invasive surgery fellowship and thus the opportunity to co-edit this book. Finally, I would like to thank all the authors and my co-editors, whose collaborative effort will help advance the field of surgery for years to come.

David B. Earle

Note From the Editors

There are two words that factor prominently in this textbook, both of which have multiple spelling options. We chose to simplify with one spelling for each word for the purposes of this text.

NOTES is an acronym trademarked with the US Patent and Trademark Office in January 2007 for the purpose of "promoting training, development and fundraising services for surgical techniques utilizing natural orifices…" The word was spelled as such reflecting the concept of crossing the lumen of a hollow viscus. The "T" in NOTES stands for translumenal, spelled with an "e" in the original white paper published in 2006 and in the trademark application in 2007. This did not follow the form of the word "intraluminal," however, and many authors have reverted to spelling the word "transluminal." We have chosen to largely sidestep this issue by utilizing the acronym NOTES wherever possible. This acronym is widely accepted and understood —a testament to the early thought leaders who chose to codify this new concept with uniformity.

Also, the word "per-oral" is often spelled with and without the hyphen and as one word or two separate ones. We are choosing to use the hyphenated form because, although it was initially spelled without the hyphen by Dr. Inoue, who first published the seminal work on POEM, most publications now routinely use the hyphenated form.

Contents

Contributors

Joseph Ramon Armengol-Miro World Institute for Digestive Endoscopy (WIDER), Barcelona, Spain; Digestive Endoscopy, Vall d'Hebron University Hospital, Barcelona, Spain

Benjamin Babic Agaplesion Markus Krankenhaus, Frankfurt am Main, Germany

Valerio Balassone Department of Surgery, University of Rome Tor Vergata Hospital, Rome, Italy

Todd H. Baron Division of Gastroenterology and Hepatology, University of North Carolina, Chapel Hill, NC, USA

Robert Bechara Division of Gastroenterology, Kingston General Hospital & Queen's University, Kingston, ON, Canada

Vikram Budhraja Gastroenterology Division, Department of Medicine, Baystate Health, Springfield, MA, USA

Majidah A. Bukhari Department of Medicine and Division of Gastroenterology and Hepatology, The Johns Hopkins Medical Institutions, Baltimore, MD, USA; Department of Gastroenterology, Baltimore, MD, USA

Ram Chuttani Department of Medicine and Division of Gastroenterology, Center for Advanced Endoscopy, Beth Israel Deaconess Medical Center, Harvard Medical School, Boston, MA, USA

Jonah Cohen Department of Medicine and Division of Gastroenterology, Center for Advanced Endoscopy, Beth Israel Deaconess Medical Center, Harvard Medical School, Boston, MA, USA

David J. Desilets Division of Gastroenterology, Department of Medicine, Baystate Health, Springfield, MA, USA

Anthony P. D'Andrea Department of Surgery, Division of Colon and Rectal Surgery, Icahn School of Medicine at Mount Sinai, New York, NY, USA

David B. Earle Lowell Surgical Associates, Lowell General Hospital, North Chelmsford, MA, USA

David Friedel Department of Gastroenterology, Hepatology and Nutrition, Winthrop University Hospital, NY, USA

Karl-Hermann Fuchs Agaplesion Markus Krankenhaus, Frankfurt am Main, Germany; Department of Surgery, Agaplesion Markus-Krankenhaus, Frankfurt am Main, Germany

Kevin L. Grimes Department of Surgery, MetroHealth Medical Center and Case Western Reserve University School of Medicine, Cleveland, OH, USA

Oz Harmanli Chief, Yale Urogynecology & Reconstructive Pelvic Surgery, Professor, OB/GYN/RS, Department of OB/GYN/RS, Yale Medical School, New Haven, CT, USA

Jeffrey Hazey Wexner Medical Center, The Ohio State University, Columbus, OH, USA

Santiago Horgan Center for the Future of Surgery, Department of Surgery, University of California at San Diego, San Diego, CA, USA

Haruhiro Inoue Digestive Disease Center, Showa University Koto-Toyosu Hospital, Tokyo, Japan

Garth R. Jacobsen Center for the Future of Surgery, Department of Surgery, University of California at San Diego, San Diego, CA, USA

Erica D. Kane Department of Surgery, Baystate Medical Center, Springfield, MA, USA

Sergey V. Kantsevoy University of Maryland School of Medicine, Baltimore, USA; Therapeutic Endoscopy, Institute for Digestive Health and Liver Diseases, Mercy Medical Center, Baltimore, MD, USA

Mouen A. Khashab Department of Medicine and Division of Gastroenterology and Hepatology, The Johns Hopkins Medical Institutions, Baltimore, MD, USA; Division of Gastroenterology and Hepatology, Johns Hopkins Hospital, Baltimore, MD, USA

Ryan Law Division of Gastroenterology and Hepatology, University of Michigan, Ann Arbor, MI, USA

Shanglei Liu Department of Surgery, UCSD Healthcare Systems, San Diego, CA, USA

John H. Marks Department of Colorectal Surgery, Lankenau Medical Center, Wynnewood, PA, USA

Mersadies Martin Department of Surgery, Kaiser Permanente, San Diego, CA, USA

Rani Modayil Department of Gastroenterology, Hepatology and Nutrition, Winthrop University Hospital, NY, USA

Anil Bernard Nagar Department of Medicine, Section of Digestive Diseases, Yale University, New Haven, CT, USA; VACT Healthcare, West Haven VA Medical Center, West Haven, CT, USA

Peter Nau University of Iowa Hospitals and Clinics, Iowa City, IA, USA

Raymond P. Onders Margaret and Walter Remen Chair of Surgical Innovation, University Hospitals Case Medical Center, Case Western Reserve University School of Medicine, Cleveland, OH, USA

Kristel Lobo Prabhu Department of Surgery, University Health Network, Toronto, ON, Canada

Kevin M. Reavis Division of Gastrointestinal and Minimally Invasive Surgery, Foregut and Bariatric Surgery, The Oregon Clinic, Portland, OR, USA

Kurt E. Roberts Department of Surgery, Yale Gastrointestinal Surgery, New Haven, CT, USA

John R. Romanelli Department of Surgery, University of Massachusetts Medical School, Baystate Medical Center, Springfield, MA, USA

Jean Salem Department of Colorectal Surgery, Lankenau Medical Center, Wynnewood, PA, USA

Payal Saxena Department of Medicine and Division of Gastroenterology and Hepatology, The Johns Hopkins Medical Institutions, Baltimore, MD, USA; Department of Medicine and Division of Gastroenterology and Hepatology, Royal Prince Alfred Hospital, Camperdown, NSW, Australia

Eran Shlomovitz Toronto General Hospital, Toronto, ON, Canada

Stavros N. Stavropoulos Department of Gastroenterology, Hepatology and Nutrition, Winthrop University Hospital, NY, USA; GI Endoscopy and Program in Advanced GI Endoscopy, Winthrop University Hospital, NY, USA; Clinical Medicine, Columbia University, New York, USA; Medicine, Temple University, Philadelphia, USA

Patricia Sylla Department of Surgery, Division of Colon and Rectal Surgery, Icahn School of Medicine at Mount Sinai, New York, NY, USA

Gabor Varga Agaplesion Markus Krankenhaus, Frankfurt am Main, Germany

Yijun Xue Department of Urology, First Affiliated Hospital of Gannan Medical University, Ganzhou, Jiangxi Province, China

Guoxi Zhang Department of Urology, First Affiliated Hospital of Gannan Medical University, Ganzhou, Jiangxi Province, China

Carsten Zornig Israelitisches Krankenhaus, Hamburg, Germany

Xiaofeng Zou Department of Urology, First Affiliated Hospital of Gannan Medical University, Ganzhou, Jiangxi Province, China

The History of NOTES

1

John R. Romanelli and David B. Earle

Abstract

Natural orifice translumenal endoscopic surgery (NOTES™) was officially born in 2005 when a forward thinking group of gastroenterologists and surgeons convened to discuss, organize, codify, and elucidate concerns about this potential new disruptive surgical idea. This meeting came on the heels of a report of "flexible transgastric peritoneoscopy" from Johns Hopkins University [1] and several subsequent experiments in animal models expanding upon the possibilities this technique represented [2]. The NOTES moniker was adopted at this meeting, as was the formation of the Natural Orifice Surgery Consortium for Assessment and Research (NOSCAR®) [2]. But a peek into the history of surgery via the natural orifice reveals that the idea was an old one, dating back into the 1800s in some cases. Many animal experiments were performed, demonstrating many new and novel techniques to commonly performed operations, and scientific investigation was undertaken to determine the safety and feasibility of these approaches. Human work began to emerge in 2005 and continues to develop; in some cases, becoming widely adopted.

J.R. Romanelli (✉)
Department of Surgery, University of Massachusetts Medical School, Baystate Medical Center, Springfield, MA 01199, USA
e-mail: john.romanelli@baystatehealth.org

D.B. Earle
Lowell Surgical Associates, Lowell General Hospital, 20 Research Place, Suite 130, North Chelmsford, MA 01863, USA
e-mail: davidearle59@gmail.com

J.R. Romanelli et al. (eds.), *NOTES and Endoluminal Surgery*,
Clinical Gastroenterology, DOI 10.1007/978-3-319-50610-4_1

Keywords
Natural orifice translumenal endoscopic surgery · NOTES · Transvaginal surgery · Transgastric surgery · Transanal surgery · Transurethral surgery · Transsphenoidal surgery · Transesophageal surgery

A Disruptive Approach to a Disruptive Approach

While physicians have peered into the depths of the human body through its natural openings for more than 100 years, natural orifice translumenal endoscopic surgery, or NOTES™, dates back to 2005. This occurred when a group of gastroenterologists and surgeons convened in an attempt to propagate this disruptive concept of minimally invasive surgery in a thoughtful, scientific, and safe manner. The meeting was catalyzed by a report of "flexible transgastric peritoneoscopy" published by Kalloo et al. in 2004. The procedure was performed in a swine model, and subsequent animal work by the same group at Johns Hopkins University demonstrated the feasibility of procedures such as transgastric ligation of fallopian tubes, cholecystectomy, gastrojejunostomy, and splenectomy [1]. The novel innovation was the use of the flexible endoscope as the operating platform.

The slow progress of utilizing a natural orifice has gone from simply looking to performing procedures adjacent to the opening, and finally to performing procedures far from the natural orifice. While all procedures were both enhanced and limited by one technological device or another, the technologic restrictions did not limit the imagination and foresight of the surgical and gastroenterological pioneers that laid the foundation for NOTES™ as we know it today.

In 2005, fourteen thought leaders, representing the Society of American Gastrointestinal Endoscopic Surgeons (SAGES) and the American Society of Gastrointestinal Endoscopy (ASGE), assembled in Phoenix, Arizona, to form a working group on this nascent field. The result of this meeting was an important white paper written by the working group published in 2006 [2]. There were three critical accomplishments from this meeting.

The first accomplishment was an agreement on nomenclature. Although the focus at the time of the meeting was on transgastric surgery, the leaders recognized that other routes of access to the abdomen, namely transvaginal or transcolonic, could also develop. The term "natural orifice translumenal endoscopic surgery" was adopted to describe this, and the acronym NOTES™ was born. It was also uniformly agreed upon that these were to be considered surgical procedures because "tissue resection and repair is the ultimate goal of accessing intraperitoneal organs." The working group named itself the Natural Orifice Surgery Consortium for Assessment and Research (NOSCAR), a clever acronym for the development of incisionless surgery. While it may seem trivial to have spent so much effort on nomenclature and taxonomy, one only needs to consider the bewildering sea of names and acronyms created to describe techniques and devices used in single-port laparoscopic surgery to realize that agreement on nomenclature is important [3].

The second accomplishment was to define criteria by which one could participate in NOSCAR, with an eye on avoiding the large increase in complications caused by the last revolution in gastrointestinal surgery: the introduction of laparoscopy. In the name of patient safety, NOSCAR outlined the following criteria for participation:

1. A multidisciplinary team, consisting of advanced laparoscopists and advanced therapeutic endoscopists
2. Membership in SAGES and/or ASGE
3. An on-site animal laboratory for both research and training

4. Must be willing to share laboratory data at NOSCAR semiannual meetings
5. Must be willing to perform all human cases under the auspices of Institutional Research Board (IRB) approval
6. Must be willing to submit cases to a society-sponsored registry.

The third accomplishment was to define the current limitations in the ability to perform NOTES™ procedures. They outlined the following eleven potential barriers to the safe introduction of NOTES™ in human patients:

1. Access to peritoneal cavity
2. Gastric (intestinal) closure
3. Prevention of infection
4. Development of a suturing device
5. Development of anastomotic (non-suturing) device
6. Spatial orientation
7. Development of a multitasking platform to accomplish procedures
8. Control of intraperitoneal hemorrhage
9. Management of iatrogenic intraperitoneal complications
10. Physiologic untoward events
11. Training other providers.

This paper immediately set into motion those interested in NOTES™ research and development, as well as the clinical introduction of these techniques.

Transvaginal Approach

Transvaginal surgery dates back to ancient times. Some claim that the first surgical procedure described in history was a vaginal hysterectomy by Themison of Athens in 50 BC. Others claim the first vaginal hysterectomy was performed by Soranus of Ephesus in 120 AD, whose treatise, gynecology, has survived into modern times (translated into English in 1956) [4, 5]. This was considered a seminal work at the time and provided a look at ancient obstetric and gynecological techniques. Soranus described a transvaginal hysterectomy for severe uterine prolapse associated with ischemia and gangrene. Morbidity and mortality, however, were almost universal. In the eleventh century, an Arabian physician, Alsaharavius, wrote of vaginal hysterectomy, and there are some who believe that these patients survived. Clearer reports of survival date back about 500 years; Berengarius da Carpi of Bologna in 1507 performed a partial vaginal hysterectomy on a patient who survived. More incredible is the case of Faith Howard, a 46-year-old peasant, who performed a vaginal hysterectomy on herself in 1670. She was said to be carrying a heavy load when her uterus prolapsed completely. Frustrated by this frequent occurrence, she grabbed her uterus, pulled as hard as possible, and cut the whole lot of it with a short knife. The bleeding soon stopped and she lived on for many years, with a persistent vesico-vaginal fistula [5, 6]. The first elective cases began to appear in the literature from France and Germany shortly after 1800—and many years before Charles Clay reported the abdominal hysterectomy in 1843, which unfortunately was unsuccessful due to an incorrect diagnosis and early postoperative mortality [5, 7]. Vaginal hysterectomy for cancer was reported in 1892 by Terrier and Hartman [8].

In the late 1800s Durhssen, Mackerodt, and Martin of Berlin, Germany, utilized anterior colpotomy to perform transvaginal operations of the tubes, ovaries, and uterus for a variety of conditions, including ectopic pregnancy, and the use of "morcellement" for the removal of very large uterine myomas. At the annual meeting of the British Medical Association in London in 1895, Martin touted the decreased morbidity compared to laparotomy as justification for the approach. He closed the colpotomy initially with silk and silver wire, but abandoned these for juniper catgut. Postoperatively, the vaginal wound was said to take only 8–10 days to heal, "so that about the twelfth day the patient may be allowed to leave bed." No local treatment was necessary, and all of his 152 cases recovered without "feverish reaction." [9].

In 1901, Russian gynecologist Dmitry Von Ott presented his work in St. Petersburg using a posterior colpotomy for a variety of gynecological operations. Unique to his approach, which he dubbed "ventroscopy," was the use of "a peanut-sized lamp and a spoon-shaped shield to protect the patient from burn," and reflected light into the cavity using metallic mirrors and a headlamp. He also utilized the Trendelenburg position and placed a cotton swab in the vagina, allowing filtered air to be vacuumed into the peritoneal cavity, creating a "natural form of insufflation." His technique was used by the Europeans into the 1920s to 1930s, and by the Americans from the 1940s to 1960s [10].

Transvaginal tubal ligation was further advanced by the Japanese in 1970 [11], and there were additional scattered case reports throughout the 1970s. Transvaginal oophorectomy (at the same time as a hysterectomy) was revisited by Nichols in 1978 [12]. He noted that access to the ovaries could be very challenging due to the constraints of the size of the colpotomy and the bony anatomy.

Transvaginal specimen extraction was first described in the early 1990s. Delvaux et al. from Brussels [13] described a case report of a laparoscopic cholecystectomy in a woman with large gallstones, where they opted for specimen removal via a posterior colpotomy rather than removal from a larger abdominal wall incision. Also in 1993, Breda et al. in Italy used a posterior colpotomy for extraction of a tuberculous left kidney after laparoscopic nephrectomy [14]. Although these reports were overlooked at the time, they were proof of concept that organs not immediately adjacent to the vagina can be safely removed via this natural orifice.

In the mid-1990s, there were two reports of transvaginal oophorectomy using an endoscope. In London Magos published a technique using a standard laparoscopic instrumentation without pneumoperitoneum, and Yuen in Hong Kong, in his published experience, commented on the difficulty of manipulating three instruments in such a small working space—a prescient statement given the subsequent development of single-site surgery and the challenges that the concept introduced [15, 16].

It was not until the turn of the twenty-first century, about 100 years since the first surgeon peered through the vaginal vault into the peritoneal cavity using a small lamp with metal mirrors that our current concept of transvaginal NOTES™ came into being.

In 2007, Scott et al. used a swine model to perform transvaginal cholecystectomy utilizing a proprietary magnetic instrument system [17]. The first report of a transvaginal cholecystectomy in the USA was presented as a video at the April 2007 annual meeting of the Society of American Gastrointestinal and Endoscopic Surgeons (SAGES). This seminal video was the first time a human NOTES™ cholecystectomy had been presented, and it utilized a hybrid approach with a transvaginal flexible endoscope and umbilical laparoscopic port and took approximately 3 h. This report was immediately criticized, with one surgeon interviewed for a New York Times article calling the procedure "repulsive," stating that "the idea of puncturing internal organs and then sewing them up was cause for concern". She further stated that "As a woman I find it very invasive, physically and emotionally. To me it's quite distasteful." [18]. The report of the video was published in December of the same year [19].

The first South American report of transvaginal cholecystectomy also appeared in the literature in 2007. Zorron et al. performed a case the same week as Bessler's group in New York, and the case was successfully completed with endoscopic instruments placed alongside the vaginal endoscope. Amazingly, the procedure lasted only 66 min, and this technique quickly gained popularity in Brazil [20].

Also in 2007, Marescaux and colleagues at IRCAD (Institut de Recherche contre les Cancers de l'Appareil Digestif; French: Institute for Research into Cancer of the Digestive System) in Strasbourg reported a hybrid transvaginal cholecystectomy using a flexible endoscope aided by a single, 2-mm, laparoscopic port in a human. The authors were careful to report that "all of the principles of cholecystectomy were strictly adhered to," and that the patient had an uneventful recovery [21]. A second human case, this one from Hamburg, was published a month later, where Zornig and colleagues performed a cholecystectomy with standard laparoscopic instrumentation (i.e., a rigid endoscope) via the vagina and one umbilical port. The authors emphasized that the vaginal access was better for closure and infection, and rigid instrumentation was easier to use than a flexible endoscope [22]. This approach became common in Europe for those who adopted the procedure.

The first case report of human transvaginal appendectomy came in 2008 from India. The report details six attempted cases: the first three failed, the next two were completed with a 3-mm laparoscope in the umbilicus, and the final case succeeded as a purely transvaginal case. In the final case, pneumoperitoneum was initiated via a transumbilical Veress needle. Hot biopsy forceps were used to divide the mesoappendix, and endoloops were used to secure the appendix. All patients in the series recovered uneventfully [23].

After these early reports there have been hundreds of articles published about transvaginal operations. While the vast majority of these focused on cholecystectomy, removal of all of the GU organs, liver, spleen, and stomach have also been reported. Exploration and specimen removal have also been reported, along with hernia repair.

Importantly, genuine concerns about the safety and appropriateness of a transvaginal approach gave rise to a host of published surveys given to patients, spouses, and healthcare workers. These surveys suggest there is no specific patient type that prefers a transvaginal approach over standard laparoscopy. Results are highly variable when examined by age, reason for operation, and BMI. Concerns regarding scarring and cosmesis were generally less important compared to issues related to safety and recovery time. In general, patients were more likely to accept a transvaginal approach compared to healthcare workers [24–33].

Transgastric Approach

The first published cases of transgastric surgery appeared in 1950, when Scovel and Holliger reported a case of transgastric pancreatocystogastrostomy [34]. In 1959, Brewer and Shumway reported transgastric catheter drainage of a pancreatic pseudocyst [35]. Although both of these cases were performed via laparotomy, they were the first cases that described crossing the lumen of a hollow organ to gain access to the operative field, an important precursor to NOTES™. Another interesting concept using a transgastric approach was published by Petropoulos in 1979, where he described a transgastric route for highly selective vagotomy to control peptic ulcer symptoms [36].

In 1980, Ponsky et al. in Cleveland described the percutaneous placement of a gastrostomy tube, rather than placement via a laparotomy incision [37]. A monumental achievement at the time, this drastically reduced the invasiveness of gastrostomy tube placement. The procedure was accomplished via a natural orifice, traversed the lumen of a hollow viscus, and utilized a flexible endoscope. One could easily argue that Ponsky's PEG tube is the very first NOTES™ procedure by today's standards.

Another use of transgastric surgery was for specimen extraction. In 1998, Gagner published a series of needlescopic cholecystectomies where a gastrotomy was performed, and the gallbladder was placed into the stomach. After laparoscopic suturing of the stomach, the gallbladder was extracted orally with an endoscope [38]. Although the work was published and successful, local criticism prompted abandonment of the idea.

Kalloo et al. published their landmark paper on transgastric peritoneoscopy in 2004, and this immediately opened the eyes of many to the potential toward intra-abdominal surgical procedures via the natural orifice, in this case, the mouth. Using a swine model, the authors created a gastrotomy using a needle knife and passed a guidewire across the opening. The gastric wall was dilated with a balloon or enlarged with a pull-type sphincterotome. The endoscope was passed into the abdominal cavity, and a liver biopsy was performed. The gastrotomy was closed using endoscopic clips. They performed 12 nonsurvival cases and later 5 survival cases [1]. This series demonstrated that deliberate perforation and subsequent closure of the gastrointestinal tract, with a minor procedure performed through the opening, was safe and repeatable. This study began to fuel the imaginations of both gastroenterologists and gastrointestinal and endoscopic surgeons about the possibilities of incisionless surgery in the abdominal cavity.

Also in 2004, a surgeon and a gastroenterologist team in Hyderabad, India, performed a human NOTES™ case. Rao and Reddy had a patient with severe burn scars on the abdominal wall who presented with acute appendicitis, so they chose a transgastric route to the abdomen [39]. Although this work has never been formally published, they presented a video of this case at both the Society of American Gastrointestinal and Endoscopic Surgeons and Digestive Disease Week annual meetings in 2005. In the operation, they used an endoscope to transit the stomach and used bipolar cautery via the endoscope to divide the mesoappendix. An endoscopic loop was utilized to ligate the appendiceal stump, and a hot snare was used to divide the appendix. Using an overtube, they withdrew the specimen through the mouth. They later reported seven successful cases using this approach in 2010 [40].

In 2005, Kalloo's group followed their initial work with a report detailing the transgastric ligation of the fallopian tubes in a swine survival study [41]. Six pigs underwent unilateral tubal ligation using endoloops, with the opposite side left intact as a control. Necropsy at two weeks revealed all ligations to be successful both radiographically (hysterosalpingogram) and histologically. There was no evidence of infection or other complications. Also in 2005, Kantsevoy and colleagues performed endoscopic gastrojejunostomy in two pigs. They utilized a prototype suturing device dubbed the "Eagle Claw" to secure a loop of jejunum to the gastrotomy site. Midway through the two-week survival period, both contrast and endoscopic examination revealed patent anastomoses with no evidence of leakage. At the two-week necropsy, there were no signs of infection, abscess, leakage, or adhesions [42]. Park and colleagues in Sweden published their swine series of nonsurvival and survival transgastric cholecystectomies in 2005 [43]. They utilized two side-by-side endoscopes, and all survival cases were successful. The gastrotomy site was closed with an endoscopic suturing technique, which they also used to successfully perform three cholecystogastrostomies. Importantly, they described the concept of utilizing a laparoscopic instrument to facilitate the procedure, which they would later refer to as "hybrid NOTES™"—a hybrid of laparoscopic and NOTES™ techniques. In 2005–2006, Thompson et al. in Boston published two reports using a survival swine model that included transgastric peritoneal explorations, oophorectomy and partial hysterectomy [44, 45]. Endoscopic clips were used for gastric closure. All cases in both studies were successful and without complications. In 2006, Gostout et al. at the Mayo clinic developed a model for appendicitis, creating inflammation of the uterine horn with an injection, followed by endoscopic transgastric resection two days later with a second procedure. This report is also important because it described gastric closure using T-tags rather than endoscopic clips [46]. In 2006, the "Apollo Group" performed transgastric splenectomy in a nonsurvival swine model. The splenic vessels were ligated with endoscopic loops and a single endoscopic clip; the vessels were divided with an endoscopic polypectomy snare. The gastrotomy was enlarged for specimen removal with a sphincterotome and closed with endoscopic clips [47].

Transgastric work on the biliary tree, mostly looking at cholecystectomy, began in the laboratory setting in 2007. These early experiments focused on feasibility and device development, recognizing the need for a flexible instrument platform that could be "rigidized." [48–54]. The first human cases of transgastric cholecystectomy were reported by Auyang et al. in 2009 [55]. Four transgastric cholecystectomies were completed via a hybrid approach—the cystic duct and artery were ligated with a laparoscopic clip applier. They noted the difficulty of performing the entire case in a retroflexed position, as has been noted by others.

Our group reported initial experience with transoral, transgastric pancreatic pseudocystgastrostomy in 2008 [56]. Our initial patient was a critically ill man with a large infected pancreatic pseudocyst, who was hemodynamically unstable. Two double-pigtail stents had previously been placed endoscopically into the infected cyst, but due to hemorrhage and the presence of debris, endoscopic drainage had failed. We removed the stents, dilated the tract with an endoscopic balloon dilator, and passed a flexible, transoral linear stapler through the opening into the cyst. Firing the stapler created a stapled pseudocystgastrostomy. Further details on this technique are discussed elsewhere in this text.

Transgastric peritoneoscopy was reported by Hazey et al. in 2008 in ten patients [57]. In this pilot series, patients that had a pancreatic mass and were to undergo diagnostic staging laparoscopy prior to potential pancreaticoduodenectomy underwent both laparoscopy and transgastric endoscopic peritoneoscopy. For patients who went on to undergo pancreaticoduodenectomy, the gastrotomy site was resected. For those were not resectable, the gastrotomy site was used for the palliative gastrojejunostomy. The findings at laparoscopy and endoscopic peritoneoscopy were in agreement in 9 of 10 patients, leading the authors to conclude that the approach was safe.

Transanal Approach

While Ponsky was working on endoscopic surgery of the upper GI tract in the early 1980s, Buess in Germany began work on the lower GI tract with a technique he coined transanal endoscopic microsurgery (TEM) [58]. In 1985, he reported twelve rectal operations with surgical suturing utilizing an operating endoscope [59]. He continued developing the technique, and over the next decade more reports by him and by others emerged. While there were scattered case reports of colectomy via a transanal approach dating back to the 1950s, its use aside from abdominoperineal resection was not popularized until after the development of the laparoscopic approach to colon surgery in the 1990s. In the early 1990s, Franklin in San Antonio began using a transanal approach for specimen extraction after laparoscopic colectomy [60].

A review from 2011 found only 19 reports from a search spanning five-and-a-half decades (1955–2011). They concluded that natural orifice specimen extraction (NOSE) was safe and feasible, but lack of a uniform technique made widespread adoption limited [61].

The evolution of TEM has utilized the same concept with newer instrumentation and a further reach. This concept has adapted the single-port devices for use in transanal operations and rebranded the technique transanal minimally invasive surgery, or TAMIS. First reported in about 2010 by Atallah and colleagues in Orlando, this technique is rapidly gaining enthusiasm among colorectal surgeons as the equipment is much easier to use compared to that used for TEM [62].

Transesophageal Approach

An interesting offshoot of the NOTES™ transgastric work was the idea of mediastinal work being done outside the lumen of the esophagus. Fritscher-Ravens et al. published nonsurvival and survival porcine studies looking at mediastinal exploration across the esophageal lumen in 2007. The esophagotomy site was chosen with endoscopic ultrasound to avoid vascular injury and was closed with both endoscopic clips or suturing. All of the pigs who were survived six weeks were found that have healed the esophagotomy sites, and none suffered from mediastinitis or leak [63].

Another important early work in the esophagus was published in 2007 by Pasricha and colleagues in Texas [64]. They used a swine model for performing a transesophageal myotomy of the lower esophageal sphincter (LES). In four animals, they made an incision in the mucosa of the esophagus 5 cm above the LES. A balloon was then used to open the submucosal plane, and a monopolar needle knife was used to divide the circular muscle fibers of the LES. The mucosa was then clipped closed. All animals survived for one week, and at necropsy, all of the closure sites had healed without evidence of infection. This seminal work led to the clinical application of a similar technique in humans, first performed in Japan by Inoue and colleagues. In their 2010 publication, they described the technique and results in their first 17 patients and coined the term per-oral endoscopic myotomy (POEM). Their extensive experience in endoscopic submucosal dissection was a significant factor in moving forward with this approach in humans [65]. A noteworthy difference in their technique was the use of dyed saline to distend the submucosal space, along with division of the connective tissue under direct vision using a monopolar triangular-shaped knife rather than a balloon. This procedure has since been performed on thousands of patients across the globe, sparking research, development, and continuing education opportunities, along with almost 200 peer-reviewed publications on the technique.

Transurethral Approach

The urethra has typically been disregarded as a viable natural orifice for utilizing NOTES™ techniques, primarily due to its diminutive diameter. Transurethral surgery has been the domain of urologists since the late 1890s. The first report of rigid cystoscopy in a male patient appeared in 1898 by Howard Kelly and remains a seminal work to this day [66]. Interestingly, illumination of the bladder came via reflection from a head mirror. By 1908, bladder tumors were routinely being removed endoscopically by urologists, albeit not without significant morbidity and mortality [67]. Transurethral resection of the prostate (TURP) began in 1926, when Stern in New York City used a novel "resectoscope." [68]. Stern later moved to Florida and was subsequently expelled from the American Urological Association (AUA) for attempting to charge urologists a $5 fee for every TURP. Stern died in 1946, never having been readmitted to the AUA [69]. Scattered case reports began to appear in the 1940s concerning ureteral instrumentation and stone extraction, which were widely reported by the late 1950s and 1960s. Wagenknecht published the first account of cystoscopy with flexible endoscopic technology in Germany in 1982 [70]. It was not until 2006 that the transurethral approach began looking and operating on organs distant from the genitourinary tract. Lima and colleagues published a series of nonsurvival and survival cases in a swine model, initially performing trans-vesical peritoneoscopy. They did not close the bladder, rather decompressed it for four days, allowing all cases to heal successfully. They subsequently published work on cholecystectomy and nephrectomy in a nonsurvival swine model using the transurethral approach in combination with a transgastric approach [71–73]. In 2009, more reports emerged utilizing a transurethral approach in an animal model to access organs outside of the urethra and bladder [74–76].

The limited size of the urethra, however, obviously restricts specimen extraction size, and this led Lima and colleagues in Portugal to experiment with endoscopic morcellation in a nonsurvival swine model for nephrectomy in 2011 [77].

Limitations of instrumentation and clinical scenarios, along with the availability of other natural orifices, make the urethra less practical for most NOTES™ applications. Continued research in this area remains important, as it may spawn the development of better techniques and instrumentation that could be applied in a wide array of applications.

Transsphenoidal Approach

Transsphenoidal pituitary gland surgery is another procedure performed via a natural orifice. The earliest known case report of a transsphenoidal approach to pituitary tumors was published by Hirsch in 1949 [78], another early account of this technique more than twenty years later from France in 1972 [79]. The first reported use of an endoscope for this technique arrived 6 years later from Germany [80]. In the latter report, high-pressure lumbar air insufflation was used in combination with an angled rigid endoscope to provide a quality view and the ability to distinguish tumor from normal pituitary tissue. The use of flexible endoscopic technology for hypophysectomy has emerged over the last decade with scattered case reports.

NOTES™ Hernia Repair

Given its purely reconstructive nature and frequent use of an implantable prosthetic, we have included hernia repair as a separate section, encompassing a variety of natural orifice approaches. Initial reports of NOTES™ hernia repair appeared in 2007. Hu and colleagues used a transgastric approach in a nonsurvival swine model to create a small (3 × 2 cm) laparotomy incision from the inside, not opening the skin. This was repaired with a prototype endoscopic suturing device, and the gastrostomy was closed with endoscopic clips [81]. Also in 2007, Thompson et al. used a transanal approach in a survival porcine model [82]. They introduced an approximately 2 × 3 cm piece of composite hernia mesh (polytetrafluoroethylene—PTFE/polypropylene—PP) into the peritoneal cavity through a small colotomy with a mesh delivery device over a guidewire. The mesh had preplaced ferro-magnetic endoscopic clips on the corners and was held on the abdominal wall with a magnet placed on the exterior surface of the abdominal wall. The mesh was then fixed with T-tags and a suture crimping device. The colotomy was initially closed with an endoscopic loop and subsequently with the same T-tag sutures used to fix the mesh. The 3 animals in the survival portion of the study all thrived for 14 days and showed no evidence of any complications.

In 2008, Bingener and colleagues simulated a ventral hernia repair using a transgastric approach in a survival swine model [83]. They placed a 2 cm^2 PP mesh using a delivery device and clipped it to the peritoneum of the abdominal wall with an endoscopic clip. The gastrotomy was successfully closed in all cases with endoscopic clips. At the two-week necropsy, there was a 36% gross infection rate of the mesh.

In 2009, Kantsevoy's group used a nonsurvival and survival swine model to use PTFE mesh to repair an iatrogenically created abdominal wall defect. After a mesh infection of the first survival animal, the subsequent four animals had the mesh placed with a sterile cover, and no infections were observed. All gastrotomy sites were successfully closed with T-bars [84].

Sherwinter in Brooklyn published his work on transgastric inguinal hernia repair in 2009–2010. In the survival study, a biological mesh was delivered through an overtube and fixed on the peritoneum at the myopectineal orifice with glue. The gastrotomy was closed with an endoscopic suturing device, and all 5 animals survived the 14-day period. Necropsy revealed no complications and all mesh to be in proper position [85, 86].

Our group also reported a similar technique with polypropylene and used a sterile mesh delivery device. The mesh was fixed to the abdominal wall with transfascial sutures and endoscopically delivered nitinol tacks [87]. Our subsequent survival model confirmed the ability to place a 10 × 15 cm PP mesh without clinical infection [88].

In 2010, reports began emerging detailing case reports of human repair of small primary and incisional ventral hernias. All have used a transvaginal approach with both biological and synthetic meshes. Long-term follow-up is still in progress, but the procedure seems to be feasible [89–92].

Conclusion

Natural orifice translumenal endoscopic surgery, no longer in its infancy, has evolved with the combination of disruptive innovative research, meticulous attention to technique development in animal models, and a collaborative environment between surgeons and gastroenterologists. New reports of human NOTES™ procedures surface frequently, and acceptance of this disruptive technology seems assured. Lessons learned from the laparoscopic revolution were applied to prevent poor outcomes. While the relative lack of development of special instrumentation for NOTES™ has hindered the widespread growth and adoption of these procedures, some of what has been learned is increasingly being applied to modern surgical patient care. Spin offs from NOTES™, including single-port laparoscopic surgery and endoluminal surgery, continue to evolve and mature as well. The future of NOTES™ seems bright, as long as pioneers in the field continue to innovate, collaborate, and push the envelope of "minimally invasive surgery" in an effort to improve the lives of our patients.

References

1. Kalloo AN, Singh VK, Jagannath SB, Niiyama H, Hill SL, Vaughn CA, et al. Flexible transgastric peritoneoscopy: a novel approach to diagnostic and therapeutic interventions in the peritoneal cavity. Gastrointest Endosc. 2004;60(1):114–7.
2. Rattner D, Kalloo, A, the SAGES/ASGE Working Group on Natural Orifice Translumenal Endoscopic Surgery. ASGE/SAGES Working Group on Natural Orifice Translumenal Endoscopic Surgery. Surg Endosc. 2006;20:329–33.
3. Romanelli JR, Earle DB. Single-port laparoscopy: an overview. Surg Endosc. 2009;23(7):1419–27.
4. Sutton C. Past, present and future of hysterectomy. J Minim Invasive Gynecol. 2010;17(4):421–35.
5. Sheth S. Vaginal hysterectomy. 2nd ed. New Delhi, India: Jaypee Brothers Medical Publishers Ltd.; 2014.
6. Sparić R, et al. Hysterectomy throughout history. IzIstorije Med. doi:10.2298/ACI1104009S.
7. Sutton C. Hysterectomy: a historical perspective. Baillieres Clin Obstet Gynaecol. 1997;11(1):1–22.
8. Lloyd S. The immediate and ultimate results of vaginal hysterectomy for cancer of the uterus. Ann Surg. 1892;16(1):83–6.
9. Martin A. Anterior colpotomy. Br Med J. 1896; 1 (1827):10–3.
10. Nezhat C. Nezhat's history of endoscopy: a historical analysis of endoscopy's ascension since antiquity. Tuttlingen, Germany: Endo Press; 2011. p. 83–4.
11. Kai I. Key points of our method of transvaginal tubal sterilization. Sanfujinka No Jissai. 1970;19(4): 408–11.
12. Nichols DH. A technique for vaginal oophorectomy. Surg Gynecol Obstet. 1978;147(5):765.
13. Delvaux G, Devroey P, De Waele B, Willems G. Transvaginal removal of gallbladders with large stones after laparoscopic cholecystectomy. Surg Laparosc Endosc. 1993;3(4):307–9.
14. Breda G, Silvestre P, Giunta A, Xaus D, Tamai A, et al. Laparoscopic nephrectomy with vaginal delivery of the intact kidney. Eur Urol. 1993;24:116–7.
15. Magos AL, Bournas N, Sinha R, Lo L, Richardson RE. Transvaginal endoscopic oophorectomy. Am J Obstet Gynecol. 1995;172(1 Pt 1):123–4.
16. Yuen PM. Transvaginal Endoscopic Oophorectomy. Am J Obstet Gynecol. 1995;173(3 Pt 1):976–7.
17. Scott DJ, Tang SJ, Fernandez R, Bergs R, Goova MT, et al. Completely transvaginal NOTES cholecystectomy using magnetically anchored instruments. Surg Endosc. 2007;21(12):2308–16.
18. Grady D. Testing scarless surgery: doctors remove a gallbladder through the vagina. The New York Times. 2007;20:A14.
19. Bessler M, Stevens PD, Milone L, Parikh M, Fowler D. Transvaginal laparoscopically assisted endoscopic cholecystectomy: a hybrid approach to natural orifice surgery. Gastrointest Endosc. 2007;66 (6):1243–5.
20. Zorrón R, Filgueiras M, Maggioni LC, Pombo L, Lopes Carvalho G, et al. NOTES. Transvaginal cholecystectomy: report of the first case. Surg Innov. 2007;14(4):279–83.
21. Marescaux J, Dallemagne B, Perretta S, Wattiez A, Mutter D, et al. Surgery without scars: report of transluminal cholecystectomy in a human being. Arch Surg. 2007;142(9):823–6; discussion 826-7.
22. Zornig C, Emmermann A, von Waldenfels HA, Mofid H. Laparoscopic cholecystectomy without visible scar: combined transvaginal and transumbilical approach. Endoscopy. 2007;39(10):913–5.
23. Palanivelu C, Rajan PS, Rangarajan M, Parthasarathi R, Senthilnathan P, et al. Transvaginal endoscopic appendectomy in humans: a unique approach to NOTES–world's first report. Surg Endosc. 2008;22(5):1343–7.
24. Peterson CY, Ramamoorthy S, Andrews B, Horgan S, Talamini M, et al. Women's positive perception of transvaginal NOTES surgery. Surg Endosc. 2009;23 (8):1770–4.
25. Fei YF, Fei L, Salazar M, Renton DB, Hazey JW. Transvaginal surgery: do women want it? J Laparoendosc Adv Surg Tech A. 2014;24(10): 676–83.
26. Gerö D, Lukovich P, Hulesch B, Pálházy T, Kecskédi B, et al. Inpatients and specialists' opinions about natural orifice translumenal endoscopic surgery. Surg Technol Int. 2010;19:79–84.
27. Li W, Xu H, Wang ZK, Fan ZN, Ba SD, et al. Natural orifice translumenal endoscopic surgery (NOTES): patients' perceptions and attitudes. Dig Dis Sci. 2011;56(8):2415–22.
28. Tsang ME, Theman K, Mercer D, Hopman WM, Hookey L. Patient perceptions of natural orifice translumenal surgery. Minim Invasive Surg. 2012;2012:317249.
29. Gerntke CI, KerstenJF Schön G, Mann O, Stark M, et al. Women's perception of transvaginal natural orifice transluminal endoscopic surgery (NOTES): results of a survey of female medical staff and literature review. World J Gastroenterol. 2012;18 (15):1800–5.
30. Hucl T, Saglova A, Benes M, Kocik M, Oliverius M, et al. Patient and physician perception of natural orifice transluminal endoscopic appendectomy. World J Gastroenterol. 2012;18(15):1800–5.
31. Strickland AD, Norwood MG, Behnia-Willison F, Olakkengil SA, Hewett PJ. Transvaginal natural orifice translumenal endoscopic surgery (NOTES): a survey of women's views on a new technique. Surg Endosc. 2010;24(10):2424–31.
32. Swanstrom LL, Volckmann E, Hungness E, Soper NJ. Patient attitudes and expectations regarding natural orifice translumenal endoscopic surgery. Surg Endosc. 2009;23(7):1519–25.
33. Gerntke CI, Kersten JF, Schön G, Mann O, Stark M, et al. Women's perception of transvaginal natural orifice transluminal endoscopic surgery (NOTES): results of a survey of female medical staff and

literature review. Surg Innov. 2015 (Epub ahead of print).
34. Scovel RE, Holliger VH. Transgastric pancreatocystogastrostomy. J Int Coll Surg. 1950;13(3):278–84.
35. Brewer WA, Shumway OL. Transgastric catheter drainage of pancreatic pseudocysts. AMA Arch Surg. 1959;78(1):79–84.
36. Petropoulos PC. Transgastric highly selective vagotomy (HSTRV) without drainage. Preliminary report of a new simplified procedure of treatment of duodenal ulcer. Langenbecks Arch Chir. 1979;350 (2):95–101.
37. Gauderer MW, PonskyJL, Izant RJ Jr. Gastrostomy without laparotomy: a percutaneous endoscopic technique. J Ped Surg. 1980;15(6):872–5.
38. Gagner M, Garcia-Ruiz A. Technical aspects of minimally invasive abdominal surgery performed with needlescopic instruments. Surg Laparosc Endosc. 1998;8(3):171–9.
39. Rao GV, Reddy DN. Personal communication.
40. Reddy DN, Rao GV, Mansard, MJ. NOTES. In: Dasgupta P, Fitzpatrick J, Kirby R, Gill IS, editors. New technologies in urology. London. Springer; 2010.
41. Jagannath SB, Kantsevoy SV, Vaughn CA, Chung SSC, Cotton PB, et al. Peroral transgastric endoscopic ligation of fallopian tubes with long-tern survival in a porcine model. Gastrointest Endosc. 2005;61(3):449–53.
42. Kantsevoy SV, Jagannath SB, Niiyama H, Chung SSC, Cotton PB, et al. Endoscopic gastrojejunostomy with survival in a porcine model. Gastroinest Endosc. 2005;62(2):287–92.
43. Park PO, Bergström M, Ikeda K, Fritscher-Ravens A, Swain P. Experimental studies of transgastric gallbladder surgery: cholecystectomy and cholecystogastric anastomosis (videos). Gastrointest Endosc. 2005;61(4):601–6.
44. Wagh MS, Merrifield BF, Thompson CC. Endoscopic transgastric abdominal exploration and organ resection: initial experience in a porcine model. Clin Gastro Hep. 2005;3(9):892–6.
45. Wagh MS, Merrifield BF, Thompson CC. Survival studies after endoscopic transgastric oophorectomy and tubectomy in a porcine model. Gastrointest Endosc. 2006;63(3):473–8.
46. Sumiyama K, Gostout CJ, Rajan E, Bakken TA, Deters JL, et al. Pilot study of the porcine uterine horn as an in vivo appendicitis model for development of endoscopic transgastric appendectomy. Gastrointest Endosc. 2006;64(5):808–12.
47. Kantsevoy SV, Hu B, Jagannath SB, Vaughn CA, Beitler DM, et al. Transgastric endoscopic splenectomy: is it possible? Surg Endosc. 2006;20(3):522–5.
48. Park PO, Bergström M, Ikeda K, Fritscher-Ravens A, Swain P. Experimental studies of transgastric gallbladder surgery: cholecystectomy and cholecystogastric anastomosis (videos). Gastrointes tEndosc. 2005;61(4):601–6.
49. Swanstrom LL, Kozarek R, Pasricha PJ, Gross S, Birkett D, et al. Development of a new access device for transgastric surgery. J Gastrointest Surg. 2005;9 (8):1129–36; discussion 1136-7.
50. Feretis C, Kalantzopoulos D, Koulouris P, Kolettas C, Archontovasilis F, et al. Endoscopic transgastric procedures in anesthetized pigs: technical challenges, complications, and survival. Endoscopy. 2007;39 (5):394–400.
51. Sumiyama K, Gostout CJ, Rajan E, Bakken TA, Knipschield MA, et al. Transgastric cholecystectomy: transgastric accessibility to the gallbladder improved with the SEMF method and a novel multibending therapeutic endoscope. Gastrointest Endosc. 2007;65(7):1028–34.
52. Perretta S, Dallemagne B, Coumaros D, Marescaux J. Natural orifice transluminal endoscopic surgery: transgastric cholecystectomy in a survival porcine model. Surg Endosc. 2008;22(4):1126–30.
53. Kouklakis G, Zezos P, Ypsilantis P, Botaitis S, Tsalikidis C, et al. Peroral transgastric endoscopic procedures in pigs: feasibility, survival, questionings, and pitfalls. Surg Endosc. 2009;23(2):394–402.
54. Astudillo JA, Sporn E, Bachman S, Miedema B, Thaler K. Transgastric cholecystectomy using a prototype endoscope with 2 deflecting working channels (with video). Gastrointest Endosc. 2009;69 (2):297–302.
55. Auyang ED, Hungness ES, Vaziri K, Martin JA, Soper NJ. Human NOTES cholecystectomy: transgastric hybrid technique. J Gastrointest Surg. 2009;13(6):1149–50.
56. Romanelli JR, Desilets DJ, Earle DB. Pancreatic pseudocystgastrostomy with a peroral, flexible stapler: a human NOTES™ anastomosis in two patients. Gastrointest Endosc. 2008;68(5):981–7.
57. Hazey JW, Narula VK, Renton DB, Reavis KM, Paul CM, et al. Natural-orifice transgastric endoscopic peritoneoscopy in humans: Initial clinical trial. Surg Endosc. 2008;22:16–20.
58. Lirici MM. In memoriam: Gerhard Friederik Buess (1948–2010). Surg Endosc. 2011;25:2405–7.
59. Buess G, Theiss R, Günther M, Hutterer F, Pichlmaier H. Endoscopic surgery in the rectum. Endoscopy. 1985;17(1):31–5.
60. Franklin ME Jr, Ramos R, Rosenthal D, Schuessler W. Laparoscopic colonic procedures. World J Surg. 1993;17(1):51–6.
61. Diana M, Wall J, Costantino F, D'agostino J, Leroy J, et al. Transanal extraction of the specimen during laparoscopic colectomy. Colorectal Dis. 2011;13 Suppl 7:23–7.
62. Atallah S, Albert M, Larach S. Transanal minimally invasive surgery: a giant leap forward. Surg Endosc. 2010;24(9):2200–5.
63. Fritscher-Ravens A, Patel K, Ghanbari A, Kahle E, von Herbay A, et al. Natural orifice transluminal endoscopic surgery (NOTES) in the mediastinum: long-term survival animal experiments in

transesophageal access, including minor surgical procedures. Endoscopy. 2007;39(10):870–5.
64. Pasricha PJ, Hawari R, Ahmed I, Chen J, Cotton PB, et al. Submucosal endoscopic esophageal myotomy: a novel experimental approach for the treatment of achalasia. Endoscopy. 2007;39(9):761–4.
65. Inoue H, Minami H, Kobayashi Y, Sato Y, Kaga M, et al. Peroral endoscopic myotomy (POEM) for esophageal achalasia. Endoscopy. 2010;42(4): 265–71.
66. Kelly H. Cystoscopy and catheterization of the ureters in the male. Ann Surg. 1898;27(4):475–86.
67. Nezhat C. Let there be light: a historical analysis of endoscopy's ascension since antiquity. Chapter 15—Endourology. Accessed at: http://laparoscopy.blogs.com/endoscopyhistory/chapter_15/.
68. http://www.baus.org.uk/_userfiles/pages/files/Museum/20%20-%20TURP.pdf. Accessed 13 Jan 2016.
69. http://www.urologichistory.museum/content/collections/uropeople/stern/p2.cfm. Accessed 13 Jan 2016.
70. Wagenknecht LV. Inspection of the urinary tract by flexible instruments. Urologe A. 1982;21(2):112–4.
71. Lima E, Rolanda C, Pêgo J, Henriques-Coelho T, Silva D, et al. Transvesical endoscopic peritoneoscopy: a novel 5 mm port for intra-abdominal scarless surgery. J Urol. 2006;176:802–5.
72. Rolanda C, Lima E, Pêgo J, Henriques-Coelho T, Silva D, et al. Third-generation cholecystectomy by natural orifices: transgastric and transvesical combined approach (with video). Gastrointest Endosc. 2007;65:111–7.
73. Lima E, Rolanda C, Pêgo JM, Henriques-Coelho T, Silva D, et al. Third-generation nephrectomy by natural orifice transluminal endoscopic surgery. J Urol. 2007;178(6):2648–54.
74. Metzelder ML, Vieten G, Gosemann J, Ure B, Kuebler JF. Rigid NOTES: the transurethral approach in female piglets. Eur J Pediatr Surg. 2009;19(6):362–5.
75. Sawyer MD, Cherullo EE, Elmunzer BJ, Schomisch S, Ponsky LE. Pure natural orifice translumenal endoscopic surgery partial cystectomy: intravesical transurethral and extravesical transgastric techniques in a porcine model. Urology. 2009;74(5):1049–53.
76. Metzelder M, Vieten G, Gosemann JH, Ure B, Kuebler JF. Endoloop closure of the urinary bladder is safe and efficient in female piglets undergoing transurethral NOTES nephrectomy. Eur J Pediatr Surg. 2009;19(6):362–5.
77. Lima E, Branco F, Parente J, Autorino R, Correia-Pinto J. Transvesical natural orifice transluminal endoscopic surgery (NOTES) nephrectomy with kidney morcellation: a proof of concept study. BJU Int. 2012;109(10):1533–7.
78. Hirsch O. The immediate and late results of the transsphenoidal and cranial methods of operation in pituitary tumors. Bull New Engl Med Cent. 1949;11(2):89–92.
79. Guiot G, Cheibani G. Risks and problems and transsphenoidal exeresis of pituitary adenomas. Nouv Presse Med. 1972;1(32):2117–9.
80. Bushe KA, Halves E. Modified technique in transsphenoidal operations of pituitary adenomas. Technical note. Acta Neurochir (Wien). 1978;41(1–3):163–75.
81. Hu B, Kalloo AN, Chung SS, Cotton PB, Gostout CJ, et al. Peroral transgastric endoscopic primary repair of a ventral hernia in a porcine model. Endoscopy. 2007;39(5):390–3.
82. Fong DG, Ryou M, Pai RD, Tavakkolizadeh A, Rattner DW, Thompson CC. Transcolonic ventral wall hernia mesh fixation in a porcine model. Endoscopy. 2007;39(10):865–9.
83. Buck L, Michalek J, Van Sickle K, Schwesinger W, Bingener J. Can gastric irrigation prevent infection during NOTES mesh placement? J Gastrointest Surg. 2008;12(11):2010–4.
84. Kantsevoy SV, Dray X, Shin EJ, Buscaglia JM, Magno P, et al. Transgastric ventral hernia repair: a controlled study in a live porcine model (with videos). Gastrointest Endosc. 2009;69(1):102–7.
85. Sherwinter DA, Eckstein JG. Feasibility study of natural orifice transluminal endoscopic surgery inguinal hernia repair. Gastrointest Endosc. 2009;70(1):126–30.
86. Sherwinter DA, Gupta A, Eckstein JG. Natural orifice translumenal endoscopic surgery inguinal hernia repair: a survival canine model. J Laparoendosc Adv Surg Tech A. 2011;21(3):209–13.
87. Earle DB, Desilets DJ, Romanelli JR. NOTES transgastric abdominal wall hernia repair in a porcine model. Hernia. 2010;14(5):517–22.
88. Mora MC, Kowalski R Desilets DJ, Romanelli JR, Earle DB. NOTES transgastric ventral hernia repair in a porcine survival model. Hernia; in press, 2016.
89. Descloux A, Pohle S, Nocito A, Keerl A. Hybrid NOTES transvaginal intraperitoneal onlay mesh in abdominal wall hernias: an alternative to traditional laparoscopic procedures. Surg Endosc. 2015;29(12):3712–6.
90. Kayaalp C, Yagci MA, Soyer V. Hybrid transvaginal incisional hernia repair. J Laparoendosc Adv Surg Tech A. 2014;24(7):497–501.
91. Wood SG, Panait L, Duffy AJ, Bell RL, Roberts KE. Pure transvaginal ventral hernia repair in humans. Surg Innov. 2014;21(2):130–6.
92. Jacobsen GR, Thompson K, Spivack A, Fischer L, Wong B, et al. Initial experience with transvaginal incisional hernia repair. Hernia. 2010;14(1):89–91.

Fundamentals of NOTES

2

David J. Desilets

Abstract

Natural orifice translumenal endoscopic surgery (NOTES) is becoming more accepted by patients and clinicians alike as new data are published and new clinical trials surface. As these studies emerge we find that there are certain features of NOTES that are common to all types of natural orifice procedures. Among these are that they must include a method of exit from the lumen, procedures for carrying out the intended operation, including methods of obtaining access, retraction, and triangulation, and finally closure of the exit site once the surgery is done. This chapter reviews these fundamentals of NOTES, with emphasis on luminal exit and closure techniques, as these are the foundation of NOTES.

Keywords

Natural orifice · Gastrotomy closure · Surgery · Myotomy · Endoscopy · Fundamentals

Abbreviations

EFTR	Endoscopic full-thickness resection
ESD	Endoscopic submucosal dissection
EUS	Endoscopic ultrasound
FNA	Fine-needle aspiration
GI	Gastrointestinal
NOTES	Natural orifice translumenal endoscopic surgery
OTSC	Over-the-scope clip
PEG	Percutaneous endoscopic gastrostomy
POEM	Per-oral endoscopic myotomy

D.J. Desilets (✉)
Division of Gastroenterology, Department of Medicine, Baystate Health, 759 Chestnut Street, Springfield, MA 01199, USA
e-mail: david.desilets@baystatehealth.org

J.R. Romanelli et al. (eds.), *NOTES and Endoluminal Surgery*, Clinical Gastroenterology, DOI 10.1007/978-3-319-50610-4_2

Introduction

Natural orifice translumenal endoscopic surgery (NOTES) is a surgical technique using a naturally occurring orifice (mouth, anus, urethra, vagina, or naris) to gain access to a body cavity or potential space beyond that orifice. When the mouth or anus is the site of entry, surgery can be carried out in the wall of the gut (e.g., per-oral endoscopic myotomy), or completely outside the gut in the mediastinum, elsewhere in the chest, in the abdomen, lesser sac, or pelvis. The surgery can take place in a true body cavity, or in a potential space such as the retroperitoneum. In all cases, one would expect to adhere to standard surgical principles that govern open or laparoscopic surgery. When first proposed, a flexible endoscope was anticipated to be the operating platform [1]. We now know that rigid surgical instruments can be used in natural orifice surgery and that this type of operation is still considered NOTES.

A natural orifice method is attractive for many theoretical reasons. It should leave no visible scars, and there is likely faster return of bowel function, shorter hospital stay (therefore, there may be a value benefit), less postoperative pain, and performance in an outpatient or ambulatory setting [2]. It has also been suggested that wound infection is potentially less of a problem (although this has not been proven in randomized trials), and that some vexing long-term postoperative problems such as incisional hernias and port site hernias would be greatly diminished. Finally, although not confirmed in randomized, prospective clinical trials, there may be a safety benefit with this most minimally invasive of surgical methods.

In this chapter, we review the fundamentals of NOTES such as getting started, devices utilized, gaining access to the surgical site through a natural orifice, and closure after the operation is completed. These are fundamental issues common to any NOTES procedure. Other topics such as individual types of surgical procedures and how to perform them (POEM, transvaginal cholecystectomy, etc.) will be dealt with elsewhere in this text.

Training, Credentialing, and Getting Started

At the time of this writing, we do not know of any formalized training programs in NOTES, and certainly none that are accredited. So if one is to begin doing NOTES, one must seek an avenue of training. This could be an apprenticeship with others actively engaged in human NOTES cases, animal laboratory training, cadaver laboratory training, or a combination of these. We recommend as much practice as possible in the animal laboratory, on both explants/models and on live animal subjects, prior to booking a first human case. Indeed, each individual hospital or institution will have local regulations regarding procedural competency and accreditation. Know the rules of your own institution and follow them to get permission to start performing NOTES. We recommend a proctor to guide you on your first few cases so that lessons learned the hard way by experts can be passed on to you before you experience the same pitfalls. More details on how to get started in NOTES have been reported by us previously [3, 4]. Also, one must consider, given the relatively experimental nature of NOTES cases at the current time, whether local Institutional Research Board approval is necessary prior to undertaking the first case.

Equipment

A multidisciplinary team is the usual approach to NOTES. In some circumstances, an individual surgeon might have training and skills in therapeutic endoscopy and could potentially do NOTES alone. However, in most cases, a surgeon well versed in laparoscopic equipment and procedures partners with an interventional endoscopist familiar with advanced therapeutic endoscopic equipment and procedures. Often,

Table 2.1 Equipment commonly used in NOTES

Equipment
Flexible endoscope and light source
Therapeutic gastroscope (2 channel)
Standard gastroscope
Transnasal thin gastroscope
Colonoscope, pediatric or adult
Linear-array echoendoscope
Laparoscopic tower and light source
Oblique and straight-viewing laparoscopes
CO_2 insufflator, laparoscopic, and endoscopic
Electrocautery
Standard laparoscopic accessories
Ports, graspers, dissectors, sump suction, hook cautery, clipping devices, stapling devices, suturing materials, etc.
Standard endoscopic accessories
Guidewires, cannulas, cold biopsy and grasping forceps, hot biopsy forceps or coagulation forceps, triangle-tip knife, hook knife, Hybrid Knife, needle knives, dilating balloons (biliary and enteric), stone-extraction balloons, rigid and screw-type dilators, endoscopic suturing devices, hemostatic clips, over-the-scope clips, Dormia baskets, snares, endoscopic overtubes, sclerotherapy needles, and FNA needles

this "cross-pollination" allows for improvisation and off-label use of devices or equipment that might not otherwise be enjoined. See Table 2.1 for a list of devices commonly used in NOTES.

Luminal Exit Techniques

Exiting the lumen of the gut can be rather a frightening experience, at least for endoscopists who have been conditioned throughout conventional GI training to stay within the lumen, and that to do otherwise constitutes a perforation and therefore a complication. When exiting the lumen, one runs the risk of injuring a nearby organ or causing bleeding from vessels on the serosal side of a hollow organ that cannot be seen when the site of exit is selected. Every effort should be made to exit in a location and a manner that minimizes these risks. Therefore, certain landmarks should be sought and rules followed when exiting a natural orifice. For example, the "triangle of safety" can be used for transvaginal access [5]. We always attempt to exit the stomach or bowel on the antimesenteric border, where blood vessels are the fewest and smallest. Some exiting techniques were specifically designed with safety in mind.

(1) Direct Incision

This is the simplest but also the least safe of exiting techniques. A needle knife or other cutting device is used to incise the hollow organ in layers to provide a full-thickness defect through which the endoscope can be passed. The risk of injury to nearby loops of bowel and/or solid organs is not negligible. But this method is simple and quick. It is often used in nonsurvival animal experiments where perforation of a nearby loop of bowel is of little consequence. This type of exit is also the most difficult to close, essentially requiring endoscopic suturing or, if the defect is not too big, over-the-scope clips (OTSCs). This is yet another reason why this method is used in nonsurvival experiments, where closure is not attempted or at least is not critical because the animal is to be sacrificed immediately afterward. Some workers initially advocated the use of endoscopic ultrasound (EUS) to provide additional safety, but they now feel that this has little added value, and most do not use EUS in an attempt to make gastric puncture/incision safer [6].

(2) Puncture and Dilate

This method comprises a blind puncture with a 19-ga EUS needle placed through the working channel of a straight endoscope followed by the passage of a guidewire into the abdominal or other cavity. Risk of puncturing another organ is low if the puncture is done smoothly and slowly. Other hollow viscera tend to float away from the needle. If solid organ anatomy is kept in mind, this can be done safely. Once a guidewire is advanced into the peritoneal cavity, the needle is removed leaving the wire in place. A standard 15- to 18-mm esophageal dilation balloon can then be advanced over the wire and used to dilate the tract. One then pushes the balloon through with the endoscope, whose tip follows it out into the abdominal cavity. An additional way of increasing the safety of this technique is to insufflate the abdomen with CO_2 prior to anterior wall gastric puncture. This helps to prevent injury to other viscera nearby at the time of the gastric puncture or incision [7].

An advantage to this method is that there is no cutting, so bleeding risk is minimized. Another advantage is that without cutting, the muscle layers stretched during the dilation tend to return to their original configuration once the endoscope is removed, and closure may be simplified. Indeed, as will be shown in the next section, Jagannath et al. did not even close the gastrotomy site (a needle knife rather than a needle was used to make the initial small puncture) in a porcine survival model after ligation and transection of the uterine horn to simulate appendectomy [8].

(3) PEG technique

This is likely the safest but also the most complicated method of entry into the abdomen. Because the method utilizes techniques normally used in PEG placement, it can only be used for gastric exit into the peritoneal cavity. The method has been described in detail by Kantsevoy et al. [9]. In brief, the method comprises endoscopic insufflation of the stomach, transcutaneous needle puncture, and guidewire insertion under endoscopic viewing and then removal of the wire out through the mouth as would normally be done for PEG placement. The wire is then back loaded into the working channel and is captured and pulled out through the biopsy port. The scope is then reinserted and used to anchor the wire in the stomach. Next, capnoperitoneum is achieved with a transabdominal Veress needle and CO_2. Finally, the wire is pushed into the abdomen from the skin side, after fixing it in place on the stomach side with the tip of the endoscope. By pushing firmly on the skin side of the wire, it has no place else to go except to "knuckle" or flex into the inflated abdomen. A through-the-scope (TTS) balloon can then be advanced along the wire and pushed along the wire across the wall, much like a push PEG technique, and then used to dilate the puncture site to allow the scope to exit into the abdominal cavity.

The advantages to this method are that it is very safe, there is no cutting, thus minimizing bleeding risk, and closure is made easier. Disadvantages are that it is a bit time-consuming and complicated compared to just cutting one's way out of the stomach, and also that only the anterior of the stomach can be exited (which may not be appropriate for some NOTES procedures). Because of its safety profile, we use the PEG technique exclusively in survival animal studies and would recommend it in human procedures as well.

(4) Tunneling Methods

Several groups have now reported on the creation of a submucosal tunnel proximal to the seromuscular incision used to exit the stomach or esophagus [10–12]. These are all variations on a theme. Briefly, saline is injected submucosally, lifting the mucosa from the muscle layers and expanding the submucosal potential space. A mucosal incision is made at one end of the saline lift. By blunt dissection with forceps or balloons, or by using electrocautery, a long submucosal tunnel is formed that allows passage of a cap-fitted endoscope. Further injections of saline and continued dissection are used to lengthen the tunnel. Then, the muscle and serosa are incised to allow the endoscope to pass into the mediastinum or peritoneal cavity. Once the extraluminal procedure is completed, the endoscope is withdrawn. The mucosotomy and myotomy are at distant sites; they do not overlap. The mucosal tunnel acts as a flap valve preventing luminal contents from exiting through the tunnel. Most investigators [10–15] will close the mucosotomy with endoscopic hemostatic clips as insurance against leakage.

An advantage to this technique is that it provides for a very easy and safe closure. In addition, the exit site can be targeted at a place on the stomach (for gastric exit) that might not be achievable with the PEG method. However, it is time-consuming, adding to the time of the procedure and therefore to its cost. It requires considerable endoscopic skill as well, and experience in endoscopic submucosal dissection (ESD) or POEM is a prerequisite.

Closure Methods

Gastrotomy or other enterotomy closure has been an area of active research since the inception of NOTES. Various devices have been designed specifically for this purpose, and others such as hemostatic clips are adapted for closure and are essentially used off-label. The actual devices (rather than the techniques of closure) have been reviewed elsewhere [16]. Many surgeons and endoscopists emphasize the importance of adherence to proper surgical principles to prevent leaks. Leakage of luminal contents into the abdomen or mediastinum would be a potential postoperative disaster, so as much research attention has been paid to closure methods as to the surgical procedures being developed.

It is beyond the scope of this chapter to review the physiology of intraluminal gut pressures and what factors may contribute to the failure of an enterotomy closure, but a few salient points should be made. Surgical dogma has long held that enterotomy closures must be able to withstand "cough pressure" or the intra-abdominal pressure changes that occur when coughing. The mean intra-abdominal pressure can be as much as 165 cm H_2O (121 mm Hg) during cough [17]. However, our group has observed that extraluminal and intraluminal pressures are nearly identical during simulated cough and that pressure changes as a cause of leak are greatly overstated [18]. Shear forces, failure to appose the edges of a defect, and breakdown of the closure (dehiscence, device failure) are all more important than simple pressure changes in the abdomen because these pressure changes are the same both inside and outside the lumen, and the pressure differential or pressure gradient across the gut wall is near zero even during cough. Clearly, something else must influence leakage rather than pressure alone. Indeed, some surgeons do not even close the gastrotomy after uterine horn resection as will be shown in the next section.

We will now briefly review the types of closures most commonly encountered (no closure, hemostatic clips, OTSC, and T-tags). An exhaustive treatment of closure methods is beyond the scope of this chapter, and the interested reader is referred to several reviews on this subject [16, 19].

(1) No Closure

Jagannath et al. did not close the gastrotomy exit site in their survival porcine model of appendectomy (transgastric uterine horn resection) [8]. Exit was made by needle-knife puncture, but the tract was dilated with a balloon prior to pushing the endoscope across the gastric wall and into the abdominal cavity. The endoscope was simply withdrawn at the end of the procedure. The animals were fasted overnight and then given standard laboratory chow the next day. There were no leaks or infections. It is theorized that a small defect is easily tolerated (we know this from EUS/FNA) and that balloon dilation of the defect serves to spread the muscle fibers but not cut them. They spring back tonically, and the gastrotomy closes rapidly after endoscope removal. To our knowledge, no one has tried this yet in humans.

(2) Clips

Clip closure was one of the first methods used in NOTES enterotomy closure. Many case reports had already been published describing effective closure of iatrogenic perforations with endoscopic hemostatic clips after EMR, polypectomy, or other endoscopic procedures. Much work was subsequently done in the animal laboratory with the closure of intentional perforations, and clips were shown to be effective. Work initially began with hemostatic clips [20–23], and later, work was done with OTSC clips [24–33].

a. Hemostatic Clips

Endoscopic hemostatic clips are titanium devices that are intended for endoscopic hemostasis of

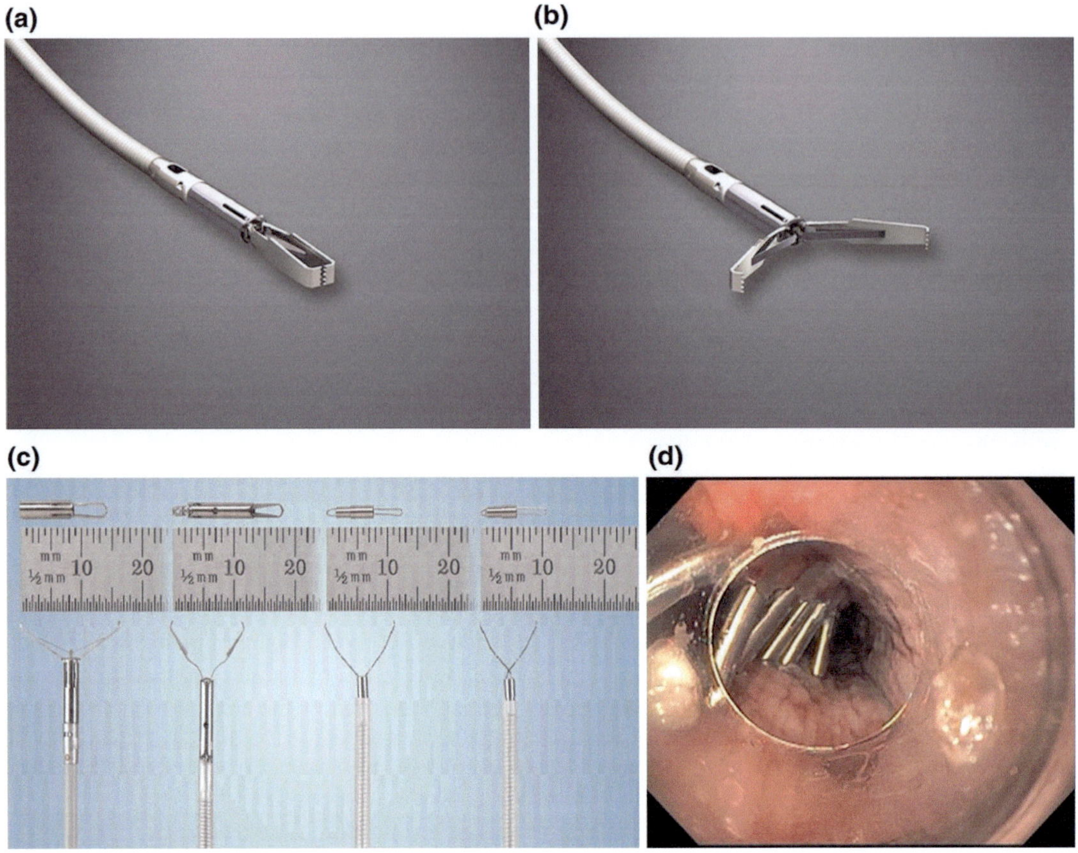

Fig. 2.1 **a** Endoscopic hemostatic clip closed. **b** Endoscopic hemostatic clip open. **c** Various types of endoscopic hemostatic clips. **d** Clip closure of the esophagus after POEM (Permission for use granted by Cook Medical Incorporated, Bloomington, Indiana)

arterial hemorrhage (Fig. 2.1). Most have two arms; some can be rotated, some can be opened and closed repeatedly, and some can do both. They are useful for peptic ulcer bleeding, Dieulafoy's lesions, postpolypectomy or postsphincterotomy bleeding, or for bleeding colonic diverticula and other lesions. However, they can also be used off-label to close a mural defect.

Raju et al. demonstrated that endoscopic hemostatic clips could be used to close small, full-thickness colon defects in a porcine model [20]. Merrifield et al. used hemostatic clips to close the gastrotomy after transgastric uterine horn resection in a survival porcine study [21]. However, 3 of the 5 experimental animals developed significant complications due to incomplete or failed gastric closure. Given this, it seems that clip closure can be risky, and strict attention must be paid to the integrity and strength of the closure. Fritscher-Ravens et al. have demonstrated effective closure of esophageal perforations in a swine NOTES model using hemostatic clips [22]. Tsunada et al. demonstrated that clip closure could be effective in human patients. Seven patients who suffered full-thickness gastric perforations after EMR had their defects closed successfully using endoscopic hemostatic clips [23]. No patient required laparotomy.

b. OTSC

The most commonly used OTSC for both NOTES and closure of defects after ESD or

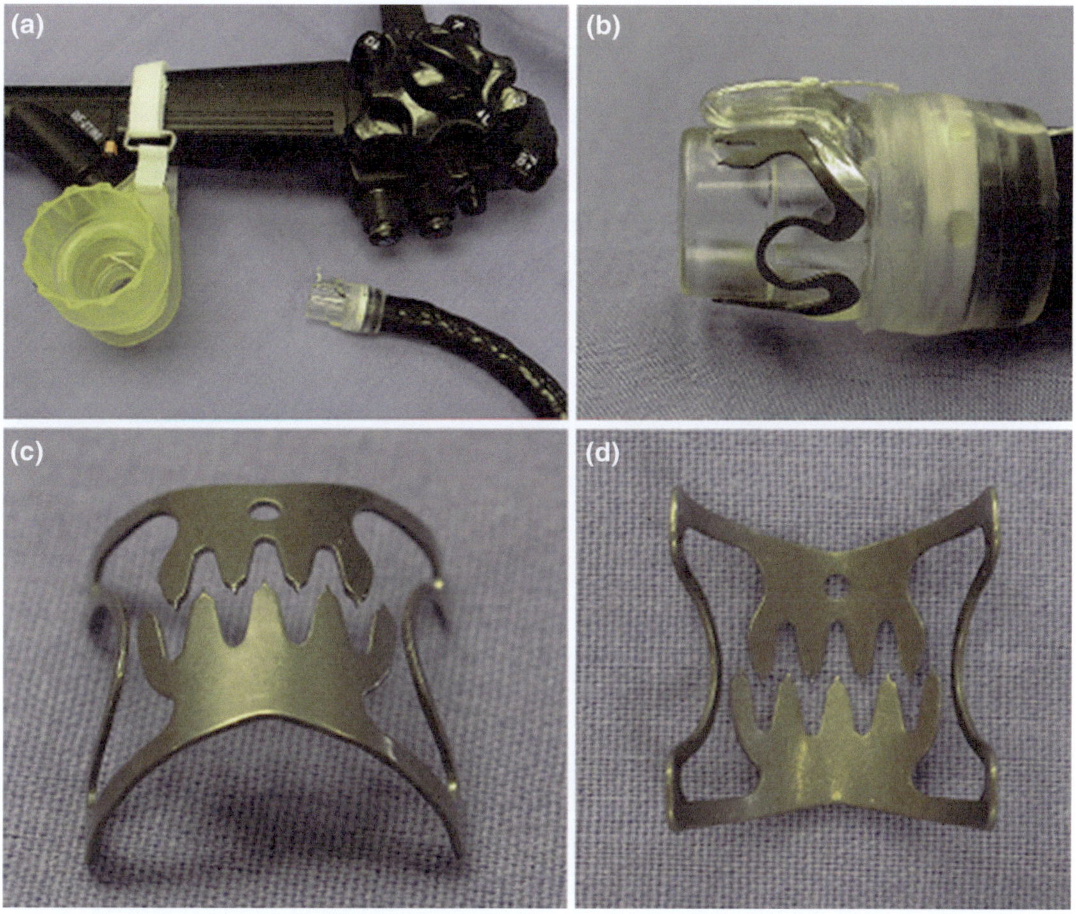

Fig. 2.2 The Ovesco over-the-scope clip. **a** Delivery system mounted on the endoscope. **b** Close-up view of open clip in transparent cap. **c** Clip in closed position, convex (serosal) side. **d** Clip in closed position, concave (mucosal) side. (Used with the permission from Ovesco Endoscopy)

EFTR (endoscopic full-thickness resection) is the OTSC® Closure system (Ovesco Endoscopy, Tübingen, Germany). These clips are made of nitinol and are in the shape of overlapping jaws or "bear claws" (Fig. 2.2). The jaws are in the closed position when manufactured, but are flexed into the open position when mounted on the tip of an endoscope. When deployed by pulling back the inner collar of the deployment pod, the device will snap shut into the closed position due to the memory properties of nitinol. This entraps the gastrotomy between the jaws of the clip, thus sealing the defect.

The feasibility of OTSC closure of defects was noted as far back as 2008 [24]. This study used the Ovesco OTSC® to close gastric defects made after needle-knife exit in a nonsurvival porcine model. Defects were primarily closed in 8 of 9 experimental subjects, but the ninth could not be closed effectively due to a 20-mm rent accidentally made in the gastric wall. In 3 of the remaining 8 animals, the closure did not withstand "burst pressures," a fact that may not be clinically significant as noted earlier [18]. Nevertheless, the feasibility of using OTSC for closure had been established.

Matthes et al. used the Ovesco OTSC to close standardized defects in explanted porcine stomachs and then burst tested them with compressed air under water to assess for strength of the closure [25]. Many similar ex vivo studies, in vivo survival and nonsurvival animal studies, and human studies have shown them to be effective as closure devices for NOTES and other iatrogenic perforations in the stomach, duodenum, colon, and esophagus [26–29].

Although used less commonly, the Padlock Clip™ OTSC (Aponos Medical, Kingston, NH) has also been used for closure of persistent fistulas, as well as transgastric and transcolonic NOTES. Originally approved for endoscopic hemostasis, this device consists of a hexagonal nitinol clip mounted in a translucent cap that fits over the endoscope. It has 6 prongs which, when deployed, gather tissue into the center of the hexagon, thus tamponading a bleeding site or, in the case of NOTES, sealing the defect (Fig. 2.3).

Our group published some of the first animal work with this device. We demonstrated in 2009, in an explant study with burst pressures, that the Padlock Clip™ could provide a secure gastric closure for NOTES [30]. Later, we reported the use of the Padlock Clip™ for gastrotomy closure in a survival study [31]. Two pigs were survived for 2 weeks, and 2 were survived for 6 weeks. All animals did well, the device appeared to be easy to use, and it provided a secure closure. So and Adler published a case report of closure of a persistent tracheoesophageal fistula in a human patient using the Padlock Clip™ [32], and Guarner-Argente et al. reported successful colonic closure with this device [33].

We have used the device a twice for closure of persistent gastrocutaneous fistulas in humans

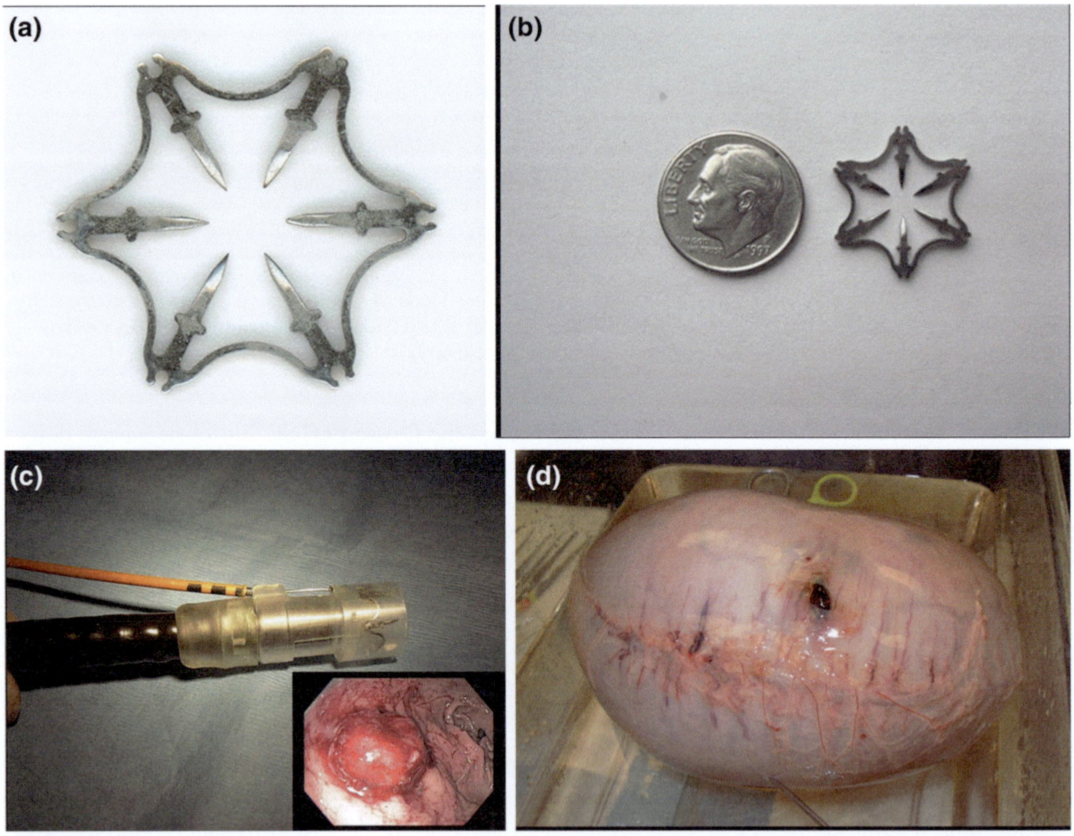

Fig. 2.3 **a** Padlock-G over-the-scope clip. **b** Actual size. **c** Padlock-G mounted on an endoscope in its delivery system. *Inset* Appearance of the Padlock-G after intragastric placement to seal a gastrocutaneous fistula post-PEG removal. **d** Burst pressure testing showing effective closure at high pressure

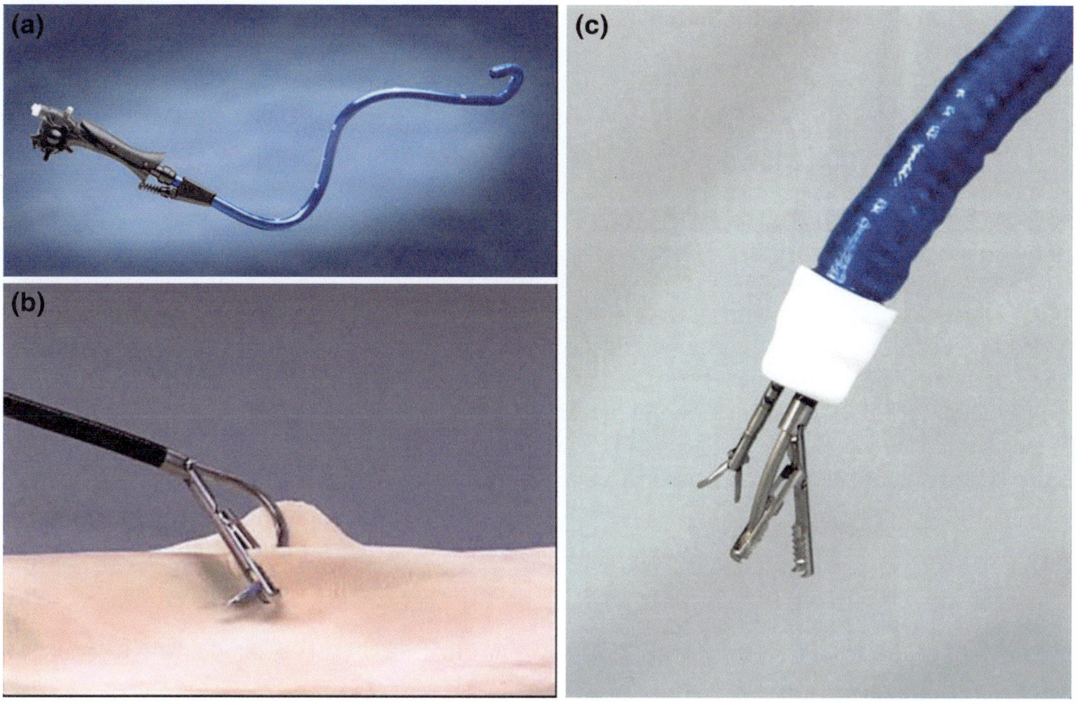

Fig. 2.4 **a** The ShapeLock™ overtube. **b** The g-Prox® device. **c** The ShapeLock™ overtube with devices inserted

after PEG removal, but we feel it suffers from design flaws in the deployment system (a trip-wire that pushes rather than pulls to deploy the device, and so this wire is prone to kinking or bending, with failed deployment). A newer deployment system is being developed.

(3) Endoscopic Suturing

Endoscopic suturing methods have been employed for gastrotomy closure since the inception of NOTES. Swanstrom and coworkers described the transport system (Transport, USGI Medical, San Capistrano, CA), which is a flexible but locking overtube that has 4 ports for insertion of graspers and other instruments for NOTES (Fig. 2.4) [34]. This group uses the g-Prox needle (USGI Medical, San Capistrano, CA) to deliver expandable tissue anchors (so-called snowshoe tissue anchors) to approximate tissue for gastrotomy closure (Fig. 2.5).

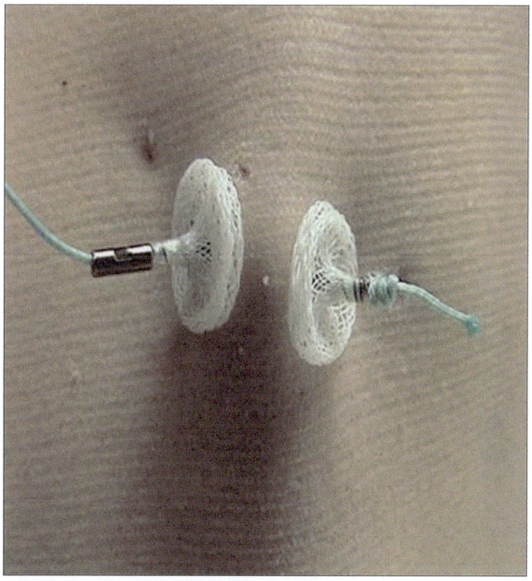

Fig. 2.5 Tissue anchor placed with g-Prox® device

Kanstevoy et al. have used the Over-Stitch suturing device (Apollo Endosurgery Inc, Austin, TX) to close a persistent gastrocutaneous fistula after PEG removal [35]. This device is the newest generation of the venerable "Eagle Claw" endoscopic suturing device [36]. Since that time, many authors have reported the use of the Overstitch device for closure of gastrotomies, colotomies, and esophagotomies after POEM and other NOTES procedures [37].

(4) T-Tags

T-tags are short (~1 cm) metal rods with a suture attached at its midpoint. These can be loaded into an 18-ga or 19-ga needle and placed transmurally, either endoscopically or percutaneously (Fig. 2.6) [38]. When traction is placed on the suture, the metal bar swings perpendicular to the axis of traction and acts as a tissue anchor.

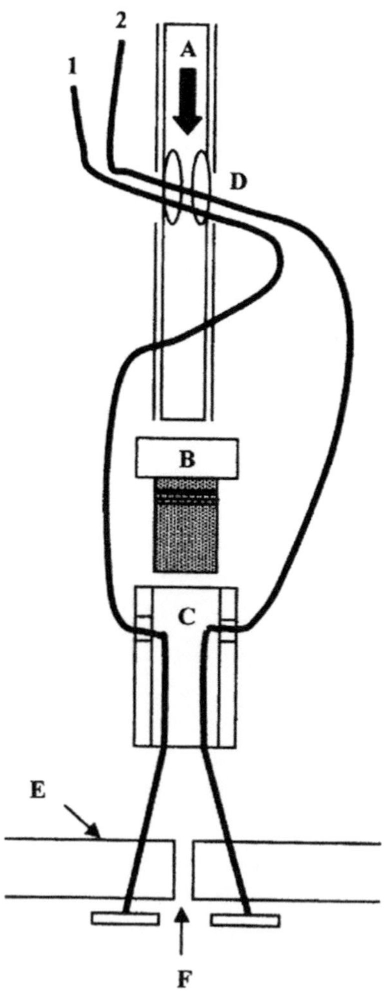

Fig. 2.6 Schematic of T-tag closure of a tissue defect

Several groups have published their results using T-tags for gastrotomy closure [21, 38, 39]. Our own group has done work along these lines and has determined that trailing sutures can become tangled, extracorporeal knots are difficult to tie, tight tissue apposition can be a challenge, and in general, T-tag closure can be problematic. We circumvented some of these problems by using multiple T-tags mounted on a single suture [40, 41]. This is accomplished by utilizing tags with a metal loop through which a suture can be threaded. The endoscopic needle must be modified to have a longitudinal slot cut into it in order to allow the looped T-tag to be loaded. When multiple such tags are placed on a single suture, and the suture is cinched tightly, the effect is similar to a purse–string suture (Figs. 2.7 and 2.8).

(5) Miscellaneous (Endoloops with Clips, Flaps, PEG, etc.)

Many other closure methods have been reported, to include endoscopic loops (detachable snares) in combination with clips [42], tunnels and mucosal flaps [10–15], PEG closure (placement of a PEG through the gastrotomy after NOTES) [43], "8-ring" device with clips [44],percutaneous suture closure of a gastrotomy [45], etc. As noted earlier, it is beyond the scope of this chapter on fundamentals to review exhaustively all closure methods. Interested readers are encouraged to start with the references listed here and to refer to technical reviews [16, 19].

Tips and Tricks, or Lessons Learned

(1) Maintaining Access

We learned early in our animal work that once capnoperitoneum has been achieved, repeat luminal exit from the stomach or colon can be a challenge. Insufflation of the abdominal cavity tends to compress the stomach or colon, and repeat location of the original exit site can be very difficult. Repeat luminal exit is even more demanding if the gastric exit was balloon-dilated

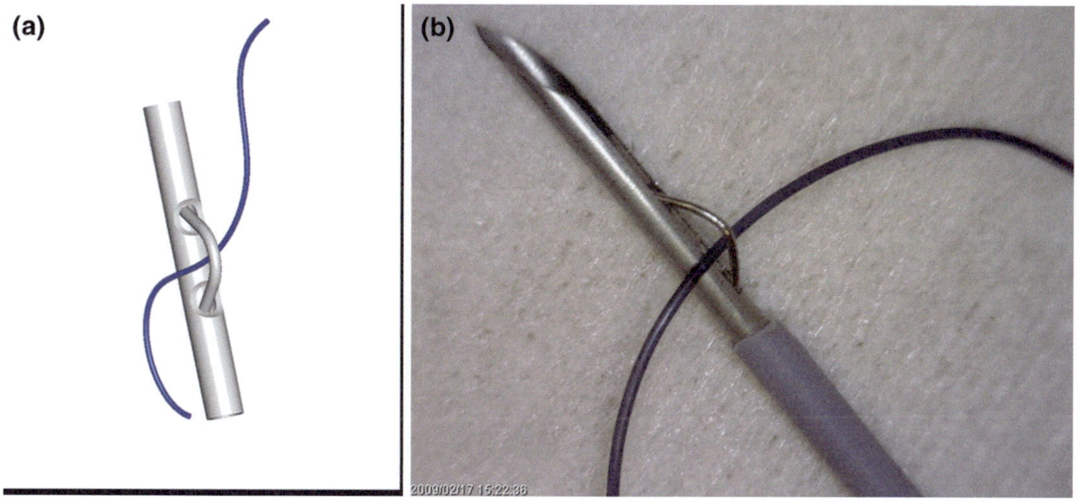

Fig. 2.7 **a** Schematic of looped T-tag. **b** Looped T-tag loaded in slotted 19-ga needle and mounted on nylon suture. (Permission for use granted by Cook Medical Incorporated, Bloomington, Indiana)

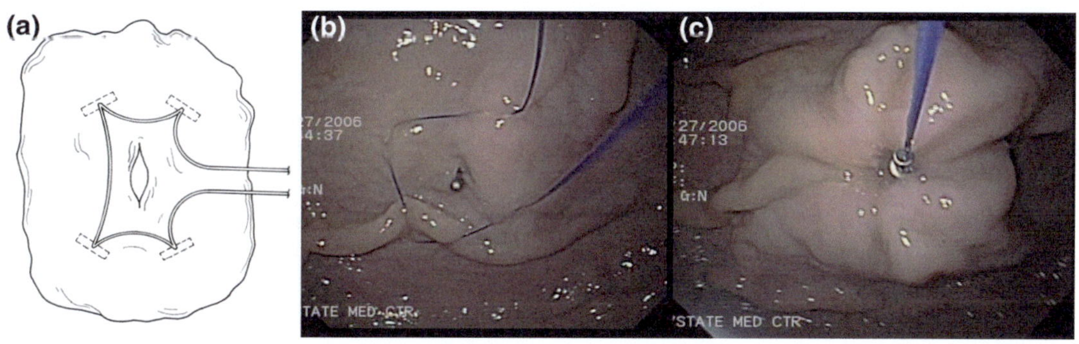

Fig. 2.8 **a** Schematic of looped T-tag closure. **b** Four looped T-tags placed in a square around gastric defect. **c** Prolene suture cinched tightly with friction-fit collar and closing gastric defect. (Permission for use granted by Cook Medical Incorporated, Bloomington, Indiana)

rather than cut. Tonic retraction of the gastric musculature tends to close the gastrotomy site very quickly, and it can be a frustrating and fruitless endeavor to find and exit the gastrotomy. Therefore, we have learned to leave a guidewire in the abdominal cavity, which can be followed endoscopically, like a trail of breadcrumbs [46] to locate the exit site. Indeed, the scope can be back loaded over the wire so that locating the exit site is assured. This can be very useful in transvaginal cholecystectomy if the endoscope must be removed for any reason. Finding one's way through the mesentery into the abdomen from the pelvis can be challenging, and leaving a wire to guide the way can be quite helpful.

We have subsequently improved on just leaving a loose wire in the abdomen. With the endoscope already in the abdomen, a needle puncture through the lower abdominal wall into the insufflated abdomen is performed under endoscopic viewing. A guidewire can then be passed to the endoscope, captured with a snare, and pulled out through the subject's mouth. The percutaneous end can be fixed with a hemostat at the skin level, and traction can be applied at the mouth. This so-called "monorail" method allows for repeated endoscope or device passage over the guidewire easily, quickly, and safely despite capnoperitoneum, and with no chance of dislodging the guidewire.

(2) Spatial Orientation

In general, spatial orientation seems to be less of a problem for endoscopists than surgeons. Endoscopists are comfortable working in retroflexion. In addition, they are utterly unable to determine true anterior, posterior, cephalad, caudad, left, or right during intraluminal endoscopy, and so they tend not to concern themselves with these parameters.

On the other hand, surgeons rely on spatial orientation much more and can easily become confused when the anatomic landmarks are not in proper orientation. We have learned to take advantage of these differences in training and experience. There are times, during transvaginal cholecystectomy for example, when paying attention to the true horizon, keeps one out of trouble. By the same token, there are times when an endoscopist's ability to work retroflexed and upside down brings a considerable advantage. Once again, we have found that having both surgeons and endoscopists on the team is of considerable value.

(3) Tissue Retraction and Triangulation

As anyone who attempts NOTES using a flexible endoscope will quickly learn, inability to perform tissue retraction is a serious constraint. Given that the accessory channel(s) of flexible endoscopes are in line with the shaft, ability to retract or triangulate is quite restricted. Blunt dissection and spreading of tissue are limited by the size of the devices that can be inserted through the working channel as well. One way to overcome such limitations is to use a laparoscopic port (so-called hybrid NOTES) for retraction or dissection. An additional endoscope can be inserted, either through the same natural orifice or from another orifice. In transvaginal cholecystectomy, multiple rigid laparoscopic instruments may be inserted alongside each other and left parallel or crossed to effect tissue retraction. These considerations may have given birth to techniques ultimately used in single-incision laparoscopic surgery (SILS). Extracorporeal magnets have also been used effectively for organ retraction, although not yet in human cases [47, 48]. Let us not forget gravity. Placing a patient in deep Trendelenburg or reverse Trendelenburg position, rotating the patient into the left or right lateral decubitus position, or even placing the patient prone may all yield effective organ or tissue "retraction" by the use of gravity.

(4) Improvising and Off-Label Use of Devices

When performing NOTES, it becomes readily apparent that the development of devices by industry has not kept pace with innovation by clinician researchers. We are left with common devices used in endoscopy and laparoscopic surgery that may need to be adapted to different uses. Endoscopic caps, guidewires (as noted above), hot and cold forceps, snares, grasping forceps, PEGs, needle knives, stents, and other devices may be used off-label to achieve desired outcomes. For example, we have modified an esophageal stent deployment system to deliver hernia mesh aseptically through the mouth to the abdomen [49]. Esophageal dilation balloons can be used to dilate gastrotomies. Closure is effected with hemostatic clips. We have also used a flexible laparoscopic stapler transorally to create a stapled cystogastrostomy to drain pancreatic pseudocysts [50, 51]. Truly, "necessity is the mother of invention" when it comes to innovation in NOTES.

Complications

As with any other surgical or endoscopic procedure, despite our best efforts, immediate or delayed adverse events will sometimes occur. These include infection, bleeding, perforated viscus, anesthesia or metabolic complications, pulmonary or cardiac complications, damage to bystander organs, bile duct or other ductal or vascular injuries, and conversion to laparoscopic or open procedure. It is beyond the scope of this chapter to address adverse events in detail, but suffice it to say that as in open or laparoscopic surgery, standard surgical attention to infection control, hemostasis, and proper technique are of critical importance in NOTES. Also, the NOTES surgeon must be prepared to recognize and react to adverse events quickly and decisively using the endoscopic or laparoscopic tools at hand. If trouble looms large, one should reach out to surgical or endoscopic colleagues for additional help when dealing with immediate or delayed complications.

Conclusion

NOTES procedures require extensive knowledge of the tools available to the advanced therapeutic endoscopist. For this reason, we still espouse the formation of a multidisciplinary team. Gastric closure remains an area of investigation for transgastric NOTES procedures, and in part due to this reason, transvaginal procedures (which are closed with simple external sutures) have become more widely adopted. An operating suite with both laparoscopic and advanced therapeutic endoscopic equipment is a must in order to perform these procedures.

References

1. Kalloo A, Rattner D, Brugge W, Gostout C, Hawes R., et al. The ASGE/SAGES working group on natural orifice translumenal endoscopic surgery white paper. Gastrointest Endosc 2006;63:199–203.
2. Moreira-Pinto J, Ferreira A, Rolanda C, Correia-Pinto J. Natural orifice transesophageal endoscopic surgery: state of the art. Minim Invas Surg 2012;2012(Article ID 896952):7. doi:10.1155/2012/896952.
3. Desilets DJ, Romanelli JR, Earle DB. Starting a peroral endoscopic myotomy program at your institution. Techn Gastrointest Endosc. 2013;15:157–9.
4. Romanelli JR, Desilets DJ. Training and credentialing in NOTES (Natural Orifice Translumenal Endoscopic Surgery). Curr Surg Rep. 2013;1:228–32.
5. Roberts K, Solomon D, Bell R, Duffy A. "Triangle of safety:" anatomic considerations in transvaginal natural orifice surgery. Surg Endosc. 2013;27:2963–5.
6. Wagh MS, Thompson CC. Surgery Insight: natural orifice transluminal endoscopic surgery—an analysis of work to date. Nature Clin Pract Gastro Hep. 2007;4:386–92.
7. Ko C-W, Shin EJ, Buscaglia JM, Clarke JO, Magno P, et al. Preliminary pneumoperitoneum facilitates transgastric access into the peritoneal cavity for natural orifice transluminal endoscopic surgery: a pilot study in a live porcine model. Endoscopy. 2007;39:845–53.
8. Jagannath SB, Kantsevoy SV, Vaughn CA, Chung SSC, Cotton PB, et al. Peroral transgastric endoscopic ligation of fallopian tubes with long-term survival in a porcine model. Gastrointest Endosc. 2005;61:449–53.
9. Kantsevoy SV, Jagannath SB, Niiyama H, Isakovich NV, Chung SSC, et al. A novel, safe approach to the peritoneal cavity for per-oral transgastric endoscopic procedures. Gastrointest Endosc 2007;65:497–500.
10. Sumiyama K, Gostout CJ, Rajan E, Bakken TA, Knipschield MA, et al. Pilot study of transesophageal endoscopic epicardial coagulation by submucosal endoscopy with the mucosal flap safety valve technique. Gastrointest Endosc. 2008;67:497–501.
11. Lee CK, Lee S-H, Chung I-K, Lee TH, Lee SH, et al. Human diagnostic transgastric peritoneoscopy with the submucosal tunnel technique performed with the patient under conscious sedation. Gastrointest Endosc. 2010;72:889–91.
12. Pauli EM, Moyer MT, Haluck RS, Mathew A. Self-approximating transluminal access technique for natural orifice transluminal endoscopic surgery: a porcine survival study. Gastrointest Endosc. 2008;67:690–7.
13. Yoshizumi F, Yasuda K, Kawaguchi K, Suzuki K, Shiraishi N, Kitano S. Submucosal tunneling using endoscopic submucosal dissection for peritoneal access and closure in natural orifice transluminal endoscopic surgery: a porcine survival study. Endoscopy. 2009;41:707–11.
14. Pauli EM, Haluck RS, Ionescu AM, Rogers AM, Shope TR, et al. Directed submucosal tunneling permits in-line endoscope positioning for transgastric natural orifice translumenal endoscopic surgery (NOTES). Surg Endosc. 2010;24:1474–81.
15. Kono Y, Yasuda K, Horoishi K, Akagi T, Kawaguchi K, et al. Transrectal peritoneal access with the submucosal tunnel technique in NOTES: a porcine survival study. Surg Endosc. 2013;27:278–85.
16. Banerjee S, Barth BA, Bhat YM, Desilets DJ, Gottlieb KT, et al. Endoscopic closure devices. Gastrointest Endosc. 2012;76:244–51.
17. Addington WR, Stephens RE, Phelipa MM, Widdicombe JG, Ockey RR. Intra-abdominal Pressures during Voluntary and Reflex Cough. Cough 2008;4 (Open-access journal). doi:10.1186/1745-9974-4-2.

18. Desilets DJ, Mader TJ, Romanelli JR, Earle DB. Gastric transmural pressure measurements in vivo: implications for natural orifice transluminal endoscopic surgery (NOTES). Gastrointest Endosc. 2010;71:583–8.
19. Raju GS. Endoscopic closure of gastrointestinal leaks. Am J Gastroenterol. 2009;104:1315–20.
20. Raju GS, Ahmed I, Brining D, Xiao SY. Endoluminal closure of large perforations of colon with clips in a porcine model. Gastrointest Endosc. 2006;64: 640–6.
21. Merrifield BF, Wagh MS, Thompson CC. Peroral transgastric organ resection: a feasibility study in pigs. Gastrointest Endosc 2006;63:693–7.
22. Fritscher-Ravens A, Hampe J, Grange P, Holland C, Olagbeye F, et al. Clip closure versus endoscopic suturing versus thoracoscopic repair of an iatrogenic esophageal perforation: a randomized, comparative, long-term survival study in a porcine model. Gastrointest Endosc. 2010;72:1020–6.
23. Tsunada S, Ogata S, Ohyama T, Ootani H, Kikkawa A, et al. Endoscopic closure of perforations caused by EMR of the stomach by application of metallic clips. Gastrointest Endosc. 2003;57:948–51.
24. Kratt T, Küper M, Traub F, Ho C, Schurr M, et al. Feasibility study for secure closure of natural orifice transluminal endoscopic surgery gastrotomies by using over-the-scope clips. Gastrointest Endosc. 2008;68:993–6.
25. Matthes K, Jung Y, Kato M, Gromski MA, Chuttani R. Efficacy of full-thickness GI perforation closure with a novel over-the-scope—clip application device: an animal study. Gastrointest Endosc. 2011;74:1369–75.
26. Von Renteln D, Schmidt A, Vassiliou MC, Gieselmann M, Caca K. Natural orifice transluminal endoscopic surgery gastrotomy closure with an over-the-scope clip: a randomized, controlled porcine study. Gastrointest Endosc 2009;70:732–9.
27. Parodi A, Repici A, Pedroni A, Blanchi S, Conio M. Endoscopic management of GI perforations with a new over-the-scope clip device. Gastrointest Endosc. 2010;72:881–6.
28. Manta R, Manno M, Bertani H, Barbera C, Pigo F, et al. Endoscopic treatment of gastrointestinal fistulas using an over-the-scope clip (OTSC) device: case series from a tertiary referral center. Endoscopy. 2011;43:545–8.
29. Mönkemüller K, Peter S, Toshniwal J, Popa D, Zabielski M, et al. Multipurpose use of the 'bear claw' (over-the-scope clip system) to treat endoluminal gastrointestinal disorders. Dig Endosc. 2014;26:350–7.
30. Romanelli JR, Desilets DJ, Earle DB. Natural orifice transluminal endoscopic surgery gastrotomy closure in porcine explants with the Padlock-G clip using the Lock-It system. Endoscopy. 2010;42:306–10.
31. Desilets DJ, Romanelli JR, Earle DB, Chapman CN. Gastrotomy closure with the lock-it system and the padlock-G clip: a survival study in a porcine model. J Laparoendosc Adv Surg Tech. 2010;20:671–6.
32. So BJ, Adler DG. Closure of a chronic, non-healing tracheoesophageal fistula with a new over-the-scope clip. ACG Case Rep J. 2014;2:18–20.
33. Guarner-Argente C, Cordova H, Martinez-Palli G, Navarro R, Cuatrecasas M, et al. Yes, we can: reliable colonic closure with the Padlock-G clip in a survival porcine study. Gastrointest Endosc. 2010;72:841–4.
34. Swanstrom LL, Whiteford M, Khajanchee Y. Developing essential tools to enable transgastric surgery. Surg Endosc. 2008;22:600–4.
35. Thuluvath PJ, Kantsevoy SV. Successful closure of a chronic refractory gastrocutaneous fistula with a new endoscopic suturing device. Gastrointest Endosc. 2012;75:688–90.
36. Hu B, Chung SC, Sun LC, Kawashima K, Yamamoto T, et al. Eagle Claw II: A novel endosuture device that uses a curve needle for major arterial bleeding: a bench study. Gastrointest Endosc. 2005;62:266–70.
37. Stavropoulos SN, Modayil R, Friedel D. Current applications of endoscopic suturing. World J Gastrointest Endosc. 2015;7:777–89.
38. Austin RCT, Mosse CA, Swain P. A novel use for T-tag sutures for the safe creation and closure of the NOTES gastrotomy using a hybrid technique. Surg Endosc. 2009;23:2827–30.
39. Trunzo JA, Cavazzola LT, Elmunzer BJ, Poulose BK, McGee MF, et al. Facilitating gastrotomy closure during natural-orifice transluminal endoscopic surgery using tissue anchors. Endoscopy. 2009;41:487–92.
40. Desilets DJ, Romanelli JR, Earle DB, Surti VC, Willingham FF, et al. Loop-anchor purse-string versus endoscopic clips for gastric closure: a natural orifice transluminal endoscopic surgery comparison study using burst pressures. Gastrointest Endosc. 2009;70:1225–30.
41. Romanelli JR, Desilets DJ, Chapman CN, Surti VC, Lovewell C, et al. Loop-anchor purse-string closure of gastrotomy in NOTES® procedures: survival studies in a porcine model. Surg Innov. 2010;17:312–7.
42. Shi Q, Chen T, Zhong Y-S, Zhou P-H, Ren Z, et al. Complete closure of large gastric defects after endoscopic full-thickness resection, using endoloop and metallic clip interrupted suture. Endoscopy. 2013;45:329–34.
43. McGee MF, Marks JM, Onders RP, Chak A, Rosen MJ, et al. Infectious implications in the porcine model of natural orifice transluminal endoscopic surgery (NOTES) with PEG-tube closure: a quantitative bacteriologic study. Gastrointest Endosc 2008;68:310–8.
44. Fujii T, Ono A, Fu K-I. A novel endoscopic suturing technique using a specially designed so-called "8-ring" in combination with resolution clips. Gastrointest Endosc. 2007;660:1215–20.

45. Sporn E, Miedema BW, Astudillo JA, Bachman SL, Loy TS, et al. Gastrotomy creation and closure for NOTES using a gastropexy technique. Gastrointest Endosc 2008;68:948–53.
46. Brothers Grimm. Hansel and Gretel. Fairy Tales, 1812.
47. Horgan S, Mintz Y, Jacobsen GR, Sandler BJ, Cullen JP, et al. Magnetic retraction for NOTES transvaginal cholecystectomy. Surg Endosc. 2010;24:2322.
48. Cho YB, Park JH, Chun H-K, Park CM, Kim HC, et al. Natural orifice transluminal endoscopic surgery applied to sigmoidectomy in survival animal models: using paired magnetic intra-luminal device. Surg Endosc. 2011;25:1319–24.
49. Earle DB, Desilets DJ, Romanelli JR. NOTES transgastric abdominal wall hernia repair in a porcine model. Hernia. 2010;14:517–22.
50. Romanelli JR, Desilets DJ, Earle DB. Pancreatic pseudocystgastrostomy with a peroral, flexible stapler: human natural orifice transluminal endoscopic surgery anastomoses in 2 patients. Gastrointest Endosc. 2008;68:981–7.
51. Pallapothu R, Earle DB, Desilets DJ, Romanelli JR. NOTES stapled cystgastrostomy: a novel approach for surgical management of pancreatic pseudocysts. Surg Endosc. 2011;25:883–9.

Endoscopic GI Surgery

3

Kevin L. Grimes, Robert Bechara, Valerio Balassone and Haruhiro Inoue

Abstract

Routine endoscopic screening programs, such as those for colonoscopy in the West or upper endoscopy in Asia, have led to an increase in the number of lesions being detected. Many of these lesions are premalignant or early-stage cancer for which surgical resection may seem excessive. As instruments and techniques evolved, the ability of endoscopists to resect lesions increased. Initial attempts at mucosal resection led to the "saline lift," the "strip biopsy," and eventually the endoscopic mucosal resection (EMR) utilizing band ligation, tubes, or transparent caps. EMR was later applied to normal mucosa in order to create an ulcer at the gastric cardia, tighten the gastroesophageal valve, and generate protection against gastroesophageal reflux as it healed. Meanwhile, advances in caps and electrical knives led to the development of the endoscopic submucosal dissection (ESD) techniques, which extended the maximum size of lesions that could be resected *en bloc*. And finally, application of ESD techniques to the creation of submucosal tunnels led to the per-oral endoscopic myotomy (POEM) and per-oral endoscopic tumor resection (POET) procedures, in which an endoscopic cardiomyotomy could be performed or a subepithelial tumor could be resected endoscopically.

K.L. Grimes (✉)
Department of Surgery, MetroHealth Medical Center and Case Western Reserve University School of Medicine, Cleveland, OH, USA
e-mail: kevin.grimes@gmail.com

R. Bechara
Division of Gastroenterology, Kingston General Hospital & Queen's University, Kingston, ON, Canada
e-mail: Bechara.robert@gmail.com

V. Balassone
Department of Surgery, University of Rome Tor Vergata Hospital, Rome, Italy
e-mail: valerio.balassone@gmail.com

H. Inoue
Digestive Disease Center, Showa University Koto-Toyosu Hospital, Tokyo, Japan
e-mail: haruinoue777@yahoo.co.jp

J.R. Romanelli et al. (eds.), *NOTES and Endoluminal Surgery*, Clinical Gastroenterology, DOI 10.1007/978-3-319-50610-4_3

Keywords
GI endoscopy · Therapeutic endoscopy · Endoscopic mucosal resection (EMR) · Endoscopic submucosal dissection (ESD) · Anti-reflux mucosectomy (ARMS) · Gastroesophageal reflux disease (GERD) · Per-oral endoscopic myotomy (POEM) · Achalasia · Per-oral endoscopic tumor resection (POET) · Subepithelial tumor (SET)

Endoscopic Mucosal Resection (EMR)

Background

The widespread use of screening endoscopy has led to an increase in the number of gastrointestinal lesions being detected, whether flat lesions or polyps of the colon and rectum, dysplastic changes arising from within Barrett's esophagus, or early neoplasms of the gastric mucosa. The presence or absence of malignancy and the depth of invasion can often only be definitely determined after resection; therefore, *en bloc* resection is preferred. A variety of techniques have been developed to increase the safety, *en bloc* resection rate, and size of mucosal lesions that can be resected. EMR is one of these, where the mucosal lesion is removed *en bloc* with a snare using either a cap-fitted endoscope and suction, saline lift, or other methods.

Indications

EMR is indicated for small (less than 10 mm) superficial squamous cell carcinomas of the esophagus if *en bloc* resection can be achieved; visible lesions in Barrett's esophagus; small (10–15 mm) gastric lesions with a low probability of advanced histology; and the majority of superficial lesions of the colon and rectum [1].

Technique

Strip Biopsy

The first reported adjunct to standard polypectomy came in 1955 when Rosenberg described the "saline lift," in which a submucosal saline injection created a buffer between the mucosa and the muscle layer, reducing the risk of perforation in the colon and rectum [2, 3]. Tada et al. extended this to the resection of gastric lesions, creating a mucosal bleb that could be resected with a wire snare [4].

Meanwhile, Martin et al. created the "lift-and-cut biopsy" in which one snare was used to grasp and elevate the mucosa, while a second snare was used to reset the specimen [5]. In a series published by Takekoshi et al., however, rates of incomplete resection were over 50% [6].

Tada et al. reported the original "strip-off" biopsy in 1984, and this was followed by the local injection of hypertonic saline by Hirao et al. [7]. Monma et al. and Makuuchi et al. reported a merging of these techniques in the Japanese literature in 1990 [8, 9]. This modified "strip biopsy" included submucosal saline injection, followed by the elevation of the mucosa with a grasper, and finally resection with a wire snare.

Band Ligation and EMR-L

Work by Chaves et al. and Masuda et al. utilized variceal ligation devices, which could convert flat lesions into "polyps" that could then be transected at the base using an electrical snare [10, 11]. The technique became known as "EMR-L" and was applied to lesions of the colon as well as the esophagus [12].

Distal Cap and EMR-C

A modification of the "life-and-cut" biopsy included the use of a transparent overtube, which improved control and increased the ability resect esophageal mucosa by grasping and snaring.

Using this technique, Inoue and Endo reported resection of large and near-circumferential segments of mucosa, though in piecemeal fashion, without damage to the underlying muscle [13].

Modifications to the overtubes, such as lateral windows that served as mucosal traps, were eventually replaced by a transparent distal attachment. First published in 1993, Inoue et al. employed the EMR-C technique, in which suction was used to draw mucosa into the transparent cap, which was then strangulated and cut using a wire snare (Fig. 3.1) [14]. This was later applied to lesions of the colon and duodenum and could theoretically be utilized anywhere that can be reached with an endoscope [15, 16].

Safety

EMR is a safe procedure, and major complications are rare. The most common complications are bleeding and perforation. The highest rates are seen in the vascular-rich stomach, where a meta-analysis of retrospective studies including nearly 2000 cases of EMR for early gastric cancer noted a bleeding rate of 8.6% and a perforation rate of 0.9% [17]. Bleeding is less common in the esophagus, colon, and rectum, with a reported rate less than 2% in large studies. Perforation is seen in less than 1% of colon and rectal cases, and in approximately 0.1% of esophageal cases [18, 19].

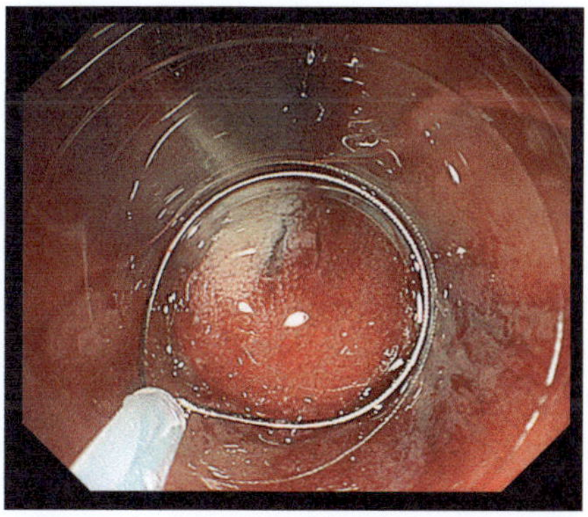

Fig. 3.1 Cap endoscopic mucosal resection (EMR-C). Following submucosal saline injection, a wire snare is positioned within a transparent distal cap. The mucosa is drawn into the cap using the scope's suction capability, and the wire snare is tightened around the mucosa, which is resected using electrocautery

Efficacy

Esophagus

In a study of 1096 patients undergoing EMR for lesions arising within Barrett's esophagus, there was failure of endoscopic treatment progressing to esophagectomy in less than 0.5%, and remission was achieved in 96%, with 15% recurrence of neoplasia at a median follow-up of about 2 years [19].

Stomach

A meta-analysis of retrospective studies analyzed nearly 2000 cases of EMR for early gastric cancer and found an *en bloc* resection rate of only 52%, though lesions larger than 20 mm were included in some studies. The local recurrence rate was 6% [17].

Colon and Rectum

In the colon and rectum, *en bloc* resection rates range from 67 to 80% as long as the tumor is less than 20 mm in size. For larger tumors, the rate of en bloc resection is significantly lower, and the risk of local recurrence may be as high as 23% at 1 year for piecemeal resection. When complete *en bloc* resection is achieved, local recurrence is higher in the rectum (4–5%) than in the colon (2%) [18].

Conclusion

EMR is a safe and effective technique for resection of superficial mucosal lesions. The main drawback is the upper limit on the size of lesions that can be resected *en bloc*, so it is best suited to small lesions and pathology in which piecemeal resection does not adversely affect oncologic outcomes.

Endoscopic Submucosal Dissection (ESD)

Background

Endoscopic submucosal dissection (ESD) is similar to EMR except that larger lesions can be removed *en bloc* by dissecting under the saline-lifted lesions rather than simple snare excision. As EMR became more commonly accepted, advances in both the technique and the equipment followed. In 1982, Hirao et al. added a "pre-cutting" step to the original "strip biopsy" by performing a submucosal injection followed by circumferential mucosal incision around the lesion using a needle knife [7]. Retraction of the specimen increased the size of the lesion that could be safely resected with a cutting snare. The technique was modified by Gotoda et al. using a knife developed by Hosokawa and Yoshida several years earlier, the Insulated Tip (IT) Knife, to minimize the risk of perforation during the pre-cutting step [20]. The upper limit of lesions that could be resected, however, remained approximately 3 cm.

Further modifications aimed at increasing en bloc resection of larger lesions included division of the submucosal fibers under direct vision using a transparent distal cap [21–23]. Development of purpose-built knives, including the HookKnife™ (Olympus America, Center Valley, PA), the FlexKnife™ (Olympus America), the Triangle Tip (TT) Knife (Olympus America), and the Flush Knife (Fujifilm, Tokyo, Japan) improved precision and allowed the submucosal dissection to proceed more safely and efficiently.

Indications

ESD is indicated for *en bloc* resection of superficial squamous cell carcinoma of the esophagus without obvious submucosal involvement; Barrett's esophagus with lesions larger than 15 mm, poorly lifting tumors, or risk of submucosal invasion; superficial gastric neoplasms with a low risk of lymph node metastasis; and colon or rectal lesions larger than 20 mm or with a high suspicion of limited submucosal invasion [1]. Of note, there is no particular upper limit to the size of lesions that can be resected *en bloc* by ESD.

Technique

ESD can be performed with a variety of endoscopic cutting instruments depending on the particulars of an individual lesion and the preferences of the endoscopist. The standard technique begins with submucosal injection to develop the potential space between the mucosa and the muscle layers, followed by pre-cutting of the mucosa, and finally division of the submucosal fibers under direct vision. In the final step, the specimen must be retracted to provide visualization, while simultaneously dissecting in the submucosal plane (Fig. 3.2). Specimen retraction can be with a second device in a double-channel endoscope, or with a variety of other novel devices such as robots, magnets, or operating platforms/overtubes.

Submucosal Tunneling

The main technical challenge of ESD is control of the specimen during dissection from the underlying muscle layer. As an alternative to the standard technique, von Delius et al. reported "endoscopy of the submucosal space" in 2007, in which they reversed the order of the mucosal incision and division of submucosal fibers [24]. In a pig model, they entered the submucosal space through a mucosotomy and created a tunnel under the lesion. Once the mucosa had been completely separated from the underlying muscle, they completed the resection by post-cutting the mucosa and were able to successfully resect lesions of various sizes, including a complete circumferential donut.

Safety

Esophagus

Overall, procedure-related bleeding and perforation were each less than 3% over 38 studies and 2223 lesions. There were no ESD-related mortalities [1].

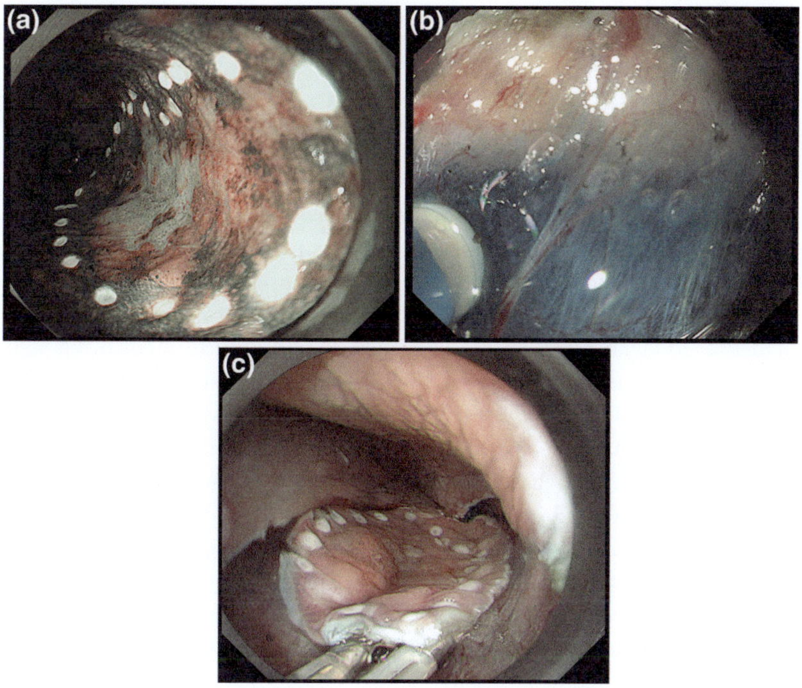

Fig. 3.2 Endoscopic submucosal dissection (ESD). **a** The lesion to be resected is marked circumferentially using electrocautery. The lesion is then lifted by submucosal saline injection, and the mucosa is incised circumferentially. **b** A transparent distal cap is used to retract the mucosa (*pink*), while a knife is used to divide the submucosal fibers (*blue*). **c** A final *en bloc* ESD specimen

Stomach

In three separate meta-analyses of 1500 or more lesions each, procedure-related bleeding ranged from 4 to 7%, while perforation ranged from 4 to 5%. There were no mortalities [17, 25, 26].

Colon and Rectum

A systematic review by Repici et al. of 2841 lesions found an overall procedure-related bleeding rate of 2% and perforation rate of 4%. There were no mortalities [27].

Efficacy

Esophagus

In a pooled analysis of 38 studies and more than 2200 lesions (including 970 squamous cell carcinoma, 346 adenocarcinoma arising in Barrett's esophagus, 678 squamous cell + adenocarcinoma, and 185 submucosal tumors), the *en bloc* resection rate ranged from 81 to 100%, with an overall average of 96%. The R0 resection rate was 85% with a local recurrence of 0.4% [1].

Stomach

In three meta-analyses of 1495, 1734, and 1916 lesions, the *en bloc* resection rate was 92%, with an R0 resection rate of 82–92%, and local recurrent of <1% [17, 25, 26].

Colon and Rectum

A systematic review by Repici et al. of 2841 lesions found an overall en bloc resection rate of 96%, R0 resection rate of 88%, and local recurrence of <0.1% [27].

Conclusion

ESD can be performed in the esophagus, stomach, colon, and rectum for superficial lesions and early cancers with a high rate of *en bloc* resection, low rates of bleeding and perforation, and no procedure-related mortalities reported to date.

Anti-reflux Mucosal Resection (ARMS)

Background

One of the known complications of EMR is the development of a stricture as the endoscopically created ulcer heals. In experimental models, the healing process involves acute inflammation, angiogenesis, fibrous hyperplasia, accumulation of dense collagen fibers in the submucosa, and atrophy of the muscularis propria [28, 29]. The risk of stricture seems to be highest when the resection involves more than two-thirds of the circumference of the esophageal lumen [30–32].

In 2003, Inoue et al. reported a case in which circumferential EMR was performed in a patient with Barrett's esophagus with high-grade dysplasia. The resected area extended for 2 cm onto the gastric cardia. Preoperatively, the patient had evidence of abnormal acid exposure on 24-h esophageal pH probe. After the patient healed his reflux symptoms resolved, he had normalization of his esophageal pH and has remained off his PPI for over 10 years [13, 33]. It was hypothesized that fibrosis of the gastric cardia resulted in reinforcement of the LES. In 2014, the group published a series of 10 patients in which they described the technique, anti-reflux mucosectomy (ARMS), for PPI-refractory GERD [34].

Indications

The ARMS procedure is currently indicated in patients with PPI-refractory GERD and objective evidence of gastroesophageal reflux, as demonstrated by esophagitis at upper endoscopy or abnormal acid exposure on esophageal pH probe. As with the first reported case, the procedure can be performed in the presence of Barrett's esophagus. The procedure has not been reported in patients with moderate or large hiatal hernias.

Technique

The mucosal resection during the ARMS procedure can be performed using any EMR or ESD technique. The mucosa is first marked along the planned resection margin, forming a crescent shape along the lesser curve of the gastric cardia (Fig. 3.3). A 2-cm portion of mucosa is spared along the greater curve to prevent the stricture from becoming too tight. Submucosal injection is performed in the standard fashion to expand the distance between the mucosal and the muscle layers and to help protect against full-thickness perforation of the stomach. The mucosa is then resected from within the marked area by either cap EMR or ESD. Hemostasis can be achieved using coagulating forceps with monopolar cautery.

Safety

Early experience with the procedure revealed that circumferential mucosal resection always resulted in tight stricture formation that required balloon dilation. Meanwhile, a 50% circumferential resection was found to produce insufficient fibrosis to alleviate reflux symptoms. All patients were managed endoscopically, and there were no significant complications reported [34].

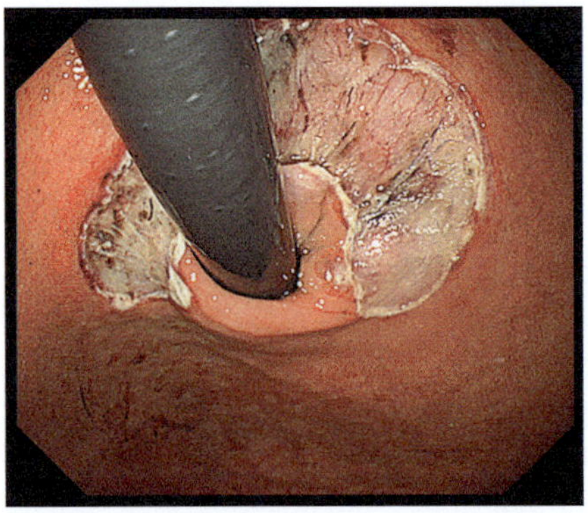

Fig. 3.3 Anti-reflux mucosectomy (ARMS). Serial bites of mucosa are excised using the EMR-C technique to create a crescent-shaped ulcer on the lesser curve of the gastric cardia

Efficacy

In the short-term follow-up, subjective outcomes were significantly improved in all patients. In addition, 24-h esophageal pH studies demonstrated improvement in both DeMeester score and mean time at a pH < 4 [34].

Conclusion

Early pilot studies in Japanese patients have shown promising results following the ARMS procedure. The procedure has the potential to be performed in any center with the ability to perform either EMR or ESD and may offer an alternative to anti-reflux surgery or to other endoscopic options that require the use of expensive purpose-built devices. Further studies are needed to confirm the early results and establish the long-term efficacy.

Per-oral Endoscopic Myotomy (POEM) of the Esophagus

Background

Achalasia is a rare esophageal motor disorder with incidence estimated between 1 and 8 per 100,000 per year. Dysfunction of inhibitory neurons leads to impaired relaxation of the LES and loss of normal esophageal peristalsis. Patients may present with dysphagia, regurgitation, chest pain, weight loss, and/or heartburn. Treatment has traditionally been limited to pneumatic balloon dilation, endoscopic injection of botulinum toxin, and surgical Heller myotomy.

The first endoscopic myotomy was reported by Ortega et al. in 1980 using a 3-mm needle knife to perform two blind 1-cm incisions just above the EGJ [35]. This was moderately successful in 17 patients, but the procedure was not widely adopted. Interest was renewed in 2004 when Kalloo et al. reported endoscopic transgastric peritoneoscopy in a pig model [36]. This was followed in 2007 with an animal model by Pasricha et al., which refined the endoscopic myotomy for achalasia [37]. They entered the submucosal space, created a submucosal a tunnel with a pneumatic balloon, and divided the circular muscle fibers under direct vision. Inoue et al. modified the porcine model to make it suitable for clinical application and performed the first human POEM in Japan in September 2008 [38]. Since that time, the procedure has been widely adopted, and thousands of cases of been performed at centers worldwide.

Indications

While there are no explicit guidelines, POEM has been successfully performed in children as young as 3 years of age and weighing as little as 15 kg [39]. The procedure has also been performed in the very elderly. Generally acknowledged contraindications include the inability to tolerate general anesthesia, portal hypertension, coagulopathy, prior radiation, ablation, or mucosal resection in the planned operative field due to an increased risk of bleeding or perforation [40].

In centers with POEM capability, the procedure can be considered first-line therapy for achalasia. It has also been successfully performed as salvage therapy in patients who have undergone prior pneumatic balloon dilation, endoscopic Botox injection, or surgical myotomy. POEM may also be effective for other motility disorders such as hypertensive LES, distal esophageal spasm, and nutcracker or jackhammer esophagus.

Technique

Preparation

POEM is generally performed using a standard-sized gastroscope with addition of an auxiliary water jet (e.g. Olympus GIF-Q260J, Tokyo, Japan) and a distal cap (FujiFilm DH-28GR or Olympus MH-588) to help maintain a clear operative field and facilitate dissection. Low- or medium-flow carbon dioxide insufflation is used due to a higher risk of complications with room air or high-flow CO_2 [41, 42].

Patients are generally placed on a liquid diet in the days prior to the procedure to minimize the residual contents and treated empirically with an antifungal due to the high rate of esophageal stasis in achalasia patients. Most centers administer perioperative antibiotics and proton pump inhibitors, and upper endoscopy is often performed immediately prior to induction of anesthesia to suction any esophageal contents and reduce the risk of aspiration.

POEM is performed under general anesthesia with a cuffed endotracheal tube, which may help protect against aspiration and may reduce the incidence of capnothorax by providing positive intrathoracic pressure. Some cases have been reported using conscious sedation, but this resulted in longer procedure times and a higher rate of complications such as bleeding, perforation, and pneumothorax [41].

The procedure can be performed in the left lateral decubitus position, though anecdotal evidence suggests this may exacerbate anatomic distortions in patients with advanced sigmoid achalasia. The supine position minimizes distortions. It also allows for monitoring of tense capnoperitoneum, which may occur in 16% or more of cases, and facilitates needle decompression if necessary [43].

Procedure

Inspection begins in the proximal esophagus, where extrinsic compression from the trachea (anterior, 12 o'clock), left main bronchus, aortic arch (anterolateral), and spine (posterior, 6 o'clock) can often be identified and used to maintain orientation. There may be a tight area with resistance to passage of the endoscope just proximal to the EGJ, and the proximal esophagus may demonstrate tertiary contractions.

The location of the EGJ is noted by measuring the distance from the incisors. Many patients will demonstrate a tight area just proximal to the EGJ, and there may be slight resistance to passage of the endoscope. Normal physiologic tightness will often be noted at the upper esophageal sphincter.

The point of entry depends on the planned myotomy length. The mean length of the total myotomy (esophageal + gastric) in published series ranges from 5.4 to 14.4 cm [41, 44]. The entry point is generally chosen 10–15 cm proximal to the EGJ, as first described by Inoue et al. [38], which allows the submucosal tunnel to extend 2–3 cm proximal to the myotomy and may protect against full-thickness perforation.

The procedure can be performed at any "clock" position, with no studies yet demonstrating a clear advantage of one location over the others. The anterior approach, as utilized in the first 500 cases by Inoue et al., avoids the gastric sling fibers and may reduce the risk of post-POEM reflux, but at the expense of an increased risk of major procedural bleeding from branches of the left gastric and left phrenic arteries [38, 39, 45]. The posterior approach avoids some of the larger blood vessels and preserves the anterior anatomy for a straightforward surgical myotomy if indicated in the future, but may disrupt the gastric fling fibers, and theoretically increase the risk of post-POEM reflux. Greater curvature myotomy has also been described, but is technically more challenging [46]. The angle of His serves as a consistent landmark (Fig. 3.4), which may be particularly useful in cases of distorted anatomy from advanced sigmoid achalasia, severe fibrosis from the previous myotomy, ESD, or repeated pneumatic balloon dilations, or inflammation from fungal esophagitis.

After the location for the mucosotomy is chosen, a "saline lift" is performed with an injection needle to expand the potential space between the mucosa and the circular muscle fibers (Fig. 3.5a). This protects against unintended full-thickness myotomy, facilitates entry of the endoscope into the submucosal space, and, if indigo carmine or methylene blue dye is used,

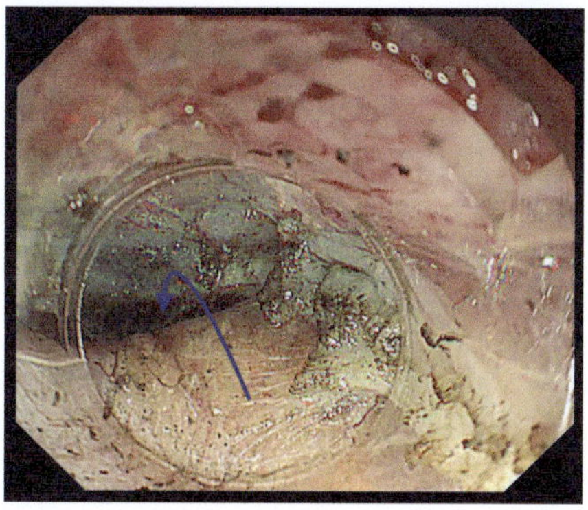

Fig. 3.4 Angle of His. Endoscopic view of the angle of His (*blue arrow*) as seen from within the submucosal tunnel during a per-oral endoscopic myotomy (POEM) procedure performed at the greater curvature (7 o'clock) location

helps to delineate the anatomy. Some centers also include epinephrine in the solution, though there is a risk of cholinergic side effects [45].

The mucosa is incised in a longitudinal direction using a cutting electrical current (Fig. 3.5b), and the submucosal fibers are dissected using spray coagulation. Creation of the submucosal tunnel can be performed using the Triangle Tip (TT) Knife (Olympus KD-640L) (see Fig. 3.5c). Multiple submucosal injections can aid in dissection. Alternate knives such as the Hybrid Knife (ERBE 20150-060, Tübingen, Germany) may reduce the need for multiple instrument exchanges and reduce the average procedure time [47]. The HookKnife™ can facilitate dissection when scarring or

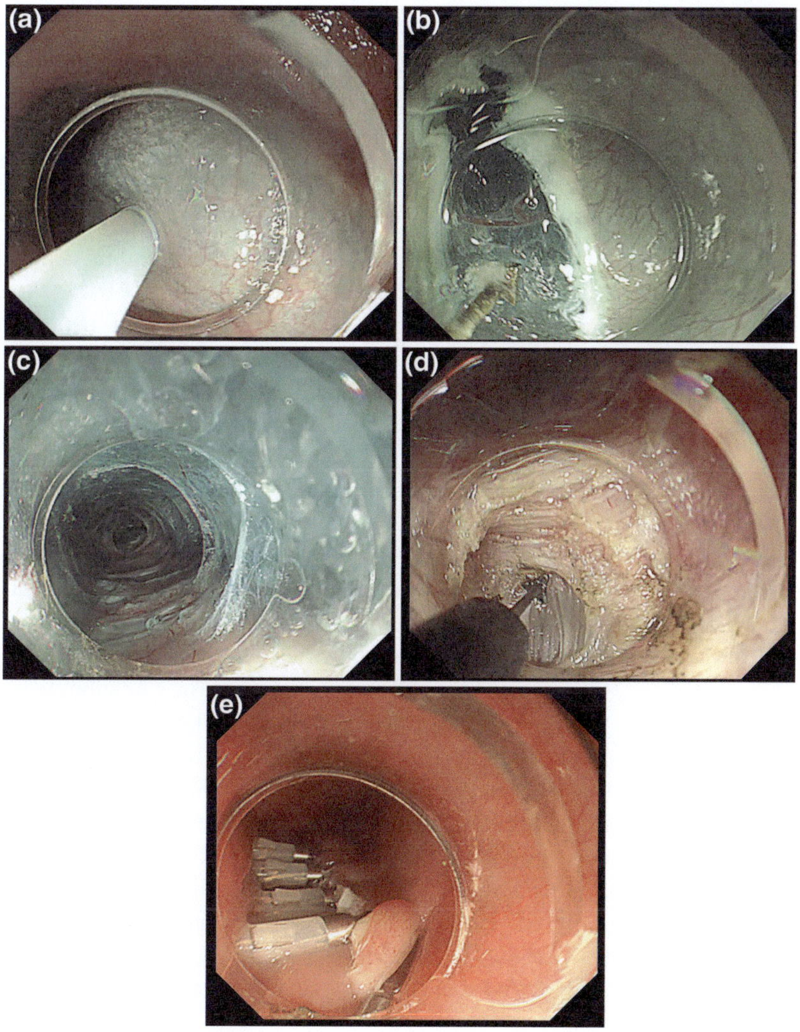

Fig. 3.5 Per-oral endoscopic myotomy (POEM). **a** Submucosal saline injection is performed to create a mucosal lift. **b** A longitudinal mucosal incision is made using the Triangle Tip Knife, exposing the submucosal fibers (*blue*). **c** A completed submucosal tunnel with the circular muscle in the 6 o'clock position (*pink*). **d** Myotomy is performed using a Triangle Tip Knife, selectively dividing the circular fibers (transverse fibers, above the tip of the knife) while leaving the longitudinal fibers (below the tip of the knife, in the 6 o'clock location) in tact. **e** Closure of the mucosal incision using hemostatic clips

inflammation is encountered. During dissection, small perforating vessels may be controlled using the dissecting knife, while larger vessels can be controlled using a coagulating forceps (Coagrasper, Olympus America).

The esophageal myotomy can be performed in anterograde or retrograde direction, with no difference in outcomes (Fig. 3.5d) [48]. The myotomy extends from 2 to 3 cm distal to the mucosal incision. This leaves a short segment of intact mucosa overlying intact muscle, protecting against full-thickness perforation in the event of mucosal closure dehiscence.

There is no clear superiority of either selective circular or full-thickness myotomy. The full-thickness approach is most similar to the surgical myotomy, in which both longitudinal and circular muscle fibers are divided; however, in an international POEM survey, only one-sixth of centers preferred the full-thickness myotomy [40]. Clinical outcomes, complication rates, and rates of post-POEM reflux appear to be similar regardless of whether both muscle layers are transected [49, 50].

The main risk factor for clinical failure of POEM is incomplete myotomy on the gastric side. A gastric myotomy length of 2–3 cm is recommended. Endoscopic landmarks of the gastric side include narrowing followed by widening of the submucosal tunnel, identification of palisade vessels (longitudinally arranged vessels that are characteristic of the gastroesophageal junction), and blue discoloration of the gastric mucosa on retroflexed view in the true lumen [40]. A number of adjuncts have been developed to ensure a complete gastric myotomy, particularly when endoscopic landmarks are likely to be inaccurate, as in cases of distorted anatomy, scarring from prior procedures, or prior esophagitis.

One technique, first described by Baldaque-Silva et al, utilizes two endoscopes to ensure adequate length of the submucosal tunnel, placing one endoscope in the tunnel and observing the transillumination with the other endoscope in retroflexed view of the gastric cardia [51]. A prospective, randomized study involving 100 patients found that the use of this technique resulted in a significant increase in average gastric myotomy length [52]. Further advantages included minimal increase in procedure time, no increases in the rate of complications, and no need for specialized equipment or additional training.

Alternate techniques include placement of a radiopaque clip to mark the EGJ followed by fluoroscopy to measure the distance from the clip to the tip of the endoscope, or the use of the EndoFLIP device to measure EGJ distensibility and guide intra-operative decision making [53–56].

After confirming adequate myotomy length and ensuring hemostasis, the mucosa is closed with hemostatic clips in the majority of cases (Fig. 3.5e). Some authors advocate the use of an antibiotic solution, which is flushed through the endoscope, prior to exiting the submucosal tunnel. Addition of endoloops, endoscopic sutures, over-the-scope clips, or fully covered metal stents may be required if the mucosa is inflamed, macerated, or otherwise difficult to close.

Post-procedure Care

Water-soluble contrast esophagram is obtained on POD #1 to exclude a leak. As many as one-third of patients may demonstrate delayed emptying in the early postoperative period, but this does not appear to correlate with treatment failure in the long term, which calls into question the true value of a contrast esophagram aside from ensuring there is not a full-thickness leak [57]. Some centers also perform upper endoscopy to assess for the development of mucosal necrosis, submucosal hematoma, or dislodgement of the hemostatic clips with dehiscence of the mucosal closure. If partial thickness mucosal necrosis or submucosal hematoma is present, oral intake is delayed until resolution can be confirmed.

Postoperative CT scans are likely to demonstrate nonspecific inflammation or collections of gas, which are considered normal postoperative findings. CT is not recommended in asymptomatic patients [58].

Clear-liquid diet is resumed on POD #1, with advancement to pureed diet on POD #2–3, and regular diet as early as POD #4. An oral PPI is prescribed for at least 1 month, though some centers continue indefinitely [39]. Patients may be discharged home as early as POD #1 [59, 60].

Follow-Up

We conduct the initial follow-up visit at 2 months postoperatively and may include upper endoscopy, high-resolution manometry, and timed barium study in the evaluation. Some centers also include an esophageal pH study. If the PPI has been discontinued, it is resumed in the presence of subjective reflux symptoms or endoscopic findings of esophagitis. Subsequent follow-up is conducted at 1 year postoperatively and then annually thereafter.

Safety

Due to heterogeneity in reporting, overall complication rates vary widely between studies but appear to be similar to LHM [43, 61]. The most common procedure-related adverse events are insufflation-related, bleeding, and perforation. Only 2 cases of significant pulmonary aspiration have been reported, and there have been no reported deaths [52, 62].

Insufflation

Events related to insufflation are relatively common, with rates as high as 30% capnoperitoneum, 11% capnothorax, 5% mediastinal emphysema, 36% subcutaneous emphysema, and one case report of tension capnopericardium (personal communication). Only 8% of patients with capnoperitoneum and 3% of patients with capnothorax require decompression, however [43, 61]. Rates also appear to be technique-dependent, with the use of air insufflation or high-flow CO_2 insufflation resulting in higher rates of adverse events than low- or medium-flow CO_2 insufflation [41, 42]. Capnothorax, capnomediastinum, and capnoperitoneum are generally self-limited. Tense capnoperitoneum may result in increased end-tidal CO_2 or increased ventilator peak pressures, with a theoretical risk of abdominal compartment syndrome. When abdominal decompression is necessary, a large-gauge angiocatheter or Veress needle can be used to decompress the peritoneal cavity. The case of tension capnopericardium required a brief period of chest compressions; however, the patient recovered without complications.

Bleeding

Minor procedural bleeding is common and can generally be controlled using a hemostatic forceps or the knife with a coagulating current. Compared to standard dissection, the Hybrid Knife may reduce the number of minor bleeding episodes [63]. Only one case of severe bleeding has been reported early in the POEM experience; this was controlled with hemostatic forceps, and there have been no reports of procedural bleeding that could not be controlled endoscopically [39].

Delayed bleeding occurs in up to 1% of cases and is generally self-limited [43, 61]. Hemodynamically stable patients can be managed with conservative treatment [44, 64–66]. In three cases, bleeding from the cut edge of the muscle was identified and controlled during EGD [67, 68]. There are no reports of delayed bleeding that required operative intervention.

Perforation

Minor mucosal perforation occurs in less than 3% of cases overall, though some centers report rates as high as 26% [43, 69]. The overwhelming majority of perforations reported to date have been managed endoscopically with clips, endoloops, fibrin glue, endoscopic stitches, or fully covered metal stents [70–73]. Minimally invasive drainage of delayed perforation has been reported in only 4 patients, and there are no reports of perforations that required open surgery [68, 74, 75].

Postoperative imaging may reveal abnormal findings in more than two-thirds of patients, including pneumoperitoneum, pneumomediastinum, subcutaneous emphysema, atelectasis, or minor pulmonary inflammation, but there does not appear to be any correlation between CT findings and development of complications. In an otherwise stable patient, these can be considered normal postoperative findings. A finding of moderate pleural effusion or ascites, however, may be predictive of severe complications, warranting further investigation [68].

Efficacy

Short-Term Outcomes

Studies from centers around the world, including two large meta-analyses, demonstrate an overall clinical success rate for POEM of greater than 90% in reducing Eckardt symptom scores and LES pressures [43, 61]. Similar results have been achieved after prior surgical myotomy, endoscopic pneumatic dilation, or Botox injection, and in patients with spastic esophageal disorders such as DES or Jackhammer esophagus [46, 76–82].

Long-Term Outcomes

Follow-up data from the first 500 cases performed in Japan by Inoue and colleagues demonstrated significant reductions in Eckardt scores and LES pressures in both short- and long-term follow-up, with an overall success rate of 89% at 3 years [39].

Post-POEM Reflux

The main concern with POEM when compared to LHM is that an anti-reflux procedure is not performed. The incidence of reflux following POEM varies widely by geographic region, with the highest rates reported in North America and Western Europe [42, 83–85]. The overall rate in pooled analyses appears to be in the range of 11–19%, which is similar to historical rates observed following LHM (9–17%) [43, 61, 86, 87]. To date, only two studies have directly compared POEM to LHM, and there was no significant difference in the observed rates of reflux [88, 89].

Of particular interest, however, is the fact that many patients may be asymptomatic despite abnormal acid exposure. A study by Jones et al. found no correlation between acid exposure and reflux symptom scores, while a more recent study by Familiari et al. identified abnormal acid exposure in 51%, and esophagitis in 21%, while only 18% reported symptoms [90, 91]. Most centers recommend either long-term PPI or ongoing endoscopic surveillance to assess for esophagitis.

Comparison to Surgical Myotomy

There have been no randomized trials comparing POEM to LHM. Multiple studies have retrospectively compared POEM to historical LHM data and have demonstrated similar safety and efficacy for both procedures. Operative time is up to 30 min faster with POEM, and there appears to be less blood loss, lower postoperative pain, shorter length of hospital stay, and faster return to normal activity [74, 75, 88, 89]. An additional 2 studies using the EndoFLIP device have demonstrated similar increases in EGJ distensibility following both POEM and LHM [92, 93].

Conclusion

A large number of POEM cases have been performed worldwide, with most studies demonstrating excellent clinical success rates and a low rate of major complications. Long-term data show that improvement in symptoms persists for at least 3 years following the procedure, and comparative data suggest equivalence with surgical Heller myotomy. A growing body of evidence also suggests that POEM may be successfully applied to other indications such as spastic esophageal disorders.

Per-oral Endoscopic Tumor (POET) Resection

Background

Upper GI tract subepithelial tumors (SETs) are an uncommon finding on routine EGD, occurring with an incidence of 0.36% [94]. While gastric SETs carry a high risk of malignancy, esophageal SETs are most commonly leiomyomas; the risk of malignancy is approximately 1% [95, 96]. Most SETs are asymptomatic incidental findings. However, larger SETs can result in dysphagia, chest pain, regurgitation, or bleeding [97, 98].

Surgical resection by an open, laparoscopic, or thoracoscopic approach is associated with significant morbidity. Following the introduction of POEM, the submucosal tunneling technique provided an endoscopic alternative for the resection of benign SETs. A description of the technique, per-oral endoscopic tumor resection (POET), was reported by Inoue et al, in 2012, and subsequently applied to the resection of SETs in the esophagus and gastric cardia [99]. Multiple series have since been published supporting its safety and efficacy.

Indications

POET resection is indicated for SETs that are symptomatic, enlarging, or for which the diagnosis is uncertain. The majority of SETs that have been excised using POET were presumed to be benign based on preoperative endoscopy, endoscopic ultrasound, or CT scan. It has also recently been reported for an esophageal bronchogenic cyst [100]. No recommendation can yet be made for endoscopic resection of malignant tumors.

Technique

Similar to POEM, POET is performed using a gastroscope with a distal cap and CO_2 insufflation. The use of air insufflation can result in high rates of pneumothorax and pneumoperitoneum [101]. POET begins with submucosal injection and mucosal incision 5 cm proximal to the tumor, and the submucosal tunnel is created in similar fashion to the POEM technique. The tunnel is continued for 1–2 cm distal to the tumor to ensure adequate space for dissection of the tumor itself. Careful circumferential dissection is performed, taking care to avoid rupture of the capsule or injury to the overlying mucosa (Fig. 3.6). Tumors that extend into the muscle layer can be safely removed with full-thickness resection of the muscle layers. Once freed, the tumor can be grasped using a snare or forceps, or suctioned into the hood and withdrawn through mucosal incision. After confirming adequate hemostasis, the mucosal incision is closed, as with POEM, using endoscopic clips, sutures, or covered stents [102–104].

Postoperatively, we manage patients similar to post-POEM patients, and so they undergo water-soluble contrast esophagram on POD #1 to rule out a leak. Some centers also check CT scans to evaluate for insufflation-related complications [105]. Diet is advanced, and patients are discharged home on the same schedule as POEM patients, generally within 1–4 days, depending on the center. Follow-up surveillance generally includes EUS and CT scans to ensure resolution and assess for tumor recurrence [101, 106].

Safety

Nearly all reported adverse events have been insufflation-related, including subcutaneous

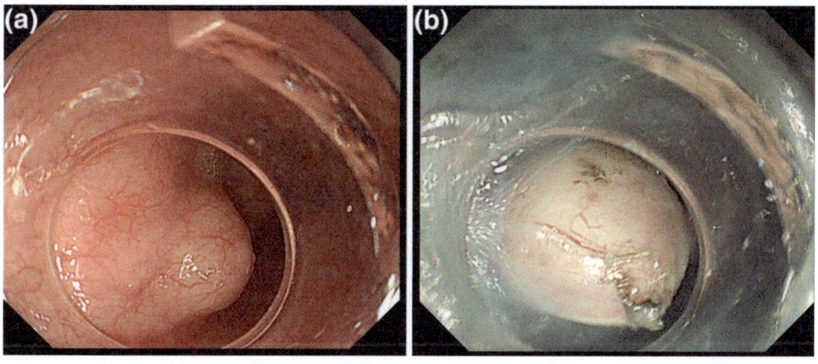

Fig. 3.6 Per-oral endoscopic tumor resection (POET). **a** Endoscopic view of a submucosal nodule. **b** A submucosal tunnel is created up to the nodule (*pink*), which is circumferentially dissected from the submucosal fibers (*blue*)

emphysema, capnoperitoneum, or capnomediastinum. As with POEM, these can be managed conservatively or with needle decompression.

Efficacy

Nearly every case series reports *en bloc* resection with an intact capsule in 100% of patients. Maintaining an intact capsule is thought to be important in the prevention of seeding if the tumor is found to be malignant or premalignant. The limiting factor for performance of POET is the size of the tumor; the largest SET to be excised endoscopically was a 6 × 2.8 × 2.2 cm leiomyoma that was removed in piecemeal fashion [103]. The upper limit for complete resection with an intact capsule appears to be 4–5 cm [99, 101, 102, 107–113].

Conclusion

SETs of the esophagus and cardia are rare and generally found incidentally on routine endoscopy or radiologic studies. The majority of esophageal SETs are benign, and POET provides an endoscopic option for the resection. POET can be performed safely and effectively, with *en bloc* resection of tumors up to 4–5 cm in size.

References

1. Pimentel-Nunes P, Dinis-Ribeiro M, Ponchon T, Repici A, Vieth M, De Ceglie A, et al. Endoscopic submucosal dissection: European Society of Gastrointestinal Endoscopy (ESGE) guideline. Endoscopy. 2015;47(9):829–54.
2. Rosenberg N. Submucosal saline wheal as safety factor in fulguration or rectal and sigmoidal polypi. Arch Surg. 1955;70(1):120–2.
3. Edmonson JM. History of the instruments for gastrointestinal endoscopy. Gastrointest Endosc. 1991;37(2 Suppl):S27–56.
4. Tada M, Murakami A, Karita M, Yanai H, Okita K. Endoscopic resection of early gastric cancer. Endoscopy. 1993;25(7):445–50.
5. Martin TR, Onstad GR, Silvis SE, Vennes JA. Lift and cut biopsy technique for submucosal sampling. Gastrointest Endosc. 1976;23(1):29–30.
6. Takekoshi T, Baba Y, Ota H, Kato Y, Yanagisawa A, Takagi K, et al. Endoscopic resection of early gastric carcinoma: results of a retrospective analysis of 308 cases. Endoscopy. 1994;26(4):352–8.
7. Hirao M, Masuda K, Asanuma T, Naka H, Noda K, Matsuura K, et al. Endoscopic resection of early gastric cancer and other tumors with local injection of hypertonic saline-epinephrine. Gastrointest Endosc. 1988;34(3):264–9.
8. Monma K, Sakaki N, Yoshida M. Endoscopic mucosectomy for precise evaluation and treatment of esophageal intraepithelial cancer. Dig Endosc. 1990;2:501–6.
9. Makuuchi H, Machimura T, Sugihara T. Endoscopic diagnosis and treatment of mucosal cancer of the esophagus. Dig Endosc. 1990;2:447–52.
10. Chaves DM, Sakai P, Mester M, Spinosa SR, Tomishige T, Ishioka S. A new endoscopic technique for the resection of flat polypoid lesions. Gastrointest Endosc. 1994;40(2 Pt 1):224–6.
11. Masuda K, Fujisaki J, Suzuki H. Endoscopic mucosal resection using a ligating device (EMRL). Dig Endosc. 1993;5:58–62.
12. Fleischer DE, Wang GQ, Dawsey S, Tio TL, Newsome J, Kidwell J, et al. Tissue band ligation followed by snare resection (band and snare): a new technique for tissue acquisition in the esophagus. Gastrointest Endosc. 1996;44(1):68–72.
13. Inoue H, Endo M. Endoscopic esophageal mucosal resection using a transparent tube. Surg Endosc. 1990;4(4):198–201.
14. Inoue H, Takeshita K, Hori H, Muraoka Y, Yoneshima H, Endo M. Endoscopic mucosal resection with a cap-fitted panendoscope for esophagus, stomach, and colon mucosal lesions. Gastrointest Endosc. 1993;39(1):58–62.
15. Tada M, Inoue H, Yabata E, Okabe S, Endo M. Colonic mucosal resection using a transparent cap-fitted endoscope. Gastrointest Endoscopy. 1996;44(1):63–5.
16. Izumi Y, Teramoto K, Ohshima M, Shin S, Yamamura A, Matsumoto M. Endoscopic resection of duodenal ampulla with a transparent plastic cap. Surgery. 1998;123(1):109–10.
17. Lian J, Chen S, Zhang Y, Qiu F. A meta-analysis of endoscopic submucosal dissection and EMR for early gastric cancer. Gastrointest Endosc. 2012;76(4):763–70.
18. Tanaka S, Kashida H, Saito Y, Yahagi N, Yamano H, Saito S, et al. JGES guidelines for colorectal endoscopic submucosal dissection/endoscopic mucosal resection. Dig Endosc. 2015;27(4):417–34.
19. Pech O, May A, Manner H, Behrens A, Pohl J, Weferling M, et al. Long-term efficacy and safety of endoscopic resection for patients with mucosal adenocarcinoma of the esophagus. Gastroenterology. 2014;146(3):652–60.e1.
20. Gotoda T, Kondo H, Ono H, Saito Y, Yamaguchi H, Saito D, et al. A new endoscopic mucosal resection

procedure using an insulation-tipped electrosurgical knife for rectal flat lesions: report of two cases. Gastrointest Endosc. 1999;50(4):560–3.
21. Yamamoto H, Koiwai H, Yube T, Isoda N, Sato Y, Sekine Y, et al. A successful single-step endoscopic resection of a 40 millimeter flat-elevated tumor in the rectum: endoscopic mucosal resection using sodium hyaluronate. Gastrointest Endosc. 1999; 50(5):701–4.
22. Yamamoto H, Sekine Y, Higashizawa T, Kihira K, Kaneko Y, Hosoya Y, et al. Successful en bloc resection of a large superficial gastric cancer by using sodium hyaluronate and electrocautery incision forceps. Gastrointest Endosc. 2001;54(5): 629–32.
23. Yamamoto H, Kawata H, Sunada K, Satoh K, Kaneko Y, Ido K, et al. Success rate of curative endoscopic mucosal resection with circumferential mucosal incision assisted by submucosal injection of sodium hyaluronate. Gastrointest Endosc. 2002;56(4):507–12.
24. von Delius S, Feussner H, Henke J, Schneider A, Hollweck R, Rosch T, et al. Submucosal endoscopy: a novel approach to en bloc endoscopic mucosal resection (with videos). Gastrointest Endosc. 2007;66(4):753–6.
25. Park YM, Cho E, Kang HY, Kim JM. The effectiveness and safety of endoscopic submucosal dissection compared with endoscopic mucosal resection for early gastric cancer: a systematic review and metaanalysis. Surg Endosc. 2011;25 (8):2666–77.
26. Facciorusso A, Antonino M, Di Maso M, Muscatiello N. Endoscopic submucosal dissection vs endoscopic mucosal resection for early gastric cancer: a meta-analysis. World J Gastrointest Endosc. 2014;6(11):555–63.
27. Repici A, Hassan C, De Paula Pessoa D, Pagano N, Arezzo A, Zullo A, et al. Efficacy and safety of endoscopic submucosal dissection for colorectal neoplasia: a systematic review. Endoscopy. 2012;44 (2):137–50.
28. Ohki T, Yamato M, Ota M, Takagi R, Murakami D, Kondo M, et al. Prevention of esophageal stricture after endoscopic submucosal dissection using tissue-engineered cell sheets. Gastroenterology. 2012;143(3):582–8.e1-2.
29. Honda M, Nakamura T, Hori Y, Shionoya Y, Nakada A, Sato T, et al. Process of healing of mucosal defects in the esophagus after endoscopic mucosal resection: histological evaluation in a dog model. Endoscopy. 2010;42(12):1092–5.
30. Qumseya B, Panossian AM, Rizk C, Cangemi D, Wolfsen C, Raimondo M, et al. Predictors of esophageal stricture formation post endoscopic mucosal resection. Clin Endosc. 2014;47(2): 155–61.
31. Sato H, Inoue H, Kobayashi Y, Maselli R, Santi EG, Hayee B, et al. Control of severe strictures after circumferential endoscopic submucosal dissection for esophageal carcinoma: oral steroid therapy with balloon dilation or balloon dilation alone. Gastrointest Endosc. 2013;78 (2):250–7.
32. Mizuta H, Nishimori I, Kuratani Y, Higashidani Y, Kohsaki T, Onishi S. Predictive factors for esophageal stenosis after endoscopic submucosal dissection for superficial esophageal cancer. Dis Esophagus. 2009;22(7):626–31.
33. Satodate H, Inoue H, Yoshida T, Usui S, Iwashita M, Fukami N, et al. Circumferential EMR of carcinoma arising in Barrett's esophagus: case report. Gastrointest Endosc. 2003;58(2):288–92.
34. Inoue H, Ito H, Ikeda H, Sato C, Sato H, Phalanusitthepha C, et al. Anti-reflux mucosectomy for gastroesophageal reflux disease in the absence of hiatus hernia: a pilot study. Ann Gstroenterol. 2014;27(4):346–51.
35. Ortega JA, Madureri V, Perez L. Endoscopic myotomy in the treatment of achalasia. Gastrointest Endosc. 1980;26(1):8–10.
36. Kalloo AN, Singh VK, Jagannath SB, Niiyama H, Hill SL, Vaughn CA, et al. Flexible transgastric peritoneoscopy: a novel approach to diagnostic and therapeutic interventions in the peritoneal cavity. Gastrointest Endosc. 2004;60(1):114–7.
37. Pasricha PJ, Hawari R, Ahmed I, Chen J, Cotton PB, Hawes RH, et al. Submucosal endoscopic esophageal myotomy: a novel experimental approach for the treatment of achalasia. Endoscopy. 2007;39 (9):761–4.
38. Inoue H, Minami H, Kobayashi Y, Sato Y, Kaga M, Suzuki M, et al. Peroral endoscopic myotomy (POEM) for esophageal achalasia. Endoscopy. 2010;42(4):265–71.
39. Inoue H, Sato H, Ikeda H, Onimaru M, Sato C, Minami H, et al. Per-oral endoscopic myotomy: a series of 500 patients. J Am Coll Surg. 2015;221 (2):256–64.
40. Stavropoulos SN, Modayil RJ, Friedel D, Savides T. The international per oral endoscopic myotomy survey (IPOEMS): a snapshot of the global POEM experience. Surg Endosc. 2013;27 (9):3322–38.
41. Wang J, Tan N, Xiao Y, Chen J, Chen B, Ma Z, et al. Safety and efficacy of the modified peroral endoscopic myotomy with shorter myotomy for achalasia patients: a prospective study. Dis Esophagus. 2015;28(8):720–7.
42. Familiari P, Gigante G, Marchese M, Boskoski I, Tringali A, Perri V, et al. peroral endoscopic myotomy for esophageal achalasia: outcomes of the first 100 patients with short-term follow-up. Ann Surg. 2016;263(1):82–7.
43. Talukdar R, Inoue H, Reddy DN. Efficacy of peroral endoscopic myotomy (POEM) in the treatment of achalasia: a systematic review and meta-analysis. Surg Endosc. 2015;29(11):3030–46.
44. Minami H, Isomoto H, Yamaguchi N, Matsushima K, Akazawa Y, Ohnita K, et al. Peroral

endoscopic myotomy for esophageal achalasia: clinical impact of 28 cases. Dig Endosc. 2014;26 (1):43–51.
45. Bechara R, Ikeda H, Inoue H. Peroral endoscopic myotomy: an evolving treatment for achalasia. Nat Rev Gastroenterol Hepatol. 2015;12(7):410–26.
46. Onimaru M, Inoue H, Ikeda H, Sato C, Sato H, Phalanusitthepha C, et al. Greater curvature myotomy is a safe and effective modified technique in per-oral endoscopic myotomy (with videos). Gastrointest Endosc. 2015;81(6):1370–7.
47. Tang X, Gong W, Deng Z, Zhou J, Ren Y, Zhang Q, et al. Comparison of conventional versus Hybrid knife peroral endoscopic myotomy methods for esophageal achalasia: a case-control study. Scand J Gastroenterol. 2016;51(4):494–500.
48. Ponsky JL, Marks JM, Orenstein SB. Retrograde myotomy: a variation in per oral endoscopic myotomy (POEM) technique. Surg Endosc. 2014;28(11):3257–9.
49. von Renteln D, Inoue H, Minami H, Werner YB, Pace A, Kersten JF, et al. Peroral endoscopic myotomy for the treatment of achalasia: a prospective single center study. Am J Gastroenterol. 2012;107(3):411–7.
50. Li QL, Chen WF, Zhou PH, Yao LQ, Xu MD, Hu JW, et al. Peroral endoscopic myotomy for the treatment of achalasia: a clinical comparative study of endoscopic full-thickness and circular muscle myotomy. J Am Coll Surg. 2013;217(3):442–51.
51. Baldaque-Silva F, Marques M, Vilas-Boas F, Maia JD, Sa F, Macedo G. New transillumination auxiliary technique for peroral endoscopic myotomy. Gastrointest Endosc. 2014;79(4):544–5.
52. Grimes KL, Inoue H, Onimaru M, Ikeda H, Tansawet A, Bechara R, et al. Double-scope per oral endoscopic myotomy (POEM): a prospective randomized controlled trial. Surg Endosc. 2016;30 (4):1344–51.
53. Kumbhari V, Besharati S, Abdelgelil A, Tieu AH, Saxena P, El-Zein MH, et al. Intraprocedural fluoroscopy to determine the extent of the cardiomyotomy during per-oral endoscopic myotomy (with video). Gastrointest Endosc. 2015;81 (6):1451–6.
54. Rohof WO, Hirsch DP, Kessing BF, Boeckxstaens GE. Efficacy of treatment for patients with achalasia depends on the distensibility of the esophagogastric junction. Gastroenterology. 2012;143(2):328–35.
55. Pandolfino JE, de Ruigh A, Nicodeme F, Xiao Y, Boris L, Kahrilas PJ. Distensibility of the esophagogastric junction assessed with the functional lumen imaging probe (FLIP) in achalasia patients. Neurogastroenterol Motil. 2013;25(6):496–501.
56. Familiari P, Gigante G, Marchese M, Boskoski I, Bove V, Tringali A, et al. EndoFLIP system for the intraoperative evaluation of peroral endoscopic myotomy. United Eur Gastroenterol J. 2014;2 (2):77–83.
57. Sternbach JM, El Khoury R, Teitelbaum EN, Soper NJ, Pandolfino JE, Hungness ES. Early esophagram in per-oral endoscopic myotomy (POEM) for achalasia does not predict long-term outcomes. Surgery. 2015;158(4):1128–35.
58. Cai MY, Zhou PH, Yao LQ, Zhu BQ, Liang L, Li QL. Thoracic CT after peroral endoscopic myotomy for the treatment of achalasia. Gastrointest Endosc. 2014;80(6):1046–55.
59. Ponsky JL, Marks JM, Pauli EM. How i do it: per-oral endoscopic myotomy (POEM). J Gastrointest Surg. 2012;16(6):1251–5.
60. Sharata A, Kurian AA, Dunst CM, Bhayani NH, Reavis KM, Swanstrom LL. Technique of per-oral endoscopic myotomy (POEM) of the esophagus (with video). Surg Endosc. 2014;28(4):1333.
61. Patel K, Abbassi-Ghadi N, Markar S, Kumar S, Jethwa P, Zaninotto G. Peroral endoscopic myotomy for the treatment of esophageal achalasia: systematic review and pooled analysis. Dis Esophagus. 2015 Jul 14 [Epub ahead of print].
62. Chiu PW, Wu JC, Teoh AY, Chan Y, Wong SK, Liu SY, et al. Peroral endoscopic myotomy for treatment of achalasia: from bench to bedside (with video). Gastrointest Endosc. 2013;77 (1):29–38.
63. Cai MY, Zhou PH, Yao LQ, Xu MD, Zhong YS, Li QL, et al. Peroral endoscopic myotomy for idiopathic achalasia: randomized comparison of water-jet assisted versus conventional dissection technique. Surg Endosc. 2014;28(4):1158–65.
64. Sharata AM, Dunst CM, Pescarus R, Shlomovitz E, Wille AJ, Reavis KM, et al. Peroral endoscopic myotomy (POEM) for esophageal primary motility disorders: analysis of 100 consecutive patients. J Gastrointest Surg. 2015;19(1):161–70 (discussion 70).
65. Von Renteln D, Fuchs KH, Fockens P, Bauerfeind P, Vassiliou MC, Werner YB, et al. Peroral endoscopic myotomy for the treatment of achalasia: an international prospective multicenter study. Gastroenterology. 2013;145(2):309–11.e1-3.
66. Kurian AA, Dunst CM, Sharata A, Bhayani NH, Reavis KM, Swanstrom LL. Peroral endoscopic esophageal myotomy: defining the learning curve. Gastrointest Endosc. 2013;77(5):719–25.
67. Li QL, Zhou PH, Yao LQ, Xu MD, Chen WF, Hu JW, et al. Early diagnosis and management of delayed bleeding in the submucosal tunnel after peroral endoscopic myotomy for achalasia (with video). Gastrointest Endosc. 2013;78 (2):370–4.
68. Yang S, Zeng MS, Zhang ZY, Zhang HL, Liang L, Zhang XW. Pneumomediastinum and pneumoperitoneum on computed tomography after peroral endoscopic myotomy (POEM): postoperative

changes or complications? Acta Radiol. 2015;56 (10):1216–21.
69. Patel KS, Calixte R, Modayil RJ, Friedel D, Brathwaite CE, Stavropoulos SN. The light at the end of the tunnel: a single-operator learning curve analysis for per oral endoscopic myotomy. Gastrointest Endosc. 2015;81(5):1181–7.
70. Kurian AA, Bhayani NH, Reavis K, Dunst C, Swanstrom L. Endoscopic suture repair of full-thickness esophagotomy during per-oral esophageal myotomy for achalasia. Surg Endosc. 2013;27(10):3910.
71. Modayil R, Friedel D, Stavropoulos SN. Endoscopic suture repair of a large mucosal perforation during peroral endoscopic myotomy for treatment of achalasia. Gastrointest Endosc. 2014;80 (6):1169–70.
72. Ling T, Pei Q, Pan J, Zhang X, Lv Y, Li W, et al. Successful use of a covered, retrievable stent to seal a ruptured mucosal flap safety valve during peroral endoscopic myotomy in a child with achalasia. Endoscopy. 2013;45(Suppl 2 UCTN):E63-4.
73. Li H, Linghu E, Wang X. Fibrin sealant for closure of mucosal penetration at the cardia during peroral endoscopic myotomy (POEM). Endoscopy. 2012;44(Suppl 2 UCTN):E215-6.
74. Hungness ES, Teitelbaum EN, Santos BF, Arafat FO, Pandolfino JE, Kahrilas PJ, et al. Comparison of perioperative outcomes between peroral esophageal myotomy (POEM) and laparoscopic Heller myotomy. J Gastrointest Surg. 2013;17(2):228–35.
75. Ujiki MB, Yetasook AK, Zapf M, Linn JG, Carbray JM, Denham W. Peroral endoscopic myotomy: A short-term comparison with the standard laparoscopic approach. Surgery. 2013;154 (4):893–7 (discussion 7-900).
76. Khashab MA, Messallam AA, Onimaru M, Teitelbaum EN, Ujiki MB, Gitelis ME, et al. International multicenter experience with peroral endoscopic myotomy for the treatment of spastic esophageal disorders refractory to medical therapy (with video). Gastrointest Endosc. 2015;81(5):1170–7.
77. Vigneswaran Y, Yetasook AK, Zhao JC, Denham W, Linn JG, Ujiki MB. Peroral endoscopic myotomy (POEM): feasible as reoperation following Heller myotomy. J Gastrointest Surg. 2014;18 (6):1071–6.
78. Zhou PH, Li QL, Yao LQ, Xu MD, Chen WF, Cai MY, et al. Peroral endoscopic remyotomy for failed Heller myotomy: a prospective single-center study. Endoscopy. 2013;45(3):161–6.
79. Orenstein SB, Raigani S, Wu YV, Pauli EM, Phillips MS, Ponsky JL, et al. Peroral endoscopic myotomy (POEM) leads to similar results in patients with and without prior endoscopic or surgical therapy. Surg Endosc. 2015;29(5): 1064–70.
80. Sharata A, Kurian AA, Dunst CM, Bhayani NH, Reavis KM, Swanstrom LL. Peroral endoscopic myotomy (POEM) is safe and effective in the setting of prior endoscopic intervention. J Gastrointest Surg. 2013;17(7):1188–92.
81. Chen WF, Li QL, Zhou PH, Yao LQ, Xu MD, Zhang YQ, et al. Long-term outcomes of peroral endoscopic myotomy for achalasia in pediatric patients: a prospective, single-center study. Gastrointest Endosc. 2015;81(1):91–100.
82. Li C, Tan Y, Wang X, Liu D. Peroral endoscopic myotomy for treatment of achalasia in children and adolescents. J Pediatr Surg. 2015;50(1):201–5.
83. Verlaan T, Rohof WO, Bredenoord AJ, Eberl S, Rosch T, Fockens P. Effect of peroral endoscopic myotomy on esophagogastric junction physiology in patients with achalasia. Gastrointest Endosc. 2013;78(1):39–44.
84. Ling TS, Guo HM, Yang T, Peng CY, Zou XP, Shi RH. Effectiveness of peroral endoscopic myotomy in the treatment of achalasia: a pilot trial in Chinese Han population with a minimum of one-year follow-up. J Dig Dis. 2014;15(7):352–8.
85. Teitelbaum EN, Soper NJ, Santos BF, Arafat FO, Pandolfino JE, Kahrilas PJ, et al. Symptomatic and physiologic outcomes one year after peroral esophageal myotomy (POEM) for treatment of achalasia. Surg Endosc. 2014;28(12):3359–65.
86. Wang L, Li YM, Li L. Meta-analysis of randomized and controlled treatment trials for achalasia. Dig Dis Sci. 2009;54(11):2303–11.
87. Yaghoobi M, Mayrand S, Martel M, Roshan-Afshar I, Bijarchi R, Barkun A. Laparoscopic Heller's myotomy versus pneumatic dilation in the treatment of idiopathic achalasia: a meta-analysis of randomized, controlled trials. Gastrointest Endosc. 2013;78 (3):468–75.
88. Bhayani NH, Kurian AA, Dunst CM, Sharata AM, Rieder E, Swanstrom LL. A comparative study on comprehensive, objective outcomes of laparoscopic Heller myotomy with per-oral endoscopic myotomy (POEM) for achalasia. Ann Surg. 2014;259 (6):1098–103.
89. Chan SM, Wu JC, Teoh AY, Yip HC, Ng EK, Lau JY, et al. Comparison of early outcomes and quality of life after laparoscopic Heller's cardiomyotomy to peroral endoscopic myotomy for treatment of achalasia. Dig Endosc. 2016;28(1):27–32.
90. Familiari P, Greco S, Gigante G, Cali A, Boskoski I, Onder G, et al. Gastro-esophageal reflux disease after per-oral endoscopic myotomy (POEM). Analysis of clinical, procedural and functional factors, associated with GERD and esophagitis. Dig Endosc. 2016;28(1):33–41.
91. Jones EL, Meara MP, Schwartz JS, Hazey JW, Perry KA. Gastroesophageal reflux symptoms do not correlate with objective pH testing after peroral endoscopic myotomy. Surg Endosc. 2016;30 (3):947–52.
92. Teitelbaum EN, Soper NJ, Pandolfino JE, Kahrilas PJ, Boris L, Nicodeme F, et al. An extended proximal esophageal myotomy is necessary to

normalize EGJ distensibility during Heller myotomy for achalasia, but not POEM. Surg Endosc. 2014;28(10):2840–7.
93. Teitelbaum EN, Boris L, Arafat FO, Nicodeme F, Lin Z, Kahrilas PJ, et al. Comparison of esophagogastric junction distensibility changes during POEM and Heller myotomy using intraoperative FLIP. Surg Endosc. 2013;27(12):4547–55.
94. Hedenbro JL, Ekelund M, Wetterberg P. Endoscopic diagnosis of submucosal gastric lesions. The results after routine endoscopy. Surg Endosc. 1991;5 (1):20–3.
95. Miettinen M, Lasota J. Gastrointestinal stromal tumors (GISTs): definition, occurrence, pathology, differential diagnosis and molecular genetics. Pol J Pathol. 2003;54(1):3–24.
96. Winant AJ, Gollub MJ, Shia J, Antonescu C, Bains MS, Levine MS. Imaging and clinicopathologic features of esophageal gastrointestinal stromal tumors. AJR Am J Roentgenol. 2014;203(2):306–14.
97. Mutrie CJ, Donahue DM, Wain JC, Wright CD, Gaissert HA, Grillo HC, et al. Esophageal leiomyoma: a 40-year experience. Ann Thorac Surg. 2005;79(4):1122–5.
98. Punpale A, Rangole A, Bhambhani N, Karimundackal G, Desai N, de Souza A, et al. Leiomyoma of esophagus. Ann Thorac Cardiovasc Surg. 2007;13(2):78–81.
99. Inoue H, Ikeda H, Hosoya T, Onimaru M, Yoshida A, Eleftheriadis N, et al. Submucosal endoscopic tumor resection for subepithelial tumors in the esophagus and cardia. Endoscopy. 2012;44 (3):225–30.
100. Bechara R, Onimaru M, Kushima M, Inoue H. Peroral endoscopic tumor resection for an esophageal bronchogenic cyst. Gastrointest Endosc. 2016;83(4):827–8.
101. Wang XY, Xu MD, Yao LQ, Zhou PH, Pleskow D, Li QL, et al. Submucosal tunneling endoscopic resection for submucosal tumors of the esophagogastric junction originating from the muscularis propria layer: a feasibility study (with videos). Surg Endosc. 2014;28(6):1971–7.
102. Wang L, Ren W, Zhang Z, Yu J, Li Y, Song Y. Retrospective study of endoscopic submucosal tunnel dissection (ESTD) for surgical resection of esophageal leiomyoma. Surg Endosc. 2013;27 (11):4259–66.
103. Kumbhari V, Saxena P, Azola A, Messallam AA, El Zein MH, Khashab MA. Submucosal tunneling endoscopic resection of a giant esophageal leiomyoma. Gastrointest Endosc. 2015;81(1):219–20.
104. Saxena P, Chavez YH, Kord Valeshabad A, Kalloo AN, Khashab MA. An alternative method for mucosal flap closure during peroral endoscopic myotomy using an over-the-scope clipping device. Endoscopy. 2013;45(7):579–81.
105. Liu BR, Song JT, Kong LJ, Pei FH, Wang XH, Du YJ. Tunneling endoscopic muscularis dissection for subepithelial tumors originating from the muscularis propria of the esophagus and gastric cardia. Surg Endosc. 2013;27(11):4354–9.
106. Ye LP, Zhang Y, Mao XL, Zhu LH, Zhou X, Chen JY. Submucosal tunneling endoscopic resection for small upper gastrointestinal subepithelial tumors originating from the muscularis propria layer. Surg Endosc. 2014;28(2):524–30.
107. Cai M, Chen J, Zhou P, Yao L. The rise of tunnel endoscopic surgery: a case report and literature review. Case Rep Gastrointest Med. 2012;2012:847640.
108. Gong W, Xiong Y, Zhi F, Liu S, Wang A, Jiang B. Preliminary experience of endoscopic submucosal tunnel dissection for upper gastrointestinal submucosal tumors. Endoscopy. 2012;44(3):231–5.
109. Xu MD, Cai MY, Zhou PH, Qin XY, Zhong YS, Chen WF, et al. Submucosal tunneling endoscopic resection: a new technique for treating upper GI submucosal tumors originating from the muscularis propria layer (with videos). Gastrointest Endosc. 2012;75(1):195–9.
110. Xu MD, Lu W, Li QL, Zhou PH, Zhong YS, Chen WF, et al. Application and evaluation of submucosal tunneling endoscopic resection of gastric submucosal tumors originating from the muscularis propria layer. Zhonghua Wei Chang Wai Ke Za Zhi. 2012;15(7):671–4.
111. Chen H, Xu Z, Huo J, Liu D. Submucosal tunneling endoscopic resection for simultaneous esophageal and cardia submucosal tumors originating from the muscularis propria layer (with video). Dig Endosc. 2015;27(1):155–8.
112. Lu J, Jiao T, Zheng M, Lu X. Endoscopic resection of submucosal tumors in muscularis propria: the choice between direct excavation and tunneling resection. Surg Endosc. 2014;28(12):3401–7.
113. Lu J, Zheng M, Jiao T, Wang Y, Lu X. Transcardiac tunneling technique for endoscopic submucosal dissection of gastric fundus tumors arising from the muscularis propria. Endoscopy. 2014;46 (10):888–92.

Endoscopic Submucosal Dissection 4

Anil Bernard Nagar

Abstract

Endoscopic submucosal dissection (ESD) is an advanced endoscopic technique pioneered by the Japanese, for *en bloc* removal of large gastrointestinal epithelial lesions. This technique involves injection of a solution into the submucosal layer, followed by dissection around and then under the lesion, with separation of the submucosal layer using an electrocautery knife. ESD technique allows the endoscopist to visualize and control the depth of dissection. Originally described for early gastric cancer, the indications and techniques have evolved to include lesions in most locations and layers of the gastrointestinal wall. Western endoscopists have recently adopted this technique as well. From a practice standpoint, ESD provides the endoscopist with the ability to remove large superficial tumors in a single piece, including ulcerated lesions, lesions with submucosal fibrosis, recurrent neoplasms, non-lifting lesions, and potentially lesions with very early submucosal invasion. *En bloc* resection and curative resection rates are high in the eastern literature, with bleeding, perforation and strictures, the most frequently reported complications. The procedure is difficult and time consuming, with a steep learning curve and significant complication rates, and therefore requires specialized training.

Keywords

Submucosal · Dissection · ESD · *En bloc* resection

A.B. Nagar (✉)
Department of Medicine, Section of Digestive Diseases, Yale University, New Haven, CT, USA
e-mail: anil.nagar@yale.edu

A.B. Nagar
VACT Healthcare, West Haven VA Medical Center, West Haven, CT, USA

J.R. Romanelli et al. (eds.), *NOTES and Endoluminal Surgery*, Clinical Gastroenterology, DOI 10.1007/978-3-319-50610-4_4

Abbreviations

EMR	Endoscopic mucosal resection
ESD	Endoscopic submucosal dissection
HGD	High-grade dysplasia
IMC	Intramucosal cancer
IT knife	Insulated-tip knife
LST	Laterally spreading tumor
NBI	Narrowband imaging
SCC	Squamous cell carcinoma
SM	Submucosal
V	Volts
W	Watts

Introduction

Endoscopic submucosal dissection (ESD) is an advanced endoscopic technique described for *en bloc* removal of large gastrointestinal epithelial lesions, allowing the endoscopist to visualize and control the depth of dissection. This technique, pioneered by the Japanese, involves injection of a solution into the submucosal layer followed by careful dissection around and then under the lesion, with separation of the submucosal layer using an electrocautery knife. Although ESD was originally performed and described for early gastric cancer, its indications and techniques have evolved to include lesions in most locations and layers of the gastrointestinal wall. Western endoscopists have now adopted this technique, but organized training programs are not available in the USA. This *en bloc* resection technique enables complete histology and pathology assessment of the local stage of the cancer, and it precisely identifies lesions cured by resection as well as those requiring further surgical management.

History

Initially described by the Japanese, ESD evolved from the technique of endoscopic mucosal resection (EMR). EMR techniques developed in Japan in the 1990s included strip biopsies, polypectomy after hypertonic saline injection, and cap-assisted EMR [1]. These EMR techniques resulted in piecemeal resection of lesions larger than 20 mm, did not precisely control for depth of resection, and were difficult to perform in depressed-type lesions. Early work by Japanese endoscopists [2–4] using special knives demonstrated that lesions larger than 30 mm could be removed in a single piece with adequate lateral and deep margins of resection. The insulated-tip knife (IT knife) (Olympus, Tokyo, Japan) developed by Hosokawa [5] was most commonly used in Japan and helped encourage the rapid growth of ESD. Adoption in the West has been slow, with encouraging initial reports using the IT knife (Olympus) [6]. An important article by Gotoda [7] defined criteria for node-negative early gastric cancer, thus identifying a subgroup of patients that can be completely cured by local ESD without a need for gastrectomy with lymph node dissection. This established and expanded the role of ESD for the treatment of early gastric cancer and resulted in the development of criteria for ESD throughout the GI tract. With the increased acceptance of ESD in the West, recent technical reviews and guidelines have been released in the USA and Europe [8, 9].

Indications for ESD

The main reason to perform ESD is to reduce the risk of local recurrence and to provide an accurate local histological staging of the lesion.

Lesions usually larger than 20 mm cannot be removed in a single EMR specimen and require piecemeal removal. ESD is developed to obtained *en bloc* and R0 resections for larger mucosal lesions. *En bloc* resection refers to the removal of a mucosal lesion in a single piece. R0 resection refers to histological assessment that documents negative lateral and vertical margins. ESD is recommended for malignant lesions when the risk of lymph node metastasis is minimal or zero. The depth of invasion of the lesions (and thus curative likelihood of ESD) can be predicted by careful mucosal examination of the lesions and the practice of classifying lesions based on the Paris classification (Table 4.1) [10] and the use of Kudo pit pattern [11]. Careful attention should be given to the location, lateral extent of lesions, presence of depression, ulceration, nodularity, and type of or absence of pit pattern and vascular pattern. Since chromoendoscopy is not routinely performed by Western endoscopists, meticulous white light examination with high-definition endoscopes, magnification endoscopy, use of virtual chromoendoscopy, such as narrowband imaging (NBI), and use of the capillary pattern classification under NBI proposed by Sano can provide similar information about the depth of invasion [12]. The use of EUS and CT should be individualized on a case-by-case basis, particularly if the endoscopic appearance is suggestive of deeper invasion, and is mainly useful to rule out local lymph node involvement rather than superficial mucosal staging.

The Vienna classification should be used to classify the histopathology of tumors [13]. ESD results in a complete removal of mucosal and submucosal layers and since lymph node metastasis is related to the depth of invasion in addition to differentiation, Japanese investigators have developed criteria for ESD versus surgical management of tumors based on tumor differentiation, ulceration, depth of invasion, vascular involvement, and lymph node invasion (Tables 4.2 and 4.3). The major indications for ESD include SCC of esophagus involving lamina propria, high-grade dysplasia (HGD), and intramucosal cancer (IMC) in Barrett's esophagus, including *en bloc* resection for accurate local staging of T1a lesion, well-differentiated early gastric cancer, and laterally spreading tumor (LST) of colon that cannot be removed by EMR. Practically, ESD provides the endoscopist with the ability to remove large superficial tumors in a single piece including lesions that may not be

Table 4.1 Paris classification of superficial mucosal neoplastic lesions based on morphology

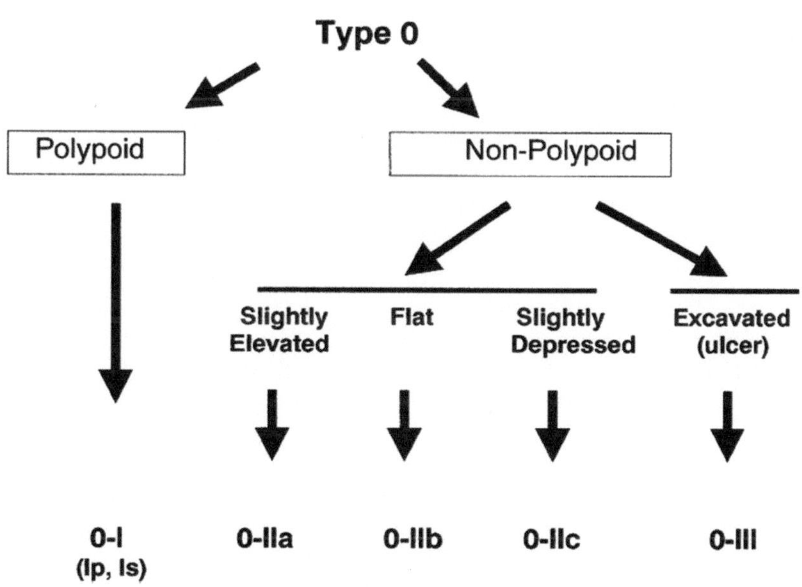

Reference Paris working group, Gastrointestinal Endoscopy 2003 [10]

Table 4.2 Indications for ESD

Esophagus	Gastric	Colon
SCC Well/moderately differentiated <20 mm M1 or M2 cancers Absent venous and lymphatic invasion	Well/moderately differentiated lla <20 mm llb <10 mm Absent venous and lymphatic invasion	Well/moderately differentiation lla <20 mm llb, llc <10 mm Superficial invasion of SM <500 micro M Laterally spreading tumors
Barrett's esophagus >20 mm HGD or IMC	Expanded criteria Any size without ulcer $\leq$ 30 mm with ulcer Minimal submucosal cancer Sml $\leq$ 30 mm	–

Table 4.3 Classifications of mucosal layer depth for the purposes of invasion and management

Mucosa
m1 epithelium
m2 lamina propria
m3 muscularis mucosa
Submucosa
Sm1 superficial
Esophagus squamous cell 200 μm
Esophagus Barrett's 500 μm
Stomach 500 μm
Colon 1000 μm
Sm2 deep

completely removable by EMR, such as ulcerated lesions, lesions with submucosal fibrosis, recurrent neoplasms, non-lifting lesions, and potentially lesions with very early submucosal invasion.

Some disadvantages of ESD include significant training requirements, prolonged procedure time, need for specialized equipment, need for an assistant during the entire procedure, and significantly higher complication rates.

Esophageal: The role of ESD in squamous cell carcinoma of the esophagus is well established in Asian studies. ESD *en bloc* resection rates of 100% with local recurrence of 1% have been reported compared to 53 and 10%, respectively, for EMR [14]. Involvement of muscularis mucosa with carcinoma increases the risk of lymph node metastasis to about 10%, and these patients will have higher recurrence rates if treated with ESD. Suggested indications for ESD for squamous cell cancer includes T1a lesions limited to lamina propria. Once the lesion invades the muscularis mucosa and infiltrates the superficial submucosa (up to 200 μm), the risk of local lymph node metastasis approaches 15%, and these patients represent a relative indication for ESD after the evaluation for local lymph nodes.

Patients with high-grade dysplasia and intramucosal cancer in the setting of Barrett's esophagus are candidates for ESD. Another indication for ESD is early adenocarcinoma lesions that are well differentiated, with less than 500-μm extension into the submucosa. Studies demonstrate 90% *en bloc* resection rates with lower R0 resection rates but with over 95% long-term cure rates [15]. When ESD is performed in the setting of Barrett's esophagus, it should be followed by radiofrequency ablation of any remaining Barrett's epithelium [16]. Based on a systematic review demonstrating a 1–2% lymph node metastasis in setting of intramucosal cancer in Barrett's, these patients are candidates for ESD given the mortality of 1–2% associated with esophagectomy [17].

Gastric: The role of ESD is best established for early gastric cancer. In large series from Asia *en bloc,* resection rates of >95% and R0 resection of >93% have been documented, with local recurrence of 1% and 5-year survival of 96–100% [18, 19]. A meta-analysis of outcomes of ESD versus EMR for early gastric cancer demonstrated higher rates of *en bloc* resection (92% vs. 52%) and R0 resection rates (82% vs. 42%) for ESD compared to EMR, although all-cause mortality did not differ between the two resection techniques [20]. Indications for ESD include lesions of any size if they have dysplasia, intramucosal well-differentiated adenocarcinoma without ulceration (<2 cm absolute indication, >2 cm expanded indication), and other expanded indications in the Japanese literature. These expanded indications include intramucosal well-differentiated adenocarcinoma with ulcer and <3 cm in size, intramucosal poorly differentiated adenocarcinoma <2 cm in size, and well-differentiated adenocarcinoma <3 cm in size and with superficial submucosal invasion, i.e., sm1 < 500 μm [21].

Colorectal: ESD in the rectum is performed by most endoscopists trained in ESD, as the rectum has a thick wall and retroflexion is easily performed. ESD for laterally spreading tumors outside of rectal area in the colon is difficult and mainly performed in Asia. A systematic review of >2800 patients, including 11% of patients with submucosal cancer, found an R0 resection rate of 88%. When compared to EMR, ESD results in less local recurrence (2% vs. 12% for EMR) [22, 23]. In one of the largest series, experienced Japanese endoscopists achieved *en bloc* and curative resections in 88 and 89% of 1111 colorectal tumors. Perforation occurred in 5% of procedures, with post-procedure bleeding in 1.5% [24]. Colorectal ESD is indicated for large adenomas that cannot be completed removed by EMR. Laterally spreading tumors (LST) are classified as granular and non-granular. Non-granular lesions have a higher likelihood of submucosal invasion. ESD may be particularly useful for larger 0-IIc lesions that do not lift with submucosal injection, lesions with scaring, and residual tumor with scar following prior EMR. ESD may be adequate resection for well-differentiated adenocarcinomas with invasion of the submucosal of <1000 μm, in the absence of lympho-vascular invasion, as the risk of lymph node metastasis in this setting is extremely low [25].

Colonic ESD outside the rectum, particularly in the right colon, is extremely difficult and challenging because of the thin wall of the colon with high risk of perforation and bleeding. Additionally, most lesions can be managed with piecemeal EMR technique with similar outcomes. Thus, colonic ESD (outside the rectum) should only be attempted by a skilled endoscopist with extensive experience performing ESD in other locations.

Instruments and Devices Used for ESD

Hybrid knife (ERBE USA, Marietta, GA): This device is a unique instrument that has a central injection port within the cutting knife, so that an ultrafine, 120-μ water jet lavage system can inject pressurized saline to lift the submucosal layer, and the 5-mm cutting knife can be used to dissect tissue without changing instruments. The knife tip is supplied in 2 configurations, the I-type (non-insulated tip) and the T-type (disk-shaped tip) (Fig. 4.1a, b). This device requires a specialized ERBE generator including a pressurized water jet.

IT knife (Olympus America, Center Valley, PA): This device, which is favored in the East for gastric ESD, features a 2.2-mm ceramic ball at the end of a 4-mm cutting knife and is used for submucosal dissection (Fig. 4.1c).

HookKnife (Olympus America: This device has an L-shaped, right-angle tip. The knife length and orientation of the hook tip can be adjusted. It is used for dissection, particularly difficult dissection, allowing for the retraction of tissue while cutting so as to avoid the burning or perforation of the serosa (Fig. 4.1d).

Injection needle catheters: These devices are available from a number of manufacturers. Typically, a 21- to 25-gauge needle catheter is used depending on the viscosity of the injectate. Injection catheters are not necessary when using a hybrid knife.

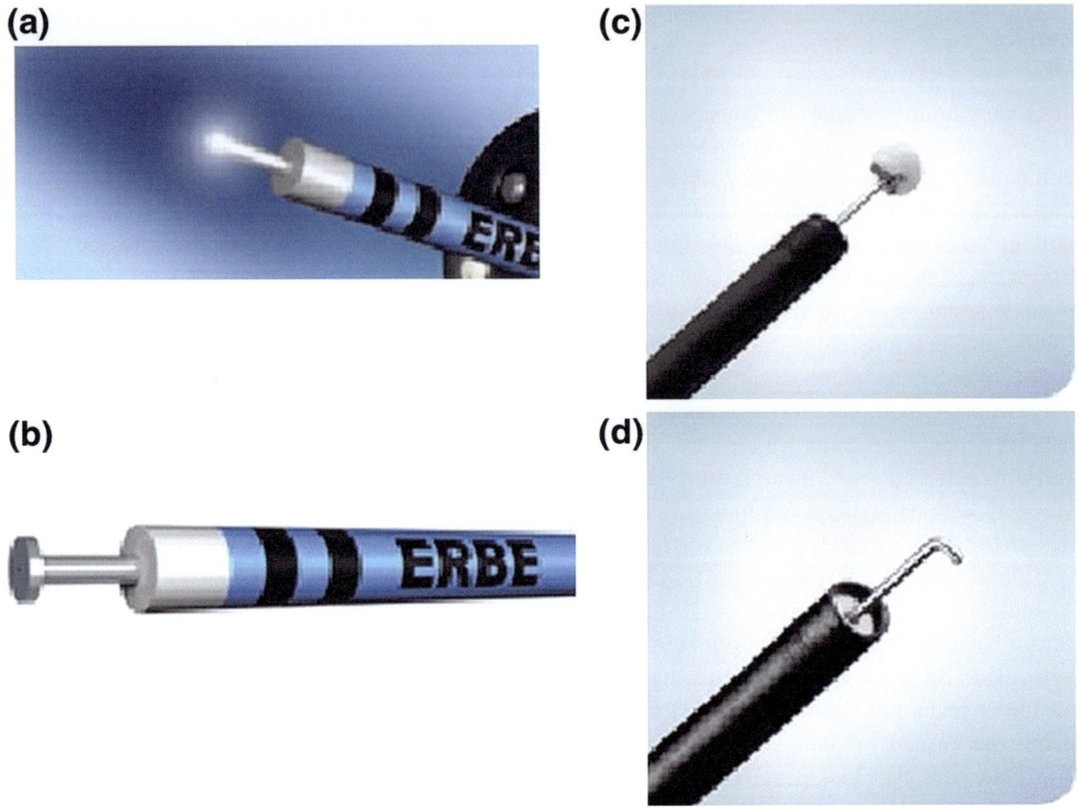

Fig. 4.1 Examples of knifes used in ESD include **a** I-type hybrid knife (ERBE USA), **b** T-type hybrid knife (ERBE USA), **c** IT knife2 (Olympus America), **d**) HookKnife (Olympus America)

Coagrasper (Olympus America, Center Valley, PA): This is a monopolar, hemostatic forceps available in gastroscope and colonoscope lengths. The forceps feature serrated jaws with either 5- or 4-mm opening to allow for targeted coagulation (Fig. 4.2).

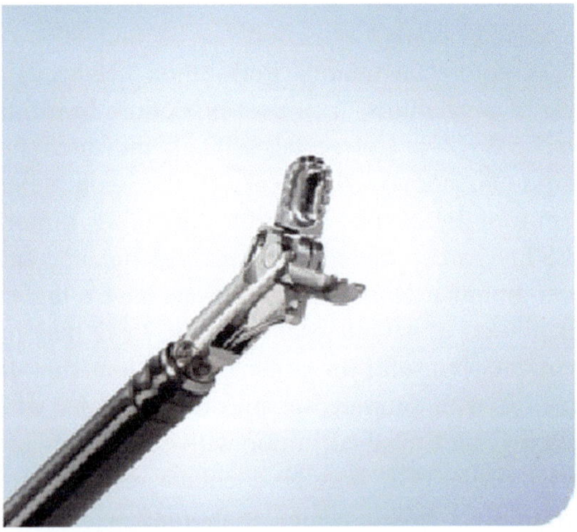

Fig. 4.2 Coagrasper used for hemostasis (Olympus America)

Endoscopy caps: Available from a variety of distributors, these disposable transparent distal attachments or caps are applied to the tip of the endoscope during dissection to maintain visualization and create tissue retraction of the submucosa, by inserting the cap under the mucosa and within the submucosal (SM) layer, thus maintaining visualization while in this layer.

Dyes, contrast agents, and injection solutions: Indigo carmine is the preferred colorant that is diluted in saline and injected into the submucosa for lifting and allows for better visualization and recognition of tissue planes and blood vessels. Methylene blue and Lugol's iodine are used as a superficial spray for chromoendoscopy, to demarcate and characterize the surface and edges of the lesions prior to resection. Normal saline plus a colorant (e.g., indigo carmine) is most commonly used for ESD as a lifting agent, although the cushion provided by saline injection is very short lasting. Epinephrine can be added to the injectate but is not recommended due to the risk of local and myocardial ischemia. Sodium hyaluronate 0.4% is used in Asian countries to provide a longer lasting "lift" to ease and accelerate dissection. 0.4% of Hydroxypropyl methylcellulose is commonly used in the West. Mesa (sodium 2-mercaptoethanesulfonate) as a submucosal injectate has been shown in a RCT to reduce submucosal dissection time and shows promise as an agent that facilitates ESD [26].

Gas insufflation: Use of CO_2 luminal insufflation is strongly recommended during ESD procedures. CO_2 is more rapidly absorbed across the intestine; since ESD may be a prolonged procedure, its use results in less discomfort and possibly reduces the likelihood of tension pneumoperitoneum in the event of a perforation. Multiple CO_2 regulators are available in the USA.

Electrosurgical units: Multiple electrosurgical units are available with newer microprocessors that sense changes in tissue resistance (impedance) and keep the voltage constant. The ERBE VIO300D unit (ERBE USA) is the most commonly used and studied in the West, and its setting for ESD use is described in detail below:

ENDO CUT® Q: This waveform is intended for applications where rapid cutting with reproducible tissue effect is paramount. It is used for mucosal incision as well as fine cutting in submucosa where hemostasis is not an issue. It also works to sculpt fibrotic tissue off muscularis propria. Typical setting used in these advanced procedures are ENDO CUT® Q **Effect 3**, cutting **duration of 1** (amount of time spark is on for 1 ms), **interval phase of 1** (length of time for soft coag phase).

DRY CUT: This waveform provides more hemostasis during cutting than ENDO CUT® Q due to increased voltage. This mode is used in areas where smaller capillaries are weeping into the dissection plane. It is useful when precise dissection with increased concurrent hemostasis (relative to ENDO CUT® Q) is needed such as well-vascularized submucosa during dissection. DRY CUT uses between 600 and 800 V, depending on the effect mode. If DRY is used, it is best to set a higher upper limit of wattage—some experts use upwards of 110 W (Effect 2), and others will routinely go to 180 W (Effect 4) in stomach.

DRY CUT is also used for mucosal incision when oozing is continuous during peripheral incision, but the downside is increased thermal insult (which can be caused by a cutting delay). Therefore, it is important to keep a wider margin from the lesion to protect the specimen's margins for pathologic readability. The salient points here are as follows: (1) Set higher power limit to allow cutting without delay (different for every patient and electrode/knife), and (2) increase Effect up to 4 to increase hemostasis.

FORCED COAG: This waveform is utilized for pinpoint coagulation, 880–1100 V depending on Effect 1 or Effect 2. It is also used with the side of the knife (increased surface area to drive more current) to pretreat larger vessels, devitalize them, and then transect. Consider injection around the vessel to tamponade and buffer surrounding structures prior coagulation being applied. Typical settings range from Effect 1 to Effect 2 (higher effect = higher voltage/thermal effect) and 25–50 W max.

SOFT COAG: This low-voltage (<200 V) coagulation waveform is used for marking around lesion for limited depth of penetration. The same waveform is used with hot coagulation graspers for vessel hemostasis. Grasp the vessel with tip of grasping forceps, tent away from the muscularis propria, and then cauterize until blanching and bubbling of target tissue is accomplished. A typical setting in Soft Coag would be Effect 5/80 W max.

SWIFT COAG: This waveform can be used for submucosal dissection and is a bit more hemostatic with less cutting ability than DRY CUT. It can be used like FORCED COAG for pinpoint hemostasis of vessels during submucosal dissection but can sometimes cut, which can be undesirable (premature transection through vessel). SWIFT COAG is slightly less hemostatic than FORCED COAG.

Clips and closure devices: Endoscopic clip devices are available from Boston Scientific (Natick, MA), Cook Endoscopy (Winston-Salem, NC), and Olympus North America. These are required in the event of inadvertent dissection through the muscularis propria and serosal layers. Clips may occasionally be necessary to treat a large bleeding submucosal blood vessel that has not responded to adequate cautery using a coagrasper.

Technique of ESD

The technique of ESD is similar in different areas of the luminal GI tract. Prior to the procedure, check all equipment, making sure that CO_2 insufflation is being used and that hemostasis and closure devices are available. Standard pre-procedure evaluation and management should be performed as with any endoscopic procedure. Anticoagulation and antiplatelet agents should be discontinued, as bleeding risk is high with ESD. Routine pre-procedure antibiotics are not recommended. Routine acid suppression is used in upper GI ESD. Conscious or deep sedation can be used, but deep sedation is recommended due to longer duration of procedure and increased discomfort from gas insufflation. The injectate solution is prepared, usually 500 cc of saline with a few drops of Indigo carmine to get a blue color.

It is preferable to position the patient so that the location of the tumor is up with respect to gravity. This facilitates submucosal dissection, since the dissected tissue "falls into the lumen" in the direction of gravity, and blood does not pool on top of the lesion, but flows away to opposite wall by gravity. It is worth repositioning the patient during the procedure to change the position of the tumor if necessary.

A cap is placed on the tip of the endoscope, and careful white light and NBI examination is performed to demarcate the lesion. The lesion should be described by location, Paris classification, and size, with image documentation. The lateral edge of the dissection field is then marked about 2–3 mm from the edge of the mucosal lesion. This is done by retracting the tip of the knife into the sheath, so that less than 1 mm is visible, then use the tip of the cautery knife and a soft coagulation current and mark cautery dots around the lesion. The two stages of ESD include circumferential mucosal incision into the submucosa followed by submucosal dissection. Both of these require repeated submucosal injections of colored saline. Begin with submucosal injection at the distal end of the lesion if possible and after a cushion is created, perform an initial cut with about 2 mm of the knife tip out. It is important to make the cut deep enough into the submucosa (but not too deep to perforate) so that the mucosal and superficial SM layers retract away from the incision and allow space to inject and begin SM dissection. The injection and circumferential incision is continued around the lesion. If the incision is deep enough, the lesion will retract toward the center. Place the tip of the knife within the incised edge of lesion and inject toward and under the lesion into the SM layer. If the incision is adequately deep, the injection will result in elevation of the lesion. Place the cap device against this elevated SM layer and begin dissection under the mucosa. Start distally (in retroflexion if necessary) and move dissection under the lesion; inject and then cut. The SM layer is identified by the appearance of loose, areolar tissue that is expanded on injection of diluted blue color. Cuts are usually 1–2 mm at a time and made by moving the tip of the scope from side to side. Change the mode of coagulation (see above) when larger vessels or bleeding are encountered. Large veins appear dark red, and arteries often appear white. Use the coagrasper to coagulate large blood vessels, either prior to cutting or after bleeding is encountered, that cannot be controlled with the knife tip coagulation. If there is brisk bleeding that is difficult to control, push the cap device gently but firmly against the bleeding area and flood with water. Then grasp the blood vessel when visualized, tent it away from the dissection, and cauterize. Movement of the endoscope tip and dissection should be careful and away from the mucosa to prevent inadvertent piecemeal resection or loss of pathologic margins due to cautery artifact. The muscularis propria layer is recognized by its white muscular bands. Care should be taken not to dissect through this layer since this will result in perforation.

The operator should use repeated submucosal injections, as much as is necessary to maintain sufficient elevation of the mucosa off the MP layer, and sufficient place to keep the cap device and endoscope in the SM layer. During the dissection of the submucosa, it is important to apply cautery only under direct endoscopic visualization of the knife and the dissection plane.

Distally, scope movement is different based on the knife. That is, the knife is not moved, but rather the endoscopist controls dissection by moving the tip of the scope laterally and vertically, mainly with torque or small dial movements. The cut direction is usually from center to periphery. When using the IT knife, the tiny porcelain hemisphere at the tip protects from unintended deep cuts. The tip is placed at the point of dissection within the submucosa and acts as a pivot to move and swing the cutting edge in a lateral and downward motion to dissect the submucosa.

Once adequate dissection has been performed distally, the lateral dissections are completed. Finally, the proximal tunnel and dissection are performed under the lesion. If fibrosis is encountered, ESD is very challenging as the SM layer does not expand with injection; careful transverse cutting should be performed in this situation, with dissection from distal and lateral end to isolate this area for final dissection. Once the dissection is complete, the site is carefully inspected for visible vessels and perforation (Figs. 4.3 and 4.4).

The specimen is then carefully retrieved in one piece, often using a retrieval net or basket. The specimen should be flattened and fixed on a thin board (styrofoam or cork board) by pinning the periphery of the lesion to the board. It is then examined and photographed for documentation. Proper orientation of the specimen allows assessment of the lateral and vertical margins and tumor depth. The pinned resected specimen is then placed in formalin. The pathologist should be informed about the technique, the importance

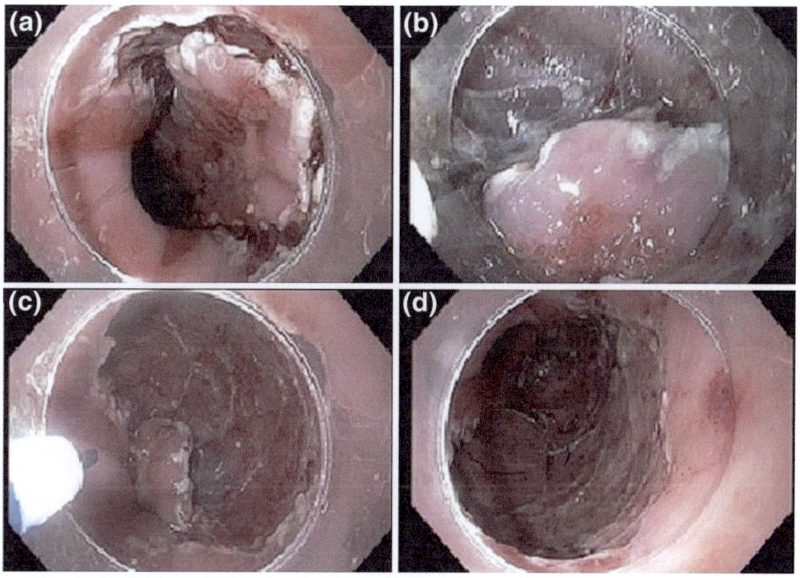

Fig. 4.3 Esophageal ESD example. **a** Marking of periphery, **b** Submucosal dissection, **c** completion of dissection, **d** Post-resection site

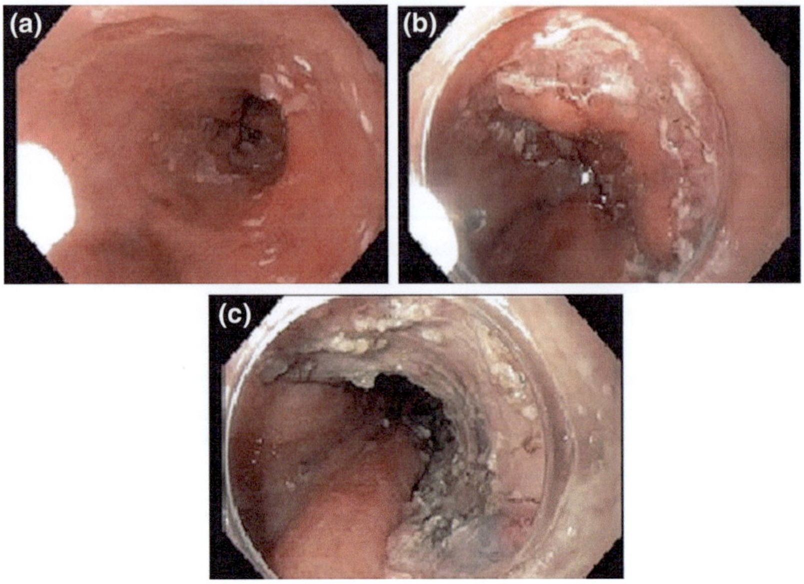

Fig. 4.4 ESD example. **a** Marking of periphery, **b** Submucosal dissection, **c** Post-resection site

of thin (2 mm) sections, and the evaluation of margins.

Post-procedure Management and Follow-Up

A standard dose of proton pump inhibitor is suggested for 8 weeks to promote ulcer healing. Patients are kept NPO for 24 h and started on a soft solid diet in the absence of complications on post-op day one. Most patients can be discharged home after 24–48 h post procedure.

Careful follow-up of biopsy results is necessary with a decision about curative ESD versus need for surgical resection in failed R0 resection. Patients should be presented at a tumor board, if available. Endoscopic follow-up is necessary to detect recurrence, usually at 3–6 months for upper GI and colon curative lesions, and an additional 1-year follow-up colonoscopy is recommended following colonic ESD. Patients with Barrett's esophagus should receive RFA following ESD to completely ablate residual Barrett's mucosa.

Management of Complications

Abdominal pain is not uncommon but is usually mild, particularly after esophageal ESD, and rarely after gastric ESD, lasting usually less than 2 days. It does not require any specific management.

Bleeding is the most common complication and occurs from 1.4 to 20% of procedures [27]. Immediate bleeding is common during the procedure, and complete hemostasis should be obtained during dissection and at the end of the procedure. This may require a combination of using soft coagulation, the coagrasper, and rarely endoscopic clip placement for brisk bleeding not responding to cautery. Immediate post-procedure bleeding is usually seen within 12 h and requires emergent endoscopy with cautery and/or clip placement on the bleeding vessel. Late bleeding can be seen at up to 30 days and is related to location (such as fundus of stomach) and large tumor resection [27].

Perforation rates for ESD are significantly higher compared to simple polypectomy and

EMR, with a risk of about 0–4% [28]. Risk of perforation is related to location and presence of ulceration and or fibrosis. When perforation is noted during the dissection, it should be closed immediately by placement of endoscopic clips [28]. Dissection can proceed if the endoscopist is comfortable that *en bloc* resection is possible and clip closure is adequate. A pneumothorax or pneumoperitoneum should be decompressed by placement of a 14-g needle or other standard techniques. Post procedure, the patient is managed with an NG tube, fasting, and antibiotics. In the setting of gastric ESD perforation with closure, the NG tube can be discontinued after 24 h and liquid oral diet resumed in 3 days. Esophageal fully covered metal stents have been used to manage iatrogenic esophageal perforation due to ESD, EMR, and other endoscopic procedures, so this option is available to the endoscopist. Surgical resection is rarely required for esophageal, gastric, or colonic perforations.

Resection of a lesion with more than one half of the circumference of the esophagus increases the risk of stricture formation, with the risk increasing significantly with resection of >2/3 circumference. Once strictures have occurred, they are very difficult to manage. Prophylactic use of oral and local corticosteroids and placement of fully covered metal stents in this setting appear promising in prevention of stricture formation [29].

Training and ESD Practice in the West

Presently, there are no dedicated and structured programs to train endoscopists for ESD in the USA, since expertise is uncommon here. Endoscopists considering ESD should be trained and be comfortable in performing advanced endoscopy. It is best to estimate the annual expected volume prior to training, since gastric cancer is uncommon in the US, and only a high expected case volume of esophageal and colon lesions would justify training in this difficult and high-risk procedure. Training on animal models is highly encouraged. It is unclear whether live models provide advantage over an explanted animal organ such as a pig stomach. In addition, there is a significant cost associated with live-model training [30]. Observation of multiple ESD procedures performed by an expert endoscopist is also essential. This usually requires travel to Japan, China, or Korea. Once adequately trained, initial ESD procedures in patients should be of lesions in the rectum or gastric antrum preferable under supervision of an expert ESD endoscopist. The mucosa is thicker in these areas, the endoscope position is also easier to control, and retroflexion is easier. Support of a gastrointestinal surgeon or a thoracic surgeon (for esophageal ESD) is also essential. The Japanese literature suggests that the performance of 30–40 gastric ESDs would provide proficiency in gastric ESD [31]. As part of any new procedure, careful records should be maintained by the endoscopist, including complications and R0 resection rates, and initial cases may need to be done with institutional review board oversight in order to obtain initial credentialing. These early outcomes should be shared with the hospital during renewal of privileges for these procedures.

Conclusion

ESD is a very useful endoscopic procedure pioneered by the Japanese for the management of early-stage luminal malignancies. In experienced hands, it results in excellent outcomes, with acceptable complication rates and with the ability to obviate the need for surgical management in selective cases. Its role is expanding, and Western endoscopists are beginning to adopt the technique. ESD is a difficult and complicated procedure and should only be performed for an accepted indication by an expert endoscopist adequately trained in the technique. Endoscopists should keep careful records on *en bloc* and R0 resection rates and complications rates for their ESD procedures.

References

1. Ono H, Kondo H, Gotoda T, Shirao K, Yamaguchi H, et al. Endoscopic mucosal resection for treatment of early gastric cancer. Gut. 2001;48:225–9.
2. Oda I, Gotoda T, Hamanaka H, et al. A novel endoscopic mucosal resection technique for early gastric cancer: submucosal dissection method with an insulation-tipped (IT) knife (abstract). Endoscopy. 2003;35 Suppl II:A43.
3. Yamamota H, Kawata H, Sunada K, Satoh K, Kaneko Y, et al. Successful *en bloc* resection of large superficial tumors in the stomach and colon using sodium hyaluronate and small-caliber-tip transparent hood. Endoscopy. 2003;35:690–4.
4. Miyamoto S, Muto M, Hamamoto Y, Boku N, Ohtsu A, et al. A new technique for endoscopic mucosal resection with an insulated-tip electrosurgical knife improves the completeness of resection of intramucosal gastric neoplasms. Gastrointest Endosc. 2002;55:576–81.
5. Hosokawa K, Yoshida S. Recent advances in endoscopic mucosal resection for early gastric cancer. Gan To Kagaku. 1998;25:476–83 (in Japanese with enlist abstract).
6. Rosch T, Sarbia M, Schumacher B, et al. Attempted endoscopic *en bloc* resection of mucosal and submucosal tumors using insulated-tip knives: a pilot series. Endoscopy. 2004;36(9):788–801.
7. Gotoda T, Yanagisawa A, Sasako M, Ono H, Nakanishi Y, et al. Incidence of lymph node metastasis from early gastric cancer: estimation with a large number of cases at two large centers. Gastric Cancer. 2000;3:219–25.
8. ASGE Technology Committee, Maple JT, Abu Dayyeh BK, Chauhan SS, Hwang JH, Komanduri S, et al. Endoscopic submucosal dissection. Gastrointest Endosc. 2015;81:1311–25.
9. Pimentel-Nunes P, Dinis-Ribeiro M, Ponchon T, Repici A, Vieth M, et al. Endoscopic submucosal dissection: European Society of Gastrointestinal Endoscopy (ESGI) guideline. Endoscopy. 2015;47: 829–54.
10. The Paris endoscopy classification of superficial neoplastic lesions: esophagus, stomach and colon: November 30 to December 1, 2002. Gastrointest Endosc. 2003;58 Suppl 6:S3–43.
11. Kudo S, Tamura S, Nakajimi T, Yamano H, Kusaka H, et al. Diagnosis of colorectal tumorous lesions by magnification endoscopy. Gastrointest Endosc. 1996;44:8–14.
12. Uraoka T, Saito Y, Ikematsu H, Yamamoto K, Sano Y. Sano's capillary pattern classification for narrow-band imaging of early colorectal lesions. Dig Endosc. 2011;Suppl 1:112–5.
13. Schlemper RJ, Riddell RH, Kato Y, Borchard F, Cooper HS, et al. The Vienna classification of gastrointestinal epithelial neoplasia. Gut. 2000;47:251–5.
14. Takahashi H, Arimura Y, Masao H, Okahara S, Tanuma T, et al. Endoscopic submucosal dissection is superior to conventional endoscopic resection as a curative treatment for early squamous cell carcinoma of the esophagus. Gastrointest Endosc. 2010;72: 255–64.
15. Hirasawa K, Kokawa A, Oka H, Yahara S, Sasaki T, et al. Superficial adenocarcinoma of the esophagogastric junction: long-term results of endoscopic submucosal dissection. Gastrointest Endosc. 2010; 72:960–6.
16. Neuhaus H, Terheggen G, Rutz EM, Vieth M, Schumacher B. Endoscopic submucosal dissection plus radiofrequency ablation of neoplastic Barrett's esophagus. Endoscopy. 2012;44:992–6.
17. Dunbar KB, Spechler SJ. The risk of lymph-node metastases in patients with high-grade dysplasia or intramucosal carcinoma in Barrett's esophagus: a systematic review. Am J Gastroenterol. 2012;107: 850–62.
18. Goto O, Fujishiro M, Kodashima S, Ono S, Omata M. Outcomes of endoscopic submucosal dissection for early gastric cancer with special reference to validation for curability criteria. Endoscopy. 2009;41:118–22.
19. Chung IK, Lee JH, Lee SH, Kim SJ, Cho JY, et al. Therapeutic outcomes in 1000 cases of endoscopic submucosal dissection for early gastric neoplasms: Korean ESD study group multicenter study. Gastrointest Endosc. 2009;69:1228–35.
20. Lian J, Chen S, Zhang Y, Qiu F. A meta-analysis of endoscopic submucosal dissection and EMR for early gastric cancer. Gastrointest Endosc. 2012;76: 763–70.
21. Gotoda T. Endoscopic resection of early gastric cancer: the Japanese perspective. Curr Opin Gastroenterol. 2006;22:561–9.
22. Repici A, Hassan C, DePaula Pessoa D, Pagano N, Arezzo A, et al. Efficacy and safety of endoscopic submucosal dissection for colorectal neoplasia: a systematic review. Endoscopy. 2012;44:137–50.
23. Saito Y, Fukuzawa M, Matsuda T, Fukunaga S, Sakamoto T, et al. Clinical outcomes of endoscopic submucosal dissection versus endoscopic mucosal resection of large colorectal tumors as determined by curative resection. Surg Endosc. 2010;24:343–52.
24. Saito Y, Uraoka T, Yamaguchi Y, Hotta K, Sakamoto N, et al. A prospective, multicenter study of 1111 colorectal endoscopic submucosal dissections. Gastrointest Endosc. 2010;72(6):1217–25.
25. Watanabe T, Itabashi M, Shimada Y, Tanaka S, Ito Y, et al. Japanese Society for Cancer of the Colon and Rectum (JSCCR) guidelines 2010 for the treatment of colorectal cancer. Int J Clin Oncol. 2012;17:1–29.
26. Olivera Ferreia A, Moleiro J, Torres J, Dinis-Robeiro M. Solutions for submucosal injection in endoscopic resection: a systematic review and meta-analysis. Endosc Int Open. 2016;04:E1–16.

27. Shiba M, Higuci K, Kadouch K, Montani A, Yamamori K, et al. Risk factors for bleeding after endoscopic mucosal resection. World J Gastroenterol. 2005;14:7335–9.
28. Minami S, Gotoda T, Ono H, Oda I, Hamanaka H. Complete endoscopic closure of gastric perforation induced by endoscopic resection of early gastric cancer using endoclips can prevent surgery. Gastrointest Endosc. 2006;63:596–601.
29. Oliveira JF, Moura EG, Bernardo WM, Ide E, Cheng S, et al. Prevention of esophageal stricture after endoscopic submucosal dissection: a systematic review and meta-analysis. Surg Endosc. 20 Oct 2015. Epub ahead of print.
30. Draganov PV, Coman RM, Gotoda T. Training for complex procedures: how to incorporate endoscopic submucosal dissection skills in the West. Expert Rev Gastroenterol Hepatol. 2014;8(2):119–21.
31. Gotoda T, Friedland S, Hamanaka H, Soetikno R. A learning curve for advanced endoscopic resection. Gastrointest Endosc. 2005;62:866–7.

Endoscopic Full-Thickness Resection 5

Sergey V. Kantsevoy and Joseph Ramon Armengol-Miro

Abstract

Flexible endoscopy was originally developed to examine and treat lesions originating from mucosal layer of gastrointestinal (GI) tract wall and located inside the lumen of hollow GI tract. Improvement in flexible endoscopes and development of new endoscopic accessories created a new endoscopic specialty—natural orifice translumenal endoscopic surgery (NOTES). Full-thickness resection of GI tract lesions is possibly one of the most promising directions in NOTES procedures. Endoscopic full-thickness resection of GI tract lesions can be done in three possible ways: via a submucosal tunnel separating the exit from GI tract lumen and the entrance into mediastinal or peritoneal cavity; the "closed" technique, allowing full-thickness resection of GI tract lesions without entering the peritoneal cavity; and the "open" technique, requiring full-thickness resection of the lesion with subsequent transmural closure of the GI tract wall defect. The OverStitch™ (Apollo EndoSurgery, Austin, TX) endoscopic suturing device allows reliable, surgical quality closure of inadvertent (perforations) and intentional (full-thickness resection) defects after endoscopic removal of GI tract lesions and truly serves as enabling technology for future NOTES procedures.

Keywords

Gastrointestinal tract · Flexible endoscopy · Perforation · Full-thickness endoscopic resection · Endoscopic submucosal dissection · Endoscopic suturing device

S.V. Kantsevoy
University of Maryland School of Medicine, Baltimore, USA

S.V. Kantsevoy (✉)
Therapeutic Endoscopy, Institute for Digestive Health and Liver Diseases, Mercy Medical Center, 301 St. Paul Place, POB 7th Floor, Suite 718, Baltimore, MD 21202, USA
e-mail: skan51@hotmail.com

S.V. Kantsevoy · J.R. Armengol-Miro
World Institute for Digestive Endoscopy (WIDER), Barcelona, Spain
e-mail: jrarmengol@gmail.com

J.R. Armengol-Miro
Digestive Endoscopy, Vall d'Hebron University Hospital, Barcelona, Spain

J.R. Romanelli et al. (eds.), *NOTES and Endoluminal Surgery*, Clinical Gastroenterology, DOI 10.1007/978-3-319-50610-4_5

Abbreviations

EFTR	Endoscopic full-thickness resection
ESD	Endoscopic submucosal dissection
GI	Gastrointestinal
NOTES	Natural orifice translumenal endoscopic surgery

Introduction

Flexible endoscopy was originally developed to examine and treat lesions originating from the mucosal layer of the gastrointestinal (GI) tract wall and located inside the lumen of the hollow GI tract. Improvement in flexible endoscopes and development of new endoscopic accessories created a new endoscopic specialty—natural orifice translumenal endoscopic surgery (NOTES) [1]. Full-thickness resection of GI tract lesions is possibly one of the most promising directions in NOTES procedures [2].

Endoscopic full-thickness resection (EFTR) of GI tract lesions can be done in 3 possible ways (Fig. 5.1).

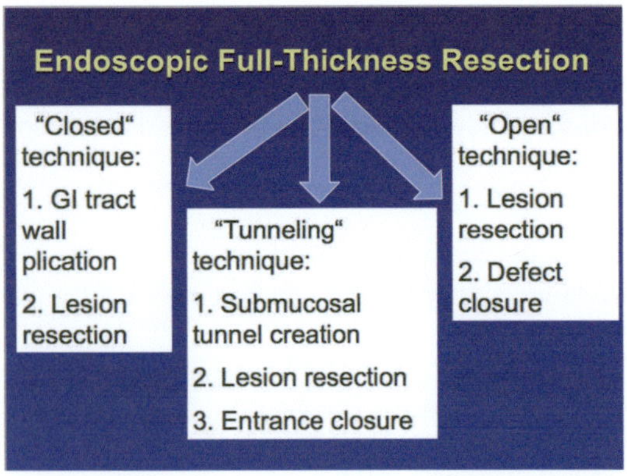

Fig. 5.1 Techniques of endoscopic full-thickness resection of GI tract lesions

Full-Thickness Resection via Submucosal Tunnel

The use of the submucosal space for NOTES procedures was first reported by Gostout et al. [3]. Full-thickness resection of GI tract lesions through the creation of a submucosal tunnel starts with submucosal injection of normal saline 20–40 mm proximal to the lesion [4]. The mucosa is incised to enter the submucosal space. The next procedural step is the creation of a submucosal tunnel toward the GI tract lesion similar to the technique utilized in per-oral endoscopic myotomy (POEM) [5–10]. The lesion is then resected inside the tunnel and removed, and the mucosal entrance to the tunnel is closed with endoscopic clips or sutures.

This technique can be used for removal of lesions originating from the submucosal or muscularis propria layers of the esophageal and gastric wall, but not the mucosa. Resection of these deeper lesions often results in the entrance into the mediastinum or peritoneal cavity. However, even in the case of resection involving the serosa, the submucosal tunnel separates the site of mucosal entrance from the exit into to the mediastinal or peritoneal space by 20–40 mm, which decreases the chance of post-procedure mediastinitis or peritonitis. After removal of the lesion, the entrance to the submucosal tunnel is usually closed with endoscopic clips or endoscopic sutures, preventing contamination of the mediastinal or peritoneal space by GI tract contents.

To clarify, submucosal tunneling resection can be used to perform deeper resections involving the serosa, and so the convention has emerged that we call these "full-thickness" resections. However, the overlying mucosa must be left intact in this method to prevent perforation. Therefore, the submucosal tunneling approach cannot be used for lesions involving mucosa and is not truly a full-thickness resection. Also, although the submucosal tunneling approach for "full-thickness" resection appears to be safe and effective, it only can be used in certain anatomic locations allowing for the creation of a submucosal tunnel (esophagus, stomach).

"Full-thickness" resection of gastric tumors (i.e., resections involving the serosa) through the submucosal tunnel technique was recently reported by Lee et al. Five lesions (3 gastrointestinal stromal tumors and 2 schwannomas) were accessed via 40-mm submucosal tunnels and resected en bloc [11]. All procedures were performed under conscious sedation, and the mean tumor size was 20.8 ± 3.27 mm. The mean hospital stay post-endoscopic submucosal tunnel full-thickness resection of gastric lesions was only 3.8 ± 1.48 days, and there were no procedure-related complications (bleeding, peritonitis, etc.) reported.

"Closed" Technique of Endoscopic Full-Thickness Resection

A "closed" approach to full-thickness resection of GI tract lesions implies plication of the GI tract wall, with subsequent resection of the lesion without entrance into the peritoneal cavity. The first clinical application of the "closed" technique was reported by Kaehler et al. [12, 13] for full-thickness resection of gastric lesions. He used a flexible endoscopic stapler to create a plication of the gastric wall, and then, the lesion was cut out of the inside of the stomach and removed without entrance into the peritoneal cavity. Unfortunately, the flexible endoscopic stapler is no longer available.

Another application of the "closed" technique was recently reported for a full-thickness resection of colonic lesions [14]. The authors used a specially designed, large OTSC® over-the-scope clip (Ovesco Endoscopy, Tübingen, Germany) mounted on the distal end of the endoscope. Colonic lesions were pulled into the full-thickness resection device; then, the clip was closed, isolating the lesion from the peritoneal cavity. The lesion could then be resected. The initial pilot study (25 patients) reported technical success in 83.3% (20/24) with complete (R0) resection in 75% (18/24) and full-thickness resection in 87.5% (21/24). Minor adverse events (bleeding, postpolypectomy syndrome) were observed in 3 patients (12%). Follow-up endoscopy revealed residual adenoma in 4 (16%) and local recurrence in 1 patient (4%).

Following this pilot study, preliminary results of a large, prospective, multicenter trial were reported during Digestive Disease Week in May 2016. Nine academic referral centers in Germany recruited 180 patients from February 2015 through April 2016 [15]. Mean lesion size was 17.6 mm. Technical success was achieved in 88.3% of patients (159/180), with complete resection (R0) in 78.1% (139/178), and confirmed full-thickness resection in 78.4% (120/153). Adverse events were observed in 9.4% of patients (17/180), including 12 major adverse events (bleeding in 5, perforation in 5, and appendicitis in 2). Surgical correction was needed in 7.2% of patients (13/180). However, follow-up in 3 months demonstrated residual or recurrent lesions in 10% (9/90) patients.

Despite the theoretical attractiveness of the "closed" full-thickness resection technique, available studies demonstrated its obvious limitations: Only relatively small lesions (mean 17.6 mm) located in favorable positions can be removed, but with a high rate of adverse events (9.4%) and high rate of residual or recurrent lesions (10.0%) [12, 13, 15].

"Open" Technique of Endoscopic Full-Thickness Resection

The first endoscopic full-thickness resection of GI tract lesions was described in a live porcine model by Ikeda et al. [16]. The authors performed full-thickness resection of the gastric wall in 4 acute and 8 survival animal experiments. Large, full-thickness defects in the gastric wall were closed endoscopically with T-tags inserted into the peritoneal cavity through blind puncture of the gastric wall with a hollow needle. Unfortunately, this closure technique could potentially damage adjacent intraperitoneal organs and is now practically abandoned [17].

Since that time, several studies demonstrated the feasibility of endoscopic full-thickness resection of GI tract lesions using the "open" technique. Huang et al. [18] reported endoscopic full-thickness resection of 13 gastric stromal tumors over 20 mm in size originating from the muscularis propria. All defects in the gastric wall were closed with endoscopic clips without any complications. Shi et al. [19] also reported full-thickness resection of gastric submucosal tumors (mean lesion size 14.7 ± 7.2 mm, range 4–30 mm) originating from the muscularis propria layer in 20 patients. All lesions were resected *en bloc* (100%), with subsequent closure of full-thickness gastric wall defects by a combination of endoloops (Olympus, Tokyo, Japan) and endoscopic metallic clips. There were no serious complications (peritonitis, abdominal abscess, etc.) after full-thickness resection, although 5 patients developed fever and slight abdominal pain on the first day after the procedure. The largest series (30 patients) of "open" full-thickness resection of gastric submucosal tumors was published by Fan et al. [20]. The mean size of the resected lesions was 19 mm, and all full-thickness defects in the gastric wall were closed with the combination of an endoloop and endoscopic clips. There were no serious complications during or after the procedure, and follow-up endoscopy 1 month after resection confirmed complete healing of the gastric wall defect.

Zhang et al. compared endoscopic "open" full-thickness resection (n = 22) of gastric stromal tumors over 20 mm in size to laparoscopic resection (n = 20) [21]. Endoscopic full-thickness resection was similar to laparoscopic resection in mean operative times (90 ± 17 min vs. 95 ± 21 min, $p > 0.05$), complete resection rates (100% vs. 95%, $p > 0.05$), and mean length of hospital stay (6.0 ± 1.8 days vs. 7.3 ± 1.7 days, $p > 0.05$). None of the patients in the endoscopic full-thickness resection group had any complications, whereas one patient in the laparoscopic resection group required conversion to laparotomy, and one experienced postoperative gastroparesis. No recurrences were observed in either group. The authors optimistically concluded that endoscopic full-thickness resection may replace surgical or laparoscopic procedures for removal of gastric stromal tumors.

Endoscopic "open" full-thickness resection of colonic lesions in a live animal model produced very heterogeneous results. Brigic et al. [22] analyzed animal studies devoted to endoscopic full-thickness resection of colonic lesions published between 1990 and 2012. A total of 113 procedures was performed on 99 porcine models, with an overall success rate of 89% and 4% mortality. The intra-operative complication rate was prohibitively high (mean = 22%; range = 0–67%). Significant heterogeneity was observed in procedure duration (median or mean 3–233 min) and size of the excised specimen (median or mean 1.7–3.6 cm). Defect closure techniques included endoscopic stapling devices, T-tags, compression closure, or closure with laparoscopic assistance. There was a high rate of failure to close the defect (5–55%) and a high incidence of abnormal findings at postmortem examination (84%). This systematic analysis clearly demonstrated that reliable closure of full-thickness colonic defects after resection could not be achieved with the previously used endoscopic closure techniques (T-tags, stapling, compression devices, etc.).

An endoscopic suturing device (OverStitch™, Apollo EndoSurgery, Austin, TX, USA) has become available for clinical use in 2011 [23–25]. It is a very versatile and user-friendly device which allows creation of separate stitches or a running suture line of variable length [26–30]. The device has already been successfully used for closure of full-thickness, colonic wall perforations with superior results compared to traditional endoscopic, through-the-scope clips [31, 32]. We have previously reported our preliminary results demonstrating safety and feasibility of "open" full-thickness endoscopic resection of GI tract lesions on a live animal model (90-kg domestic pigs) [2, 33]. Purely endoscopic full-thickness resection of the gastric and colonic wall was successfully achieved in all 9 animals [2, 34]. All defects after resection were easily and reliably closed using the OverStitch. Postmortem examination revealed good full-thickness healing of the GI tract wall at the sites of resection. After successful completion of initial animal experiments, we performed purely endoscopic full-thickness resection of an actively bleeding 2 × 4 cm colon cancer located at the hepatic flexure. In another patient, we accomplished purely endoscopic, full-thickness resection of a 2 × 5 cm recurrent gastric stromal tumor [2, 33, 34]. In both patients, colonic or gastric wall defects were completely closed with a continuous suture line. Both patients tolerated EFTR well, had no pain post-procedure, and were discharged home in 3 days. Follow-up endoscopy at 3, 6, and 12 months revealed good healing of resection sites without any residual lesions or strictures.

Our technique of NOTES "open" full-thickness resection of GI tract lesions consists of several consecutive steps (Figs. 5.2, 5.3, 5.4, 5.5, 5.6, 5.7, 5.8, 5.9, 5.10, 5.11, 5.12, 5.13, 5.13, 5.14, 5.15 and 5.16) [35, 36]. We start *en bloc* removal of the lesion (Fig. 5.2) with endoscopic submucosal dissection (ESD) utilizing dedicated ESD accessories—DualKnife™ and HookKnife™ (Olympus America, Center Valley, PA) or Hybrid Knife® (ERBE USA Inc, Marietta, GA). If the submucosal space is obliterated by extensive fibrosis (after previous unsuccessful attempts of piecemeal resection), or if cancer involves the muscularis layer, we convert ESD into a full-thickness resection (Figs. 5.3 and 5.4). After *en bloc* full-thickness resection of the lesion (Fig. 5.5), a double-channel upper endoscope (GIF 2T180, Olympus America, Center Valley, PA, USA) preloaded with the OverStitch is advanced toward the full-thickness resection site (Fig. 5.6). The suturing arm of the device is opened and then closed delivering a needle through the proximal edge of the full-thickness colonic wall defect (Fig. 5.7). The needle is transferred back onto the suturing arm (Fig. 5.8), the suturing arm is reopened (Fig. 5.9), and the device is moved toward the distal edge of the full-thickness defect. Then, the suturing arm is closed again, advancing the needle through the distal edge of the full-thickness colonic wall defect, and the needle reloaded back onto the suturing arm (Fig. 5.10). The needle is driven sequentially through the proximal (Fig. 5.11) and distal (Fig. 5.12) edges of the full-thickness defect

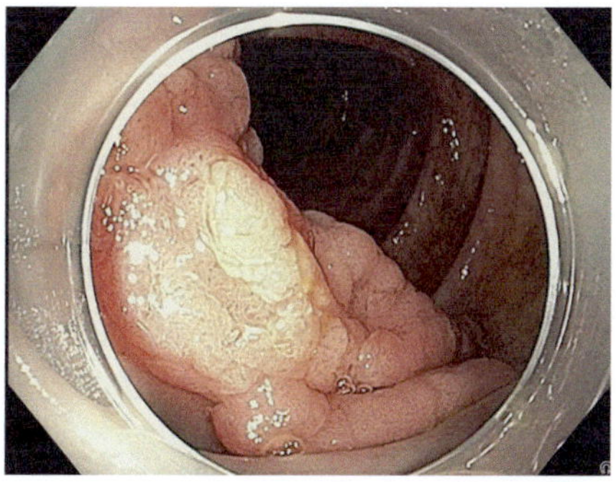

Fig. 5.2 Large, flat, sessile colonic polyp in transverse colon with extensive submucosal fibrosis after previous unsuccessful attempt of piecemeal resection in another institution

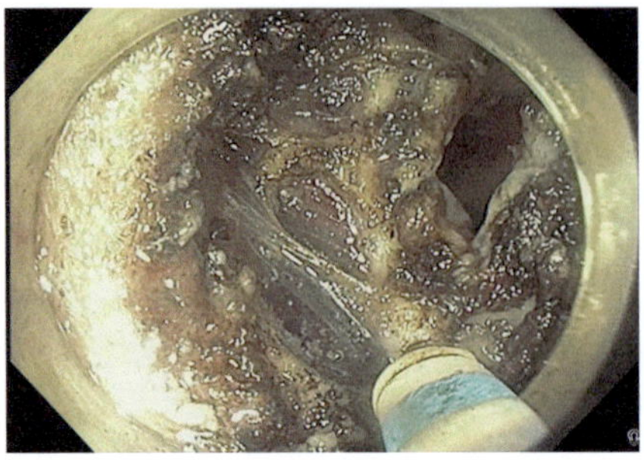

Fig. 5.3 Endoscopic full-thickness resection is performed with DualKnife

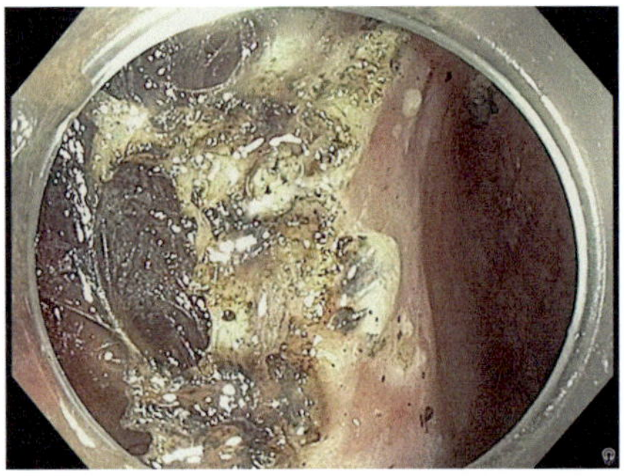

Fig. 5.4 Full-thickness endoscopic resection is completed

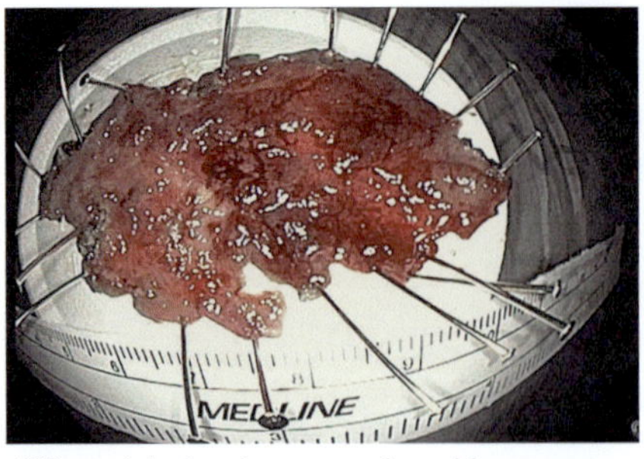

Fig. 5.5 Large (60 mm) lesion is removed *en bloc*

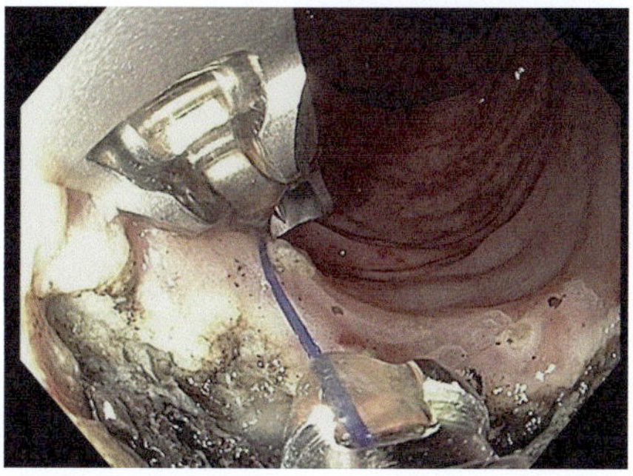

Fig. 5.6 OverStitch endoscopic suturing device is delivered toward the proximal edge of the full-thickness defect. The suturing arm is opened

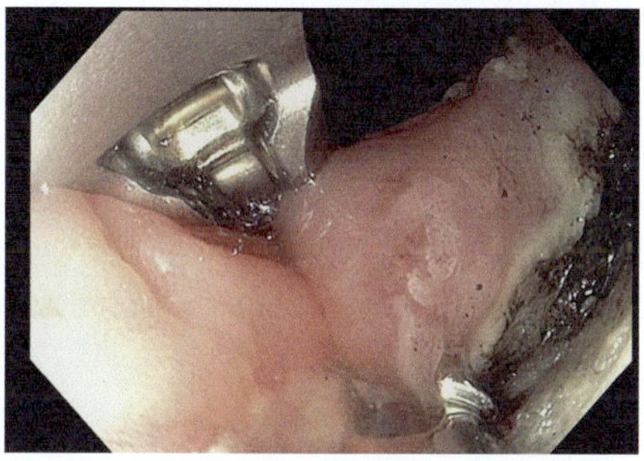

Fig. 5.7 Suturing arm is closed, delivering the needle through the proximal edge of the full-thickness, colonic wall defect

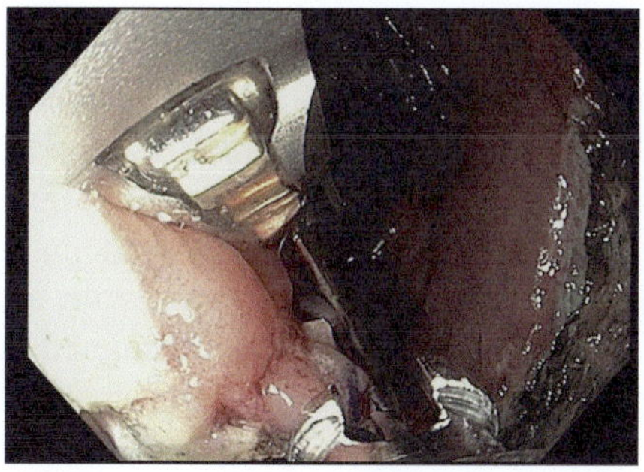

Fig. 5.8 Needle is loaded back onto the suturing arm

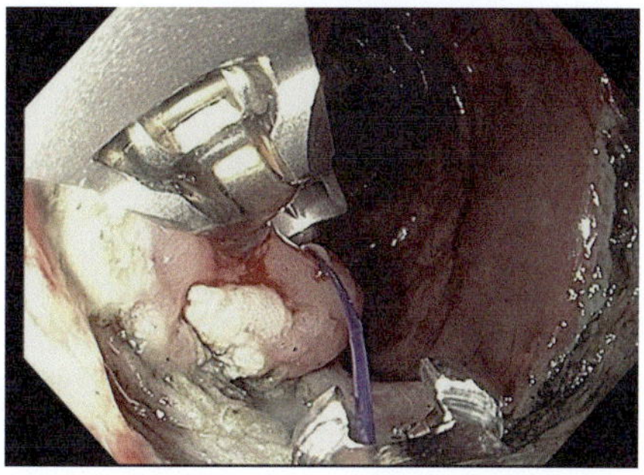

Fig. 5.9 Suturing arm is reopened and suturing device is moved toward the distal edge of the full-thickness colonic wall defect

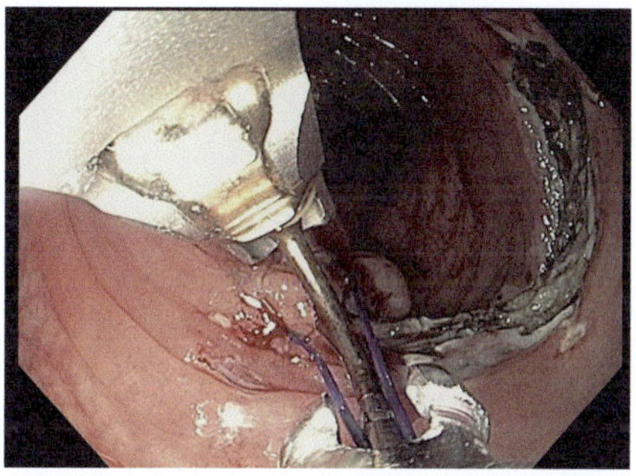

Fig. 5.10 Needle is advanced through the distal edge of the colonic wall defect and then reloaded back onto the suturing arm

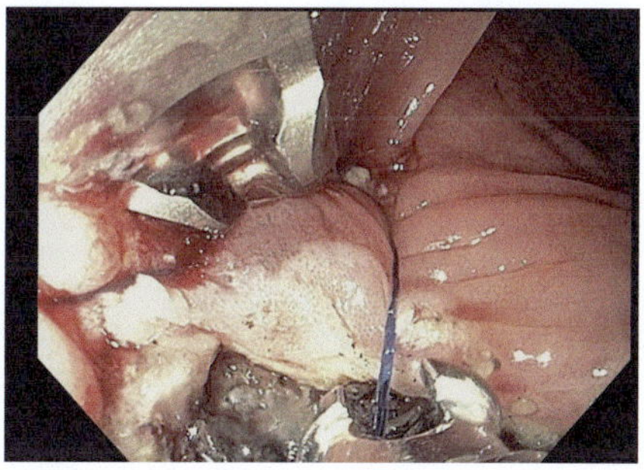

Fig. 5.11 Needle is again directed through the proximal edge of the colonic wall defect

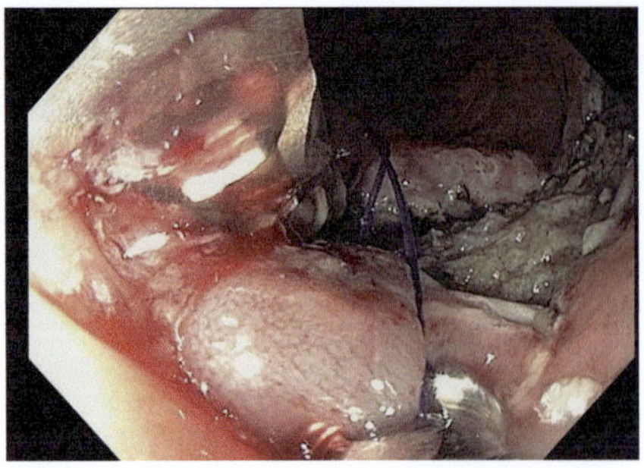

Fig. 5.12 Needle is transferred back onto the suturing arm and then guided through the distal edge of the colonic wall defect

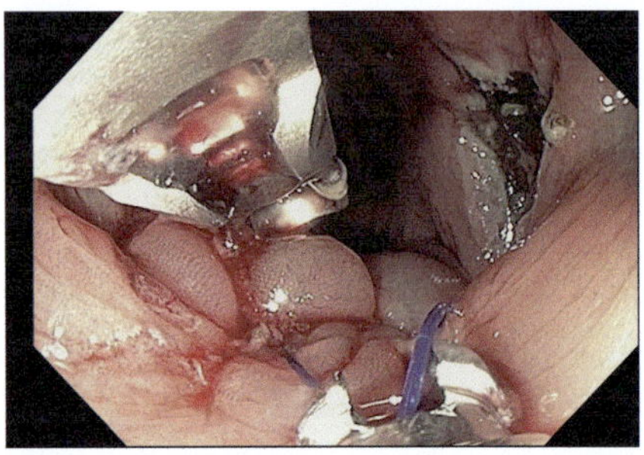

Fig. 5.13 Above steps are repeated, creating a continuous suture line, closing most of the defect post-endoscopic removal of the colonic lesion

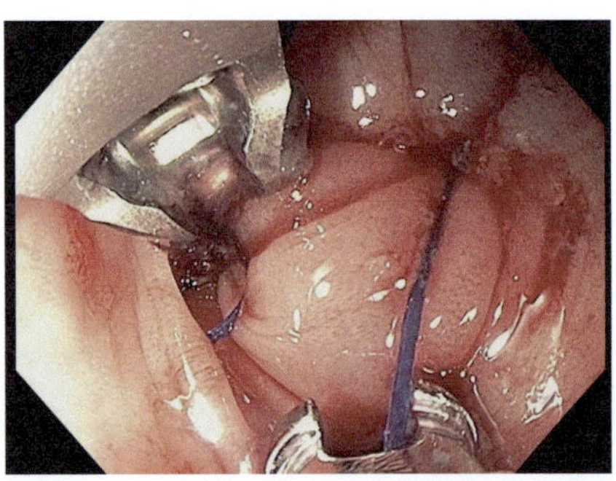

Fig. 5.14 Last needle passage is made, completely sealing colonic wall defect

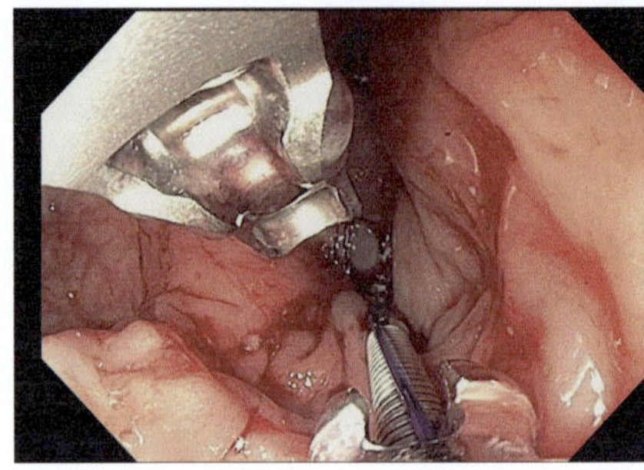

Fig. 5.15 Suture line is tightened and locked with deployment of a specially designed cinching mechanism

until it is fully closed (Figs. 5.13 and 5.14). The special cinching mechanism is then deployed (Fig. 5.15), tightening and finishing the creation of the continuous suture line, completely closing the full-thickness colonic wall defect (Fig. 5.16).

The OverStitch allows reliable, surgical quality closure of inadvertent (perforations) and intentional (full-thickness resection) defects post-endoscopic removal of GI tract lesions and truly serves as enabling technology for future NOTES procedures.

Conclusion

Endoscopic full-thickness resection of GI tract lesions has become more amenable given new tools that are developing, such as endoscopic suturing devices. While perforation of the GI tract was previously considered anathema to the endoscopist, deliberate perforation with a planned closure method is now considered not a complication, but an innovative approach to resection of small GI tract lesions.

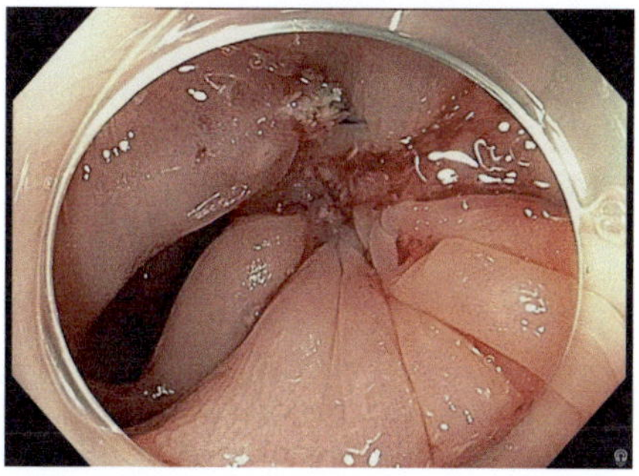

Fig. 5.16 Complete closure of the full-thickness, colonic wall defect is achieved with one continuous suture line

References

1. Rattner D, Kalloo A. ASGE/SAGES Working Group on Natural Orifice Translumenal Endoscopic Surgery. October 2005. Surg Endosc. 2006;20:329–33.
2. Armengol-Miro JR, Dot Bach J, Suboh Abadia MA, et al. Natural orifice translumenal endoscopic surgery (NOTES) for G.I. tract neoplasia. In: Testoni PA, Arcidiacono PG, Mariani A, editors. Endoscopic management of gastrointestinal cancer and precancerous conditions. Turin, Italy: Edizioni Minerva Medica; 2015, p. 277–83.
3. Sumiyama K, Gostout CJ, Rajan E, et al. Transgastric cholecystectomy: transgastric accessibility to the gallbladder improved with the SEMF method and a novel multibending therapeutic endoscope. Gastrointest Endosc. 2007;65:1028–34.
4. Liu BR, Song JT, Kong LJ, Pei FH, Wang XH, Du YJ. Tunneling endoscopic muscularis dissection for subepithelial tumors originating from the muscularis propria of the esophagus and gastric cardia. Surg Endosc. 2013;27(11):4354–9.
5. Pasricha PJ, Hawari R, Ahmed I, et al. Submucosal endoscopic esophageal myotomy: a novel experimental approach for the treatment of achalasia. Endoscopy. 2007;39:761–4.
6. Inoue H, Minami H, Kobayashi Y, et al. Peroral endoscopic myotomy (POEM) for esophageal achalasia. Endoscopy. 2010;42:265–71.
7. Inoue H, Tianle KM, Ikeda H, et al. Peroral endoscopic myotomy for esophageal achalasia: technique, indication, and outcomes. Thorac Surg Clin. 2011;21:519–25.
8. Zhou PH, Cai MY, Yao LQ. Peroral endoscopic myotomy for esophageal achalasia: report of 42 cases. Zhonghua Wei Chang Wai Ke Za Zhi. 2011;14:705–8.
9. Stavropoulos SN, Harris MD, Hida S, Brathwaite C, Demetriou C, Grendell J. Endoscopic submucosal myotomy for the treatment of achalasia (with video). Gastrointest Endosc. 2010;72:1309–11.
10. Stavropoulos SN, Friedel D, Modayil R, Iqbal S, Grendell JH. Endoscopic approaches to treatment of achalasia. Therap Adv Gastroenterol. 2013;6:115–35.
11. Lee SH, Kim SJ, Lee TH, Chung IK, Park SH, et al. Human applications of submucosal endoscopy under conscious sedation for pure natural orifice transluminal endoscopic surgery. Surg Endosc. 2013;27(8):3016–20.
12. Kaehler G, Grobholz R, Langner C, Suchan K, Post S. A new technique of endoscopic full-thickness resection using a flexible stapler. Endoscopy. 2006;38:86–9.
13. Kaehler GF, Langner C, Suchan KL, Freudenberg S, Post S. Endoscopic full-thickness resection of the stomach: an experimental approach. Surg Endosc. 2006;20:519–21.
14. Schmidt A, Bauerfeind P, Gubler C, Damm M, Bauder M, Caca K. Endoscopic full-thickness resection in the colorectum with a novel over-the-scope device: first experience. Endoscopy. 2015;47:719–25.
15. Schmidt AR, Meining A, Birk M, et al. Endoscopic full-thickness resection in the lower gastrointestinal tract using an over-the-scope device—interim results of a prospective multicenter trial. Gastrointest Endosc. 2016;83:AB119.
16. Ikeda K, Mosse CA, Park PO, et al. Endoscopic full-thickness resection: circumferential cutting method. Gastrointest Endosc. 2006;64:82–9.
17. Kantsevoy SV. Endoscopic full-thickness resection: new minimally invasive therapeutic alternative for GI-tract lesions. Gastrointest Endosc. 2006;64:90–1.
18. Huang LY, Cui J, Liu YX, Wu CR, Yi DL. Endoscopic therapy for gastric stromal tumors originating from the muscularis propria. World J Gastrenterolol 2012;18:3465–71.

19. Shi Q, Chen T, Zhong YS, et al. Complete closure of large gastric defects after endoscopic full-thickness resection, using endoloop and metallic clip interrupted suture. Endoscopy. 2013;45:329–34.
20. Zhang Y, Wang X, Xiong G, Qian Y, Wang H, et al. Complete defect closure of gastric submucosal tumors with purse-string sutures. Surg Endosc. 2014;28(6):1844–51.
21. Zhang B, Huang LY, Wu CR, Cui J, Jiang LX, Zheng HT. Endoscopic full-thickness resection of gastric stromal tumor arising from the muscularis propria. Chin Med J (Engl). 2013;126:2435–9.
22. Brigic A, Symons NR, Faiz O, Fraser C, Clark SK, Kennedy RH. A systematic review regarding the feasibility and safety of endoscopic full thickness resection (EFTR) for colonic lesions. Surg Endosc. 2013;27(10):3520–9.
23. Kantsevoy SV, Bitner M. Esophageal stent fixation with endoscopic suturing device (with video). Gastrointest Endosc. 2012;76:1251–5.
24. Kantsevoy SV, Thuluvath PJ. Successful closure of a chronic refractory gastrocutaneous fistula with a new endoscopic suturing device (with video). Gastrointest Endosc. 2012;75:688–90.
25. Armengol-Miro JR, Dot J, Abu-Suboh Abadia M, et al. New endoscopic suturing device for closure of chronic gastrocutaneous fistula in an immunocompromised patient. Endoscopy. 2012;43(Suppl 2 UCTN):E403–4.
26. Bonin EA, Wong Kee Song LM, Gostout ZS, Bingener J, Gostout CJ. Closure of a persistent esophagopleural fistula assisted by a novel endoscopic suturing system. Endoscopy. 2012;44(Suppl 2 UCTN):E8–9.
27. Jirapinyo P, Watson RR, Thompson CC. Use of a novel endoscopic suturing device to treat recalcitrant marginal ulceration (with video). Gastrointest Endosc. 2012;76:435–9.
28. Kantsevoy SV, Bitner M, Mitrakov AA, Thuluvath PJ. Endoscopic suturing closure of large mucosal defects after endoscopic submucosal dissection is technically feasible, fast, and eliminates the need for hospitalization (with videos). Gastrointest Endosc. 2013;79:503–7.
29. Rieder E, Dunst CM, Martinec DV, Cassera MA, Swanstrom LL. Endoscopic suture fixation of gastrointestinal stents: proof of biomechanical principles and early clinical experience. Endoscopy. 2012;44:1121–6.
30. Stavropoulos SN, Modayil R, Friedel D. Current applications of endoscopic suturing. World J Gastrointest Endosc. 2015;7:777–89.
31. Kantsevoy SV, Bitner M, Davis JM, Hajiyeva G, Thuluvath PJ, Gushchin V. Endoscopic suturing closure of large iatrogenic colonic perforation. Gastrointest Endosc. 2015;82:754–5.
32. Kantsevoy SV, Bitner M, Hajiyeva G, Mirovski PM, Cox ME, et al. Endoscopic management of colonic perforations: clips versus suturing closure (with videos). Gastrointest Endosc. 2015 (Epub ahead of print).
33. Armengol-Miro JR, Dot J, Abu-Suboh Abadia M, et al. Full-thickness purely endoscopic resection of colon cancer. Gastrointest Endosc. 2012;75:AB114–AB5.
34. Armengol-Miro JR, Abu-Suboh Abadia M, Dot J, et al. Full-thickness endoscopic resection of gastrointestinal cancer: from animal experiments to humans. Gastrointest Endosc. 2013;77:AB458.
35. Kantsevoy SV. Endoscopic suturing devices. In: Testoni PA, Arcidiacono PG, Mariani A, editors. Endoscopic management of gastrointestinal cancer and precancerous conditions. Turin, Italy: Edizioni Minerva Medica; 2015. p. 249–55.
36. Kantsevoy SV. Endoscopic suturing for closure of transmural defects. Techniques in Gastrointest Endosc. 2015;17:136–40.

Per-oral Endoscopic Myotomy

6

Stavros N. Stavropoulos, Rani Modayil and David Friedel

Abstract

Per-oral endoscopic myotomy, or POEM, has emerged as the most innovative therapy in achalasia after its introduction in 2008 and the most successful application of NOTES to date. Moreover, it is the prototype for the burgeoning field of tunnel endoscopy. It represents the endoscopic equivalent of laparoscopic Heller myotomy (LHM). POEM has been well validated in terms of impressive efficacy and notable safety and is being now performed all over the world by both surgeons and gastroenterologists. We will describe POEM development, patient evaluation, technique, postprocedural care, complications, accumulating longer-term data, comparison with other achalasia therapy, training concerns, and perspectives for the future.

Keywords

POEM · Achalasia · NOTES · Endoscopic myotomy · Heller myotomy · Submucosal tunnel

Abbreviations

AEs	Adverse events
ASGE	American Society for Gastrointestinal Endoscopy
CSA	Cross-sectional area
EFTR	Endoscopic full-thickness resection

S.N. Stavropoulos · R. Modayil · D. Friedel
Department of Gastroenterology, Hepatology and Nutrition, Winthrop University Hospital, 222 Station Plaza North Suite 429 Mineola, NY 11501, USA

S.N. Stavropoulos (✉)
GI Endoscopy and Program in Advanced GI Endoscopy, Winthrop University Hospital, 222 Station Plaza North, Suite 429, Mineola, NY 11501, USA
e-mail: sstavropoulos@winthrop.org

S.N. Stavropoulos
Clinical Medicine, Columbia University, New York, USA

S.N. Stavropoulos
Medicine, Temple University, Philadelphia, USA

J.R. Romanelli et al. (eds.), *NOTES and Endoluminal Surgery*, Clinical Gastroenterology, DOI 10.1007/978-3-319-50610-4_6

EMR	Endoscopic mucosal resection
ESD	Endoscopic submucosal dissection
GEJ	Gastroesophageal junction
GERD	Gastroesophageal reflux disease
HK	Hybrid knife
HM	Heller myotomy
LES	Lower esophageal sphincter
LHM	Laparoscopic Heller myotomy
MCT	Multicenter trial
NOTES	Natural orifice translumenal endoscopic surgery
PBD	Pneumatic balloon dilation
PIVI	Preservation and Incorporation of Valuable Endoscopic Innovations
POEM	Per-oral endoscopic myotomy
POET	Per-oral endoscopic tumor resection
POP	Per-oral pyloromyotomy
PPI	Proton pump inhibitor
STER	Submucosal tunnel endoscopic resection
TT	Triangle-tip

Introduction

Achalasia occurs about equally in both genders and across the age spectrum, with a reported annual incidence and prevalence of about 1/100,000 and 10/100,000 persons, respectively [1]. Patients typically have failure of relaxation of the lower esophageal sphincter (LES) and loss of peristalsis in the esophageal body. This results in dysphagia for liquids and solids, and variable chest pain, regurgitation, and weight loss. The diagnosis is suggested by a typical "bird's-beak" appearance on esophageal barium study and is usually confirmed by esophageal manometry, revealing abnormal relaxation of the LES and variable abnormalities of esophageal body peristalsis.

Development of POEM

Medical treatment of achalasia is generally ineffective and short-lived. More effective therapies are geared toward the weakening or ablation of the LES, achieved by endoscopy (botulinum toxin injection and large-diameter balloon dilation), surgery (Heller myotomy), or endoscopic surgery (POEM). Until the introduction of per-oral endoscopic myotomy (POEM), Heller myotomy (HM) had been considered the most durable option in achalasia therapy, with a single anterior myotomy extending to the gastric cardia [2]. HM may be performed both laparoscopically and thoracoscopically and is usually combined with fundoplication [3].

Ortega first described a direct endoscopic myotomy in 1980 [4], but this was not adopted by others, perhaps related to concerns about reproducibility and safety. The Apollo group, a group that had been formed in the early 2000s to study NOTES applications, described endoscopic myotomy in a porcine model utilizing a needle knife to selectively cut the esophageal circular muscle layer after an initial mucosal incision 5 cm above the gastroesophageal junction (GEJ) after creation of a submucosal tunnel using a dilation balloon [5].

Inoue performed the first POEM in a human in 2008 and coined the term "POEM." His first series of 17 subjects noted relief of dysphagia in most subjects with diminished LES pressure and no notable complications [6]. POEM was first performed outside Japan (at Winthrop University Hospital in the USA) in 2009 [7] and subsequently spread to many parts of the world. This was documented by the IPOEMS survey, an international survey sponsored by the Natural Orifice Surgery Consortium for Advancement and Research (NOSCAR) in 2012 [8]. Twenty centers were performing POEM worldwide in 2012. Sixteen of these centers (80%), including all high-volume centers (>30 POEMs), 7 from North America, 5 from Asia, and 4 from Europe, with a total number of 841 POEMs, participated in a comprehensive survey that detailed all aspects of POEM. The documented success led to a burgeoning increase in POEM operators and volume such that an estimated 4000 POEMs have been performed, with two Asian centers performing over 1000 each [9–11].

Within a few years of POEM's initial introduction, the NOSCAR POEM White Paper and the ASGE POEM PIVI (Preservation and Incorporation of Valuable Endoscopic Innovations) were published [12, 13]. These publications establish POEM not only as a primary therapy for achalasia patients without antecedent treatment, but also for those achalasia patients with prior endoscopic intervention (botulinum toxin injection and pneumatic dilation), prior HM, or previous POEM [14]. It was also determined that POEM was appropriate therapy for patients with spastic disorders of the esophagus and even "end-stage" achalasia patients with a sigmoid esophagus. A 2016 ASGE technology status evaluation report on POEM followed the comprehensive 2014 White Paper and 2015 PIVI documents, extending the literature review and assessment further to the current state of the art for this procedure [15].

Patient Evaluation

Patients should be evaluated and prepared as they would be for any elective surgery. Optimally, their esophageal motor disorder is well categorized by a high-resolution esophageal manometry and a timed barium swallow. Upper endoscopy should be performed earlier to exclude malignancy and again at the time of POEM to ensure esophageal clearance and allow lavage with topical antibiotics. Contraindications to the procedure include coagulopathy, severe pulmonary disease, evidence of mediastinal disease inflammation, prior thoracic-esophageal irradiation, and prior esophageal endoscopic mucosal resection (EMR)/endoscopic submucosal dissection (ESD) [8]. Patients should be prepared to stay at least overnight in the hospital.

POEM Technique

A suggested equipment list is presented in Table 6.1. Typically, a diagnostic gastroscope with accessory irrigation channel is used. Although Inoue initially advocated the use of an overtube and an oblique transparent distal cap attachment, most operators presently do not use an overtube routinely, and many utilize a conventional straight ESD cap (Fig. 6.1).

POEM represents an incisionless method to duplicate the traditional surgical myotomy by the ingenious concept of creating a submucosal tunnel that allows one temporary access to the mediastinum and esophageal muscle, including the LES, before the tunnel entrance is securely closed. Thus, the elements of POEM technique are as follows: (1) mucosal incision, (2) submucosal tunnel creation, (3) esophageal myotomy, (4) LES myotomy, and (5) entry point closure (Figs. 6.2 and 6.3). The entry point site varies depending on the indication, but is typically 10–15 cm proximal to the GEJ [6].

As demonstrated in the IPOEMS study, there is no consensus regarding orientation [8]. Some centers perform POEM anteriorly at the 2 o'clock position (in the usual convention of the posterior wall centered at 6 o'clock) as initially advocated by Inoue, although he appears to have recently changed his preferred approach to a posterior approach [11]. Other centers, such as Winthrop in New York and Zongshan in Shanghai, have favored a posterior orientation at

Table 6.1 POEM equipment

Equipment	Model No.
Vio 300D/200D (ERBE Tubingen, Germany) ERBE Jet Pump cartridge	20150-300
Hemostasis Coag grasper (4 mm) (Olympus, Center Valley, PA) Forceps hemostatic (5 mm) (Olympus, Center Valley, PA)	 FD-411UR FD-410LR
Injector single use (Max Force, Olympus, Center Valley, PA)	NM-400U0423
Disposable distal cap attachment 12.4 mm (Olympus)	D-201-11804
Endoscopic knife Triangle-tip knife (Olympus, Center Valley, PA) I-type hybrid knife (ERBE Tubingen, Germany) T-type hybrid knife(ERBE Tubingen, Germany)	 KD640-L 20150-261 20150-260
Decompression 14-gauge IV angiocath catheter Veress needle	
Submucosal injectate Indigo carmine Methylene blue	
Endoscopic suturing device (Overstitch, Austin Tx) Overstitch endoscopic suture system Overstitch cinch Overstitch polypropylene suture Overstitch tissue helix	 ESS-G02-160 CNH-GO1-000 PLY-G02-020 THX-165-028
Hemostatic clips Resolution 360 clip (Boston Scientific, Marlborough, MA) Resolution clip (Boston Scientific, Marlborough, MA) Instinct (Cook Medical, Winston Salem, NC) Quick Clip Pro (Olympus Center Valley, PA) Quick Clip 2 (Olympus Center Valley, PA)	 M00521230 M00522610 INSC-7230S HX-202UR HX-201UR-135
Endoflip catheter (EndoFLIP, Crospon Ltd, Galway, Ireland)	EF-325 N

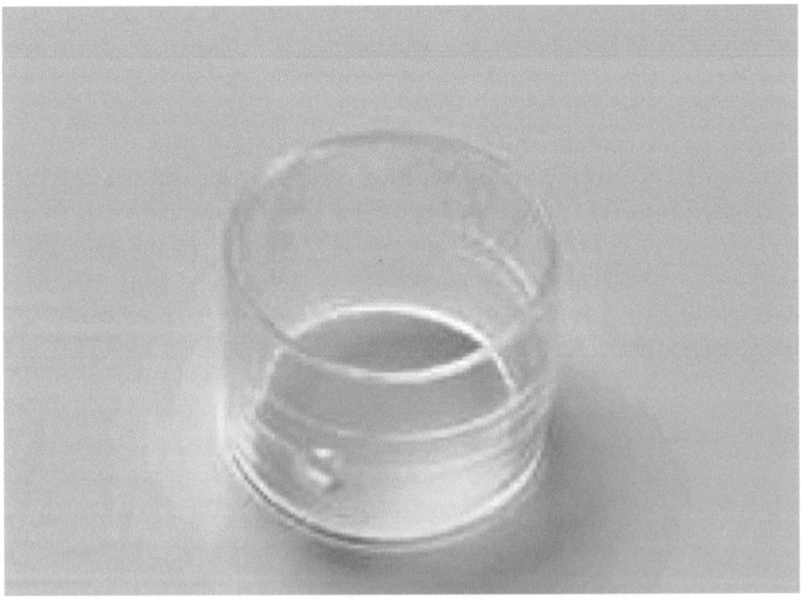

Fig. 6.1 Disposable distal cap attachment courtesy Olympus America (Center Valley, PA)

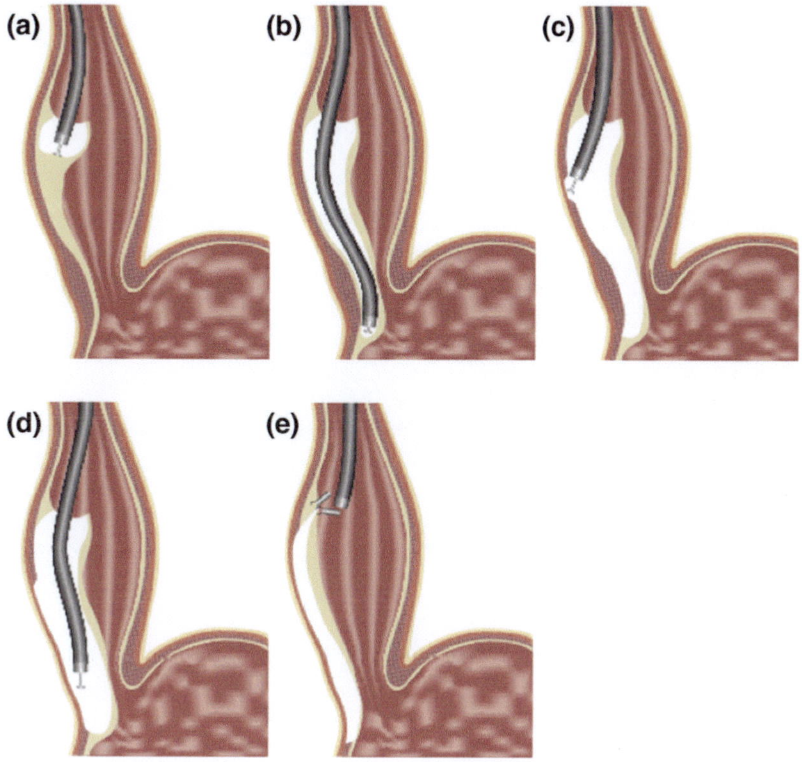

Fig. 6.2 Per-oral endoscopic myotomy technique (© S.N. Stavropoulos, Winthrop University Hospital, 2012). **a** Submucosal injection, and mucosal entry. **b** Creation of the submucosal tunnel. **c** Esophageal myotomy. **d** Lower esophageal sphincter and gastric cardia myotomy. **e** Closure of the mucosal incision

the 5 o'clock position. Various theoretical advantages have been proposed for one approach over the other. Since the posterior approach may cut some of the more powerful sling fibers of the LES compared to anterior myotomy, which is limited to the shorter and weaker clasp fibers, we have argued as early as 2013 that "one could speculate that centers employing a posterolateral approach (5 o'clock orientation), thus cutting a portion of the posterior sling fibers, may achieve higher efficacy in dysphagia relief but possibly at the cost of increased reflux" [8, 16].

It should be noted that in certain situations an anterior or posterior orientation is forced by a prior HM (in which case a posterior approach is selected to avoid postsurgical changes/scarring), or lesions such as ulcerations due to food stasis, pulsion diverticula, and severe angulation of the lumen. No prospective, randomized, comparative data have been published to date. Our group is currently near completion of enrollment of patients in a single-center, randomized study comparing anterior and posterior orientation.

We recently presented preliminary data from a retrospective comparison of anterior and posterior POEMs in our large, single-operator series using data from a prospectively maintained database [17]. In this study, we analyzed all POEMs performed at our center from October 2009 to October/2015, 248 consecutive POEMs (120 anterior, 128 posterior), all successfully completed, with no aborted POEMs or surgical conversions. No learning curve bias was expected as we performed a similar percentage of anterior POEMs in the first 3 years of our series (48/91, 53%), as in the last 2 years (72/157 46%). There were no differences in the Eckardt score, including failures (post-POEM Eckardt score >3, 5/110 anterior vs. 4/117 posterior, p = NS), accidental mucosal injuries (including non-transmural minor blanching, 29% vs. 23%), or prolonged stay of >5 days (one patient in each group). There was no difference in significant adverse events (AEs), but it should be noted that there was a paucity of such events in our series, with no leaks, no tunnel bleeds, and no

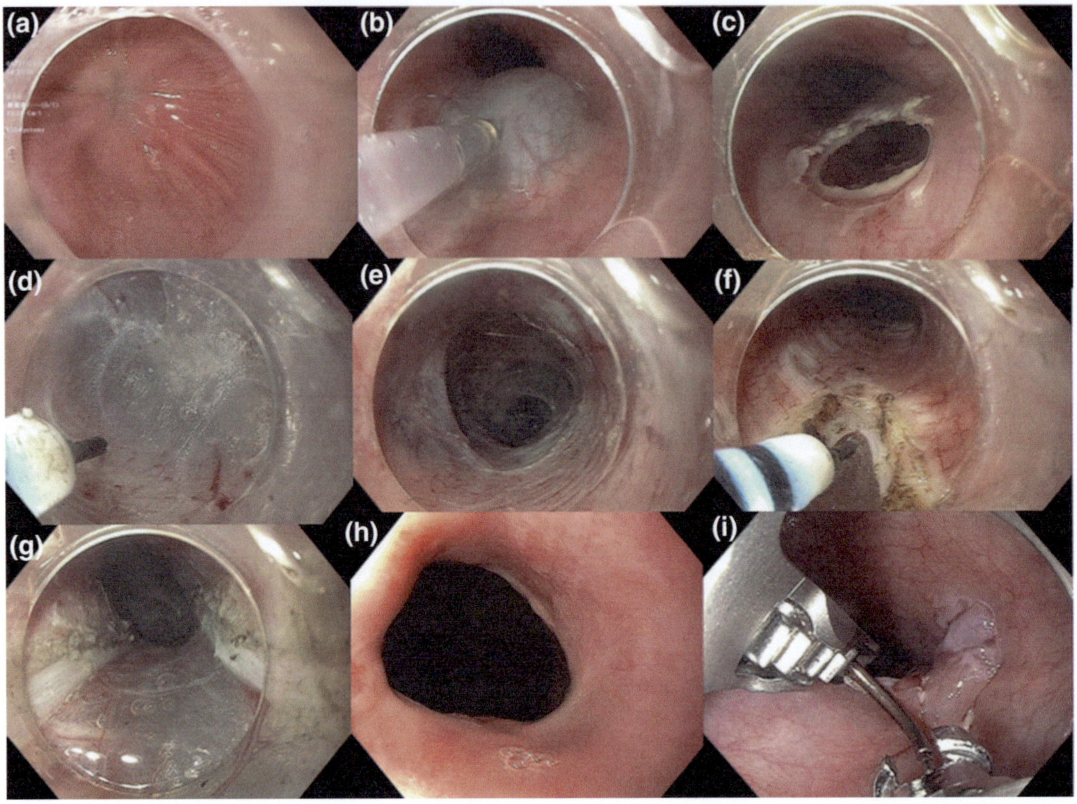

Fig. 6.3 Per-oral endoscopic myotomy endoscopic steps. **a** Tight GEJ prior to POEM. **b** Submucosal injection is performed with saline stained with methylene blue. **c** Mucosotomy is performed along the right posterior wall of the esophagus in the 5 o' clock orientation. **d** Submucosal dissection is performed with hybrid knife. **e** Submucosal tunnel is extended into the gastric cardia, and a completed submucosal tunnel is seen. **f** Myotomy is initiated 2 cm below site of mucosotomy. **g** Complete full-thickness myotomy is performed. **h** Patulous GEJ after POEM. **i** Mucosotomy closed with endoscopic suturing device

surgical/IR interventions. Posterior POEM was significantly faster overall (97 min anterior, 79 min posterior, $p = 0.0007$) including a faster closure (suturing 177, clips 71) (9.6 min anterior, 7.9 min posterior, $p = 0.02$). More patients had pain requiring narcotics in posterior POEM (17% anterior vs. 27% posterior, $p = 0.007$). There was a trend for less acid exposure in anterior POEM: +BRAVO studies (21/58 (36%) anterior vs. 29/58 (50%) posterior, $p = 0.13$) and reflux esophagitis (22/57 (38%) anterior vs. 33/60 (55%) posterior, $p = 0.076$).

Once orientation and location is selected, the submucosal space is expanded by saline injection to allow the endoscope to enter. An incision is made in the esophageal mucosa over this saline cushion, and a tunnel is begun with an electrosurgical knife inserted through the instrument channel. When the tunnel is deep and wide enough to permit introduction of the cap-fitted endoscope, it is then inserted and tunneling is continued with electrocautery distally toward the stomach. Usually, epinephrine is not utilized to avoid ischemia of the mucosal flap that may lead to necrosis. The endoscope is advanced as submucosal dissection is continued, and a tunnel is created within the submucosa from the middle esophagus to the gastric cardia. Meticulous care is taken not to tear the mucosal "roof" (or "floor," depending on the approach) of the submucosal tunnel.

The myotomy is generally performed after the tunnel creation, but recently, a technique has

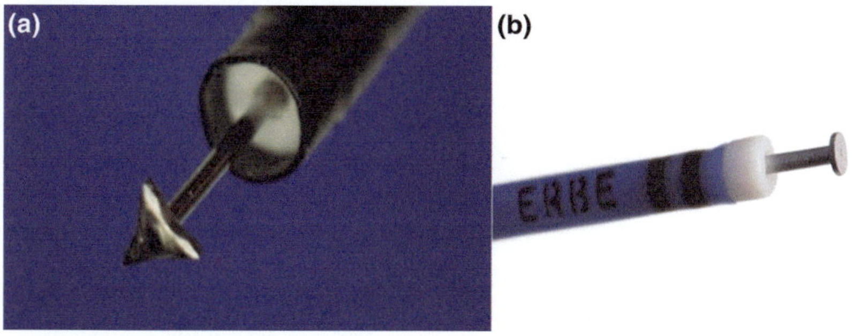

Fig. 6.4 **a** Triangle-tip knife. Courtesy Olympus America (Center Valley, PA). **b** Hybrid knife. Courtesy ERBE (Tubingen, Germany)

been described where the submucosa and muscularis are dissected simultaneously, possibly resulting in shorter procedure times [18, 19]. Some operators prefer the triangle-tip (TT) knife (Olympus, Center Valley, PA, Fig. 6.4a), while others, such as our group at Winthrop and the Shanghai group, prefer the multifunctional hybrid knife (HK) that can perform submucosal injection and dissection (ERBE, Tubingen, Germany, Fig. 6.4b). In their randomized controlled trial of 100 patients comparing POEM performed with the TT knife versus the HK [20], the Shanghai group reported that the HK produced significant decreases in POEM procedure time (22.9 vs. 35.9 min) ($p < 0.0001$) and fewer minor bleeding episodes, with no differences in complications or treatment success. This improvement in procedure times was mostly attributed to fewer exchanges of accessories. Similar results were also reported in a case–control study comparing the TT knife and the HK [21].

The incision site may be closed effectively with either clips or endoscopic sutures. Our group published data of a retrospective comparison of clips and suturing indicating similar closure times and cost for suturing versus clips [22]. Another US surgical group using much smaller numbers in a retrospective analysis of only 5 cases per group reported very long closure times with suturing (mean of 33 min), which, in their analysis, resulted in higher overall cost for suturing despite similar equipment cost to clips [23].

Infection is prevented by meticulous removal of retained food from the esophagus prior to beginning the tunnel, secure closure of the esophagotomy, and prophylactic systemic antibiotics. Many centers also perform antibiotic lavage of the tunnel prior to closure as recommended by Inoue [6].

There is significant variation in technique between POEM operators in terms of entry point (site and orientation), myotomy length, submucosal injection, mode of dissection, myotomy depth, and closure methods, all of which may vary depending upon procedure indication, operator preference, local expertise, etc. In addition, ancillary procedures to confirm adequate myotomy length may vary [24]. For instance, a myotomy of 5 cm length should suffice for most patients with Chicago Classification Achalasia types I and II, but an extended myotomy ranging to at least 15 cm may be necessary in type III achalasia patients, diffuse esophageal spasm, and jackhammer esophagus [25, 26].

A greater curvature (extended gastric) myotomy may be considered in subjects with prior HM or POEM [27]. Extension of the myotomy to the cardia is important, even without prior Heller procedure, to ensure complete LES ablation. A variety of indicators that suggest that the GEJ or cardia has been reached include the following: (1) endoscopic measurements (using the markers on the endoscope to measure depth of insertion from the incisors); (2) narrowing of the submucosal space at the GEJ with resistance to endoscope insertion caused by the LES, followed by prompt expansion of the submucosal space in the cardia with increased overall vascularity of the submucosa; (3) slender palisade vessels along the mucosal flap, indicating the distal-most aspect of the esophagus; (4) spindle-like veins on the surface of the muscularis propria near the GEJ; (5) large-caliber, arborizing, perforating vessels in the cardia (usually branches of the left gastric artery); (6) aberrant inner longitudinal muscle bundles at the GEJ originating from circular muscle fibers and inserting into circular muscle fibers after a short course of 2–3 cm; and (7) visualization of a blue hue on intraluminal inspection of the mucosa of the cardia (due to the blue color of the injectate) [12].

A transillumination auxiliary technique, initially described by Baldaque-Silva and colleagues, allows confirmation that the tunnel was extended into the cardia by inserting an ultrathin endoscope transnasally in parallel with the orally inserted gastroscope used to perform the POEM procedure. The ultrathin scope is advanced to the level of the stomach and placed in the retroflexed position with visualization of the cardia, while the gastroscope is kept within the tunnel with its tip at the tunnel terminus. The light intensity of the thin endoscope is diminished, and the light from the gastroscope within the submucosal tunnel is identified, thereby confirming its position in the cardia [28]. Inoue's group compared this technique to conventional identification of the cardia by the indicators listed above in a prospective randomized controlled trial with 100 consecutive achalasia patients undergoing POEM. POEM was completed with high rates of technical and clinical success in both groups, with low adverse events, but the double-scope transillumination group had myotomy extension in 34% of cases, which led to an increase in the length of the cardiomyotomy from 2.6 to 3.2 cm (p = 0.01) [29]. Despite the extension of the myotomy in a third of the patients in the transillumination group, suggesting that the final length of the cardiomyotomy of the control group may have not been of adequate length in a third of patients, there were no differences in clinical success rates, and no differences in postprocedure gastroesophageal reflux disease (GERD), thus raising doubts about the clinical utility of the double-scope method. Some drawbacks of this technique are that it may require two operators, is cumbersome, requires a second endoscopy tower and endoscope, and adds significant time to the procedure (17 min in this study). However, this technique may be beneficial for difficult cases such as those on patients with sigmoid end-stage achalasia or for operators early on the POEM learning curve.

Another technique for reliably identifying an adequate myotomy extension into the cardia involves the use of fluoroscopy. Kumbhari reported using either a hemoclip attached to the GEJ or the fluoroscopically guided placement of a 19-gauge needle on the skin at the level of the GEJ to help accurately assess the length of the myotomy in 24 consecutive patients undergoing the POEM procedure. Based on the fluoroscopic information, the submucosal tunnel was extended in 21% of patients, with minor increases in procedure time (4 min for the hemoclip group and 2 min for the 19-gauge needle group) [30]. Another group has also reported on the use of fluoroscopy to ensure proper orientation and extension of the tunnel into the cardia particularly in challenging cases with sigmoid esophagus [31].

Adequacy of LES ablation may also be assessed by real-time measurement of the GEJ distensibility with a balloon-based imaging probe (EndoFLIP, Crospon Ltd, Galway, Ireland) that uses impedance planimetry and can been used during the procedure to assess the adequacy of the myotomy via measurements that include GEJ cross-sectional area (CSA), minimal diameter, compliance, and distensibility [32–36].

Patients are kept nil per os until a water-soluble contrast study is performed when the patient is awake to exclude a leak, though it has little bearing on ultimate efficacy [37]. Most patients can be discharged soon after the tolerance of food.

POEM Efficacy

The NOSCAR POEM White Paper compiled results from 14 early series through early 2014 with follow-up periods ranging from 3 to

Table 6.2 POEM series with efficacy data

Location	Year	# of patients	Mean age (years)	Mean follow-up (months)	Eckardt score (pre/post)	LES pressure (pre/post) (mmHg)	Post-POEM ctimed barium esophagram	Efficacy (%)
Portland, Oregon [41]	2014	100	58 (18–83)	21.5	6/1	44.3/19.6	In 55 pts Median emptying at 1 min 93%: 100% emptying 100%: 80%–100% emptying	96
Chicago, Illinois [42]	2014	41	45	15	7/1	28/11	In 16 pts Median height 1 min 6 ± 4 cm 2 min 6 ± 4 cm 5 min 5 ± 3 cm ($p < 0.001$)	92
Rome, Italy [43]	2014	100	48 (18–75)	11	8.1/1.1	41.4/19		94.5
Mineola, New York [40]	2015	93	52 (18–93)	22	78/0.44	43/18		96
Europe MCT [44]	2015	80	44.9 (9–88)	29	7.7/1.5	31.9/10.1	In 32 pts 93.75%: >70% emptying at 5 min	78.5

12 months, with generally excellent results [12]. There was a significant decrease in the Eckardt score to ≤ 3 in 90–100% of patients, the primary clinical success criterion traditionally used in achalasia trials. Somewhat more modest 12-month results were reported by an early European multicenter series which noted only an 82% clinical response, perhaps reflecting early learning curves, since there were a small number of early procedures submitted by each of the participating centers [38].

A meta-analysis of more than 1000 patients showed POEM short-term success of 93% in terms of Eckardt scores and LES pressures [39]. Four more recent Western series from pioneering centers reflected excellent early midterm results, with a 90+% efficacy at 11- to 22-month follow-up (Table 6.2) [40–43]. Another attempt to present midterm POEM results utilized a multicenter methodology combining patients from 3 centers (Hamburg, Rome, Portland) that had completed a minimum of 24 months of follow-up (mean 29 months) [44]. This was a small study with only 79 patients and likely included patients from Hamburg that had also been included in the multicenter European series reviewed above. This 3-center study demonstrated similar modest efficacy results, with an initial high clinical success of 94% at 3–6 months, decreasing to 88% at 12–18 months and to 78% at ≥ 2 years (mean 29 mos, range 24–41). As was the case with the European multicenter trial (MCT) reviewed above, these more modest results were attributed by the authors to a learning curve effect, since half of the failures occurred in the first 10 patients from each of the 3 contributing centers.

In a recent publication of outcomes from the series with the longest follow-up to date, Inoue's series of 500 patients, 88% clinical success was reported at 3 years post-POEM [30]. However, it should be noted that there were substantial missing follow-up data (Eckardt score available in only 61 out of the 105 patients that had completed at least 3 years of follow-up) and that the patient population in this Asian series, as compared to US series, consisted of significantly younger patients with much less advanced/end-stage disease and prior Botox or Heller treatments, conditions that can result in more complicated POEM procedures [45].

GEJ-integrated relaxation pressures and barium passage have been shown to be improved post-POEM correlating with clinical parameters

[46]. POEM has demonstrated success for achalasia patients of all ages, those with prior endoscopic and surgical interventions, sigmoid esophagus, and spastic esophageal disorders [8, 11, 14, 26, 27, 39–44, 47]. POEM appears effective in relieving chest pain as well as dysphagia in achalasia and non-achalasia esophageal motility disorders, but POEM results may be somewhat more modest in spastic disorders compared to classic achalasia [26, 41, 48].

POEM Adverse Events

POEM has a superlative safety record with only one death attributed to POEM as a late complication (cachexia) reported in a recent systematic review of AEs [49]. Adverse events are uncommon and typically diminish with experience [8, 12, 13]. In the recent large series of 500 POEMs reported by Inoue, the AE rate was 3.2%, and all were mild/moderate [47]. These results were identical to the rate of AEs reported in the IPOEMS survey of pioneering centers [8].

The unusually high rate of AEs reported in an early POEM series that uniquely employed air rather than CO_2 for insufflation, particularly insufflation-related AEs such as symptomatic pneumothorax requiring decompression, tense pneumoperitoneum, and symptomatic subcutaneous emphysema, emphasizes the importance of using CO_2 for insufflation [50]. If CO_2 insufflation is used, insufflation AEs are rare, generally limited to the early learning curve, and mostly consist of capnoperitoneum that can be easily vented during the procedure with an angiocath or Veress needle without any sequelae or morbidity.

Episodes of intraprocedural hemorrhage diminish with experience and are usually easily managed with hemostatic forceps. Accidental mucosal injuries also decrease with experience [51]. They can occur in 10–20% of cases and are usually easily managed with endoscopic closure with minimal or no patient morbidity. Occasionally, closure can be difficult due to large size of the defect, difficult location, or poor tissue characteristics. In such cases, specialized techniques may be required to achieve closure and avoid risk of leak and mediastinal sepsis [52, 53]. Delayed hemorrhage within the submucosal tunnel has been reported in less than 1–2% of cases and may require reintervention such as reexploration of the tunnel and endoscopic hemostasis or, as has been reported, balloon tamponade [54].

Anesthesia complications are infrequent and usually self-limited. Attention should be paid to avoiding aspiration during induction of anesthesia and intubation, particularly in patients with a very dilated esophagus. Rapid induction should be performed with simultaneous vigorous cricoid pressure in order to avoid aspiration with resultant pulmonary infectious complications.

The most serious AE probably involves leaks, which may result in mediastinal sepsis, and which usually require emergent surgical intervention. Such leaks have been infrequently reported by a small number of centers early in their experience [42, 45, 46]. Tension capnopericardium has also been reported as a complication of POEM, resulting in cardiac arrest and premature termination of the procedure [55]. This patient survived without sequelae and went on to have a Heller–Dor procedure six months later.

GERD After POEM

A concern with POEM is that unlike laparoscopic Heller myotomy, a concomitant reflux procedure is not performed. It is now apparent that GERD is common after POEM, with GERD symptoms in 12–24%, esophagitis in 20–59%, and positive pH studies in 31–50% (Table 6.3) [41, 42, 56]. In fact, dysphagia relief is clearly correlated to LES ablation and subsequent tendency toward GERD as demonstrated in a recent multicenter study [44]. In this study concentrating on longer-term data from subjects with two-year follow-up, 37% had erosive esophagitis, and 37% were on a proton pump inhibitor (PPI) at ≥ 2 year follow-up (mean 29 months, range 24–41). The presence of GERD was the strongest predictor of POEM efficacy. GERD assessment can be complicated by the fact that up to half of the patients with GERD-like symptoms

Table 6.3 POEM series with GERD data including pH studies

Location	GERD symptoms	Erosive esophagitis	+pH study
Chicago, Illinois [42]	15/41 (15%)	13/22 (59%)	4/13 (31%)
Portland, Oregon [41]	12/100 (15%)	20/73 (27%)	26/68 (38%)
Rome, Italy [43]	19/103 (18%)	21/103 (20%)	52/103 (50%)
Mineola, New York [78]	40/174 (23%)	29/86 (34%)	29/84 (36%)

may not have a positive pH study, and conversely, a significant percentage of patients with a positive pH study may not have symptoms. In some of these patients, a falsely positive pH study may result due to stasis or fermentation [57, 58]. The Rome group proposed the term "clinically relevant GERD" for patients who, in addition to having a positive pH study, also have typical GERD symptoms and/or reflux esophagitis. Using this definition, in their comprehensive study of 103 patients, even though 50% had a positive pH study, only 29% had "clinically relevant GERD" [56].

Most patients' GERD is well controlled with PPIs, and the trade-off for dysphagia relief is seemingly worthwhile in terms of overall quality of life [59]. With regard to comparing GERD after POEM to GERD after laparoscopic Heller myotomy (LHM), in a recent retrospective comparison of 64 LHMs and 37 POEMs performed by the same surgical group in Portland, no significant difference was found in positive pH studies (32% in LHM, 39% in POEM).

It should be noted here that the Dor or Toupet "loose" fundoplications performed in achalasia patients in conjunction with a LHM have only modest efficacy. High-quality studies from expert LHM centers have shown abnormal acid exposure rates in 18–42% of patients after LHM with fundoplication [60–62], rates not too dissimilar to those after POEM. Furthermore, these pH data were collected only 6–12 months postoperatively and may be even less favorable on long-term follow-up. One may reasonably wonder why the rate of GERD after POEM is not substantially greater than that after LHM combined with a fundoplication. The explanation may lie in the lack of hiatal dissection during POEM compared to extensive dissection of the hiatus during a standard LHM. This extensive dissection disrupts important "suspensory ligaments" of the esophagus, notably the phrenoesophageal membrane, which thought to contribute to the maintenance of the angle of His and to have an important antireflux function separate from the esophageal sphincter itself. Two recent studies lend support to this hypothesis by demonstrating that a modified LHM with as limited dissection of the hiatus as possible results in much lower rates of GERD even without a fundoplication (9 and 31%, respectively) [63, 64].

Comparative Analysis

There are no published randomized trials to date comparing POEM to LHM or POEM against endoscopic therapies. There are MCTs underway in Europe between POEM, LHM, and pneumatic balloon dilation (PBD). Four studies utilized historical LHM controls to compare with POEM and found comparable excellent clinical results and few complications [45, 65–67]. These studies demonstrated shorter operative times and less blood loss for POEM, less postoperative pain, shorter length of hospital stay, and more rapid return to usual activities. Two meta-analyses with one-year follow-up found similar results, with no notable differences between POEM and LHM [68, 69]. Barium column height was comparable between POEM and LHM subjects [60]. Quality-of-life improvement is comparable between LHM and POEM [59]. A multicenter retrospective comparison of POEM and LHM for type III achalasia noted that POEM allows for a longer myotomy than LHM and found a trend toward better clinical results with POEM [70].

Training

POEM operator numbers have increased greatly since the procedure was introduced, but its performance is still largely limited to larger centers. Questions have been raised as to what constitutes adequate training and performance [8, 12, 13]. Our group's analysis of the first 93 POEMs performed by a single operator found that efficacy was attained at 40 procedures and mastery at 60 [40]. The Portland group found "mastery of POEM technique to be after 20 procedures" (as denoted by decreased procedure time and decreased rate of accidental mucosotomies) [51]. On the other hand, the Northwestern group reported a "learning rate" of 7 POEMs for completing just the submucosal access and myotomy portions of the procedure (insufficient data were reported regarding the entire procedure) [71]. Both of these analyses were by the surgical groups in Portland and Northwestern and were based on 40 or fewer POEMs by multiple operators, raising methodological questions. Another group reported on the importance of preclinical training before performing POEM in humans [72–74]. While it remains unclear exactly how many cases constitute the learning curve for POEM, it is clear that the technical difficulty of the procedure is such that significant experience is required to attain consistent results. This line of thinking may contribute to the observed performance of POEM primarily in larger centers, where this type of experience is more readily available.

Future and Offshoots

The future of POEM appears bright, and garnering longer-term data will likely further validate its dominant niche in achalasia therapy. More importantly, however, POEM has led to an exciting rebirth of NOTES in the form of "short-range," intramural, endoscopic interventions of the GI tract: interventions such as POEM, STER (submucosal tunnel endoscopic resection), EFTR (endoscopic full-thickness resection), and POP (per-oral pyloromyotomy). Whereas traditional NOTES, with its grand vision of deep incursions into the abdominal and chest cavities and major organ resections, failed to gain wide adoption, it planted the seeds for the "new NOTES" procedures, which are thriving and enjoying rapid growth. These "new NOTES" interventions are finally delivering on the great promise of NOTES, replacing traditional surgical procedures with more minimally invasive, scarless ones [73].

POEM developed as a fortuitous offshoot of early traditional NOTES work, but now arguably represents the most successful application of NOTES to date [73, 75]. Two especially promising "new NOTES" applications of submucosal endoscopy are a technique for R0 full-thickness resection of deep seated subepithelial tumors named "POET" for per-oral endoscopic tumor resection by Inoue and colleagues, or "STER" (submucosal tunnel endoscopic resection) by the Shanghai group [76–78]. Another technique has developed as an offshoot of POEM called per-oral pyloromyotomy (POP, also termed by some G-POEM) for the therapy of gastroparesis [79].

Conclusion

POEM was initially performed in 2008 as a novel therapy for achalasia, derived from the evolution of NOTES work, and is now performed globally. POEM is well validated as an achalasia therapy, with documented excellent efficacy and safety. Moreover, it can be equally successful in those with prior intervention, including LHM, and is applicable in a wide range of esophageal motility disorders beyond achalasia, including diffuse esophageal spasm and jackhammer esophagus. Longer-term data, including randomized trials of POEM versus pneumatic dilation and Heller, are awaited. These are expected to confirm the uniformly excellent efficacy of POEM reported by a large number of prospective series, including several series with early midterm data at 1- to 3-year follow-up. The burgeoning field of submucosal endoscopy "new NOTES" interventions is largely predicated upon the spectacular success of POEM.

References

1. Sadowski DC, Ackah F, Jiang B, Svenson LW. Achalasia: incidence, prevalence and survival: a population-based study. Neurogastroenterol Motil. 2010;22(9):e256–61.
2. Fisichella PM, Patti MG. From Heller to POEM (1914–2014): a 100-year history of surgery for achalasia. J Gastrointest Surg. 2014;18(10):1870–5.
3. Bencini L, Moraldi L, Bartolini I, Coratti A. Esophageal surgery in minimally invasive era. World J Gastrointest Surg. 2016;8(1):52–64.
4. Ortega JA, Madureri V, Perez L. Endoscopic myotomy in the treatment of achalasia. Gastrointest Endosc. 1980;26:8–10.
5. Pasricha PJ, Hawari R, Ahmed I, Chen J, Cotton PB, et al. Submucosal endoscopic esophageal myotomy: a novel experimental approach for the treatment of achalasia. Endoscopy. 2007;39:761–7.
6. Inoue H, Minami H, Kobayashi Y, Sato Y, Kaga M, et al. Peroral endoscopic myotomy (POEM) for esophageal achalasia. Endoscopy. 2010;42(4):265–71.
7. Stavropoulos SN, Harris MD, Hida S, Brathwaite C, Demetriou C, et al. Endoscopic submucosal myotomy for the treatment of achalasia (with video). Gastrointest Endosc. 2010;72:1309–11.
8. Stavropoulos SN, Modayil RJ, Friedel D, Savides T. The international per oral endoscopic myotomy survey (IPOEMS): a snapshot of the global POEM experience. Surg Endosc. 2013;27(9):3322–38.
9. Eleftheriadis N, Inoue H, Ikeda H, Onimaru M, Maselli R, et al. Submucosal tunnel endoscopy: peroral endoscopic myotomy and peroral endoscopic tumor resection. World J Gastrointest Endosc. 2016;8(2):86–103.
10. Li QL, Zhou PH. Perspective on peroral endoscopic myotomy for achalasia: Zhongshan experience. Gut Liver. 2015;9(2):152–8.
11. Bechara R, Ikeda H, Onimaru M, Inoue H. Peroral endoscopic myotomy, 1000 cases later: pearls, pitfalls, and practical considerations. Gastrointest Endosc. 2016;25(16):01763–6 (pii: S0016–5107).
12. Noscar POEM White, Committee Paper, Stavropoulos SN, Desilets DJ, Fuchs KH, Gostout CJ, Haber G, et al. Per-oral endoscopic myotomy white paper summary. Gastrointest Endosc. 2014;80(1):1–15.
13. ASGE PIVI Committee, Chandrasekhara V, Desilets D, Falk GW, Inoue H, Romanelli JR, et al. The American Society for gastrointestinal endoscopy PIVI (Preservation and incorporation of valuable endoscopic innovations) on peroral endoscopic myotomy. Gastrointest Endosc. 2015;81(5):1087–100.e1.
14. Fumagalli U, Rosati R, De Pascale S, Porta M, Carlani E, et al. Repeated surgical or endoscopic myotomy for recurrent dysphagia in patients after previous myotomy for achalasia. J Gastrointest Surg. 2016;20(3):494–9.
15. Technology Committee ASGE, Pannala R, Abu Dayyeh BK, Aslanian HR, Enestvedt BK, Komanduri S, et al. Per-oral endoscopic myotomy (with video). Gastrointest Endosc. 2016;83(6):1051–60.
16. Stavropoulos SN, Modayil R, Friedel D. Achalasia. Gastrointest Endosc Clin N Am. 2013;23(1):53–75.
17. Stavropoulos SN, Modayil R, Brathwaite C, et al. Anterior vs. posterior peroral endoscopic myotomy (POEM): is there a difference in outcomes? Gastrointestinal Endoscopy. 2016;83(5S):Supp AB 145.
18. Liu BR, Song JT, Omar Jan M. Video of the month. Modified peroral endoscopic myotomy. Am J Gastroenterol. 2015;110(4):499.
19. Philips GM, Dacha S, Keilin SA. Concurrent myotomy and tunneling after establishment of a half tunnel instead of myotomy after establishment of a full tunnel: a more efficient method of peroral endoscopic myotomy. Endosc Int Open. 2016;4(4):403–8.
20. Cai MY, Zhou PH, Yao LQ, Xu MD, Zhong YS, et al. Peroral endoscopic myotomy for idiopathic achalasia: randomized comparison of water-jet assisted versus conventional dissection technique. Surg Endosc. 2014;28:1158–65.
21. Tang X, Gong W, Deng Z, Zhou J, Ren Y, et al. Comparison of conventional versus Hybrid knife peroral endoscopic myotomy methods for esophageal achalasia: a case-control study. Scand J Gastroenterol. 2016;51(4):494–500.
22. Stavropoulos SN, Modayil R, Friedel D. Current applications of endoscopic suturing. World J Gastrointest Endosc. 2015;7(8):777–89.
23. Pescarus R, Shlomovitz E, Sharata AM, Cassera MA, Reavis KM, et al. Endoscopic suturing versus endoscopic clip closure of the mucosotomy during a per-oral endoscopic myotomy (POEM): a case-control study. Surg Endosc. 2016;30(5):2132–5.
24. Grimes KL, Inoue H. Per oral endoscopic myotomy for achalasia: a detailed description of the technique and review of the literature. Thorac Surg Clin. 2016;26(2):147–62.
25. Teitelbaum EN, Soper NJ, Pandolfino JE, Kahrilas PJ, Boris L, et al. An extended proximal esophageal myotomy is necessary to normalize EGJ distensibility during Heller myotomy for achalasia, but not POEM. Surg Endosc. 2014;28(10):2840–7.
26. Khashab MA, Messallam AA, Onimaru M, Teitelbaum EM, Ujiki MB, et al. International multicenter experience with peroral endoscopic myotomy for the treatment of spastic esophageal disorders refractory to medical therapy (with video). Gastrointest Endosc. 2015;81(5):1170–7.
27. Onimaru M, Inoue H, Ikeda H, Sato C, Sato H, et al. Greater curvature myotomy is a safe and effective modified technique in per-oral endoscopic myotomy (with videos). Gastrointest Endosc. 2015;81(6):1370–7.
28. Baldaque-Silva F, Marques M, Vilas-Boas F, Maia JD, Sa F, et al. New transillumination auxiliary technique for peroral endoscopic myotomy. Gastrointest Endosc. 2014;79:544–5.

29. Grimes KL, Inoue H, Onimaru M, Ikeda H, Tansawet A, et al. Double-scope per oral endoscopic myotomy (POEM): a prospective randomized controlled trial. Surg Endosc. 2016;30(4):1344–51.
30. Kumbhari V, Besharati S, Abdelgelil A, Tieu AH, Saxena P, et al. Intraprocedural fluoroscopy to determine the extent of the cardiomyotomy during per-oral endoscopic myotomy (with video). Gastrointest Endosc. 2015;81:1451–6.
31. Ramchandani M, Reddy DN, Darisetty S, Kotla R, Chavan R, et al. Peroral endoscopic myotomy for achalasia cardia: treatment analysis and follow up of over 200 consecutive patients at a single center. Dig Endosc. 2016;28(1):19–26.
32. Familiari P, Gigante G, Marchese M, Boskoski I, Bove V, et al. EndoFLIP system for the intraoperative evaluation of peroral endoscopic myotomy. European Gastroenterol J. 2014;2(2):77–83.
33. Rieder E, Swanstrom LL, Perretta S, Lenglinger J, Riegler M, et al. Intraoperative assessment of esophagogastric junction distensibility during per oral endoscopic myotomy (POEM) for esophageal motility disorders. Surg Endosc. 2013;27:400–5.
34. Verlaan T, Rohof WO, Bredenoord AJ, Eberl S, Rosch T, et al. Effect of peroral endoscopic myotomy on esophagogastric junction physiology in patients with achalasia. Gastrointest Endosc. 2013;78:39–44.
35. Teitelbaum EN, Boris L, Arafat FO, Nicodème F, Lin Z, et al. Comparison of esophagogastric junction distensibility changes during POEM and Heller myotomy using intraoperative FLIP. Surg Endosc. 2013;27:4547–55.
36. Teitelbaum EN, Sternbach JM, El Khoury R, et al. The effect of incremental distal gastric myotomy lengths on EGJ distensibility during POEM for achalasia. Surg Endosc. 2016;30:745–50.
37. Sternbach JM, El Khoury R, Teitelbaum EN, Soper NJ, Pandolfino JE, et al. Early esophagram in per-oral endoscopic myotomy (POEM) for achalasia does not predict long-term outcomes. Surgery. 2015;158(4):1128–35.
38. von Renteln D, Fuchs KH, Fockens P, Bauerfiend P, Vassiliou MC, et al. Peroral endoscopic myotomy for the Treatment of Achalasia: an international prospective multicenter study. Gastroenterology. 2013;145 (2):309–11.
39. Talukdar R, Inoue H, Reddy DN. Efficacy of peroral endoscopic myotomy (POEM) in the treatment of achalasia: a systematic review and meta-analysis. Surg Endosc. 2015;29(11):3030–46.
40. Patel KS, Calixte R, Modayil RJ, Friedel D, Brathwaite CE, et al. The light at the end of the tunnel: a single-operator learning curve analysis for per oral endoscopic myotomy. Gastrointest Endosc. 2015;81 (5):1181–7.
41. Sharata AM, Dunst CM, Pescarus R, Shlomowitz E, Wille AJ, et al. Peroral endoscopic myotomy (POEM) for esophageal primary motility disorders: analysis of 100 consecutive patients. J Gastrointest Surg. 2015;19(1):161–70; discussion 170.
42. Teitelbaum EN, Soper NJ, Santos BF, Arafat FO, Pandolfino JE, et al. Symptomatic and physiologic outcomes one year after peroral esophageal myotomy (POEM) for treatment of achalasia. Surg Endosc. 2014;28(12):3359–65.
43. Familiari P, Gigante G, Marchese M, Boskoski I, Tringali A, et al. Peroral endoscopic myotomy for esophageal achalasia: outcomes of the first 100 patients with short-term follow-up. I. 2016;263(1):82–7.
44. Werner YB, Costamagna G, Swanström LL, von Renteln D, Familiari P, et al. Clinical response to peroral endoscopic myotomy in patients with idiopathic achalasia at a minimum follow-up of 2 years. Gut. 2016;65(6):899–906.
45. Ujiki MB, Yetasook AK, Zapf M, Linn JG, Carbray JM, et al. Peroral endoscopic myotomy: a short-term comparison with the standard laparoscopic approach. Surgery. 2013;154(4):893–7.
46. Pannu D, Draganov PV. CT esophagram findings after POEM procedure. Gastrointest Endosc. 2015;81 (6):1502.
47. Inoue H, Sato H, Ikeda H, Onimaru M, Sato C, et al. Per-oral endoscopic myotomy: a series of 500 patients. J Am Coll Surg. 2015;221(2):256–64.
48. Hoppo T, Thakkar SJ, Schumacher LY, Komatsu Y, Choe S, et al. A utility of peroral endoscopic myotomy (POEM) across the spectrum of esophageal motility disorders. Surg Endosc. 2016;30(1): 233–44.
49. Patel K, Abbassi-Ghadi N, Markar S, Kumar S, Jethwa P, et al. Peroral endoscopic myotomy for the treatment of esophageal achalasia: systematic review and pooled analysis. Dis esophagus. 2015 July 14 [Epub ahead of print].
50. Ren Z, Zhong Y, Zhou P, Xu M, Cai M, et al. Perioperative management and treatment for complications during and after peroral endoscopic myotomy (POEM) for esophageal achalasia (EA) (data from 119 cases). Surg Endosc. 2012;26(11):3267–72.
51. Kurian AA, Dunst CM, Sharata A, Bhayani NH, REavis KM, et al. Peroral endoscopic esophageal myotomy: defining the learning curve. Gastrointest Endosc. 2013;77(5):719–25.
52. Modayil R, Friedel D, Stavropoulos SN. Endoscopic suture repair of a large mucosal perforation during peroral endoscopic myotomy for treatment of achalasia. Gastrointest Endosc. 2014;80(6):1169–70.
53. Yang D, Zhang Q, Draganov PV. Successful placement of a fully covered esophageal stent to bridge a difficult-to-close mucosal incision during peroral endoscopic myotomy. *Endoscopy*. 2014;46 Suppl 1 UCTN: E467-8.
54. Li QL, Zhou PH, Yao LQ, Xu MD, Chen WF, et al. Early diagnosis and management of delayed bleeding in the submucosal tunnel after peroral endoscopic myotomy for achalasia (with video). Gastrointest Endosc. 2013;78(2):370–4.
55. Banks-Venegoni AL, Desilets DJ, Romanelli JR, Earle DB. Tension capnopericardium and cardiac arrest as an unexpected adverse event of peroral

endoscopic myotomy (with video). Gastrointest Endosc. 2015;82(6):1137–9.
56. Familiari P., Greco S., Gigante G., Cali A, Boškoski I, et al. Gastro-esophageal reflux disease after per-oral endoscopic myotomy (POEM). Analysis of clinical, procedural and functional factors, associated with GERD and esophagitis. Dig Endosc. 2016;28 (1):33–41.
57. Crookes PF, Corkill S, DeMeester TR. Gastroesophageal reflux in achalasia. When is reflux really reflux? Dig Dis Sci. 1997;42(7):1354–61.
58. Malik Z, Saadi M, Modayil R, et al. Bravo pH monitoring after per oral endoscopic myotomy (POEM) overestimates true acid reflux. Gastrointest Endosc. 2016;83(5S):Supp AB 627.
59. Vigneswaran Y, Tanaka R, Gitelis M, Carbray J, Ujiki MB, et al. Quality of life assessment after peroral endoscopic myotomy. Surg Endosc. 2015;29 (5):1198–202.
60. Kumagai K, Tsai JA, Thorell A, Lundell L, Håkanson B, et al. Per-oral endoscopic myotomy for achalasia. Are results comparable to laparoscopic Heller myotomy? Scand J Gastroenterol. 2015;50(5):505–12.
61. Khajanchee YS, Kanneganti S, Leatherwood AE, Hansen PD, Swanström LL, et al. Laparoscopic Heller myotomy with Toupet fundoplication: outcomes predictors in 121 consecutive patients. Arch Surg. 2005;140:827–33.
62. Rawlings A, Soper NJ, Oelschlager B, Swanstrom L, Matthews BD, et al. Laparoscopic Dor versus Toupet fundoplication following Heller myotomy for achalasia: results of a multicenter, prospective, randomized-controlled trial. Surg Endosc. 2012;26:18–26.
63. Simić AP, Radovanović NS, Skrobić OM, Raznatović ZJ, Pesko PM. et al. Significance of limited hiatal dissection in surgery for achalasia. J Gastrointest Surg. 2010;14:587–93.
64. Zurita Macías Valadez LC, Pescarus R, Hsieh T, Wasserman L, Apriasz I, et al. Laparoscopic limited Heller myotomy without anti-reflux procedure does not induce significant long-term gastroesophageal reflux. Surg Endosc. 2015;29:1462–8.
65. Bhayani NH, Kurian AA, Dunst CM, Sharata AM, Rieder E, et al. A comparative study on comprehensive, objective outcomes of laparoscopic Heller myotomy with per-oral endoscopic myotomy (POEM) for achalasia. Ann Surg. 2014;259(6):1098–103.
66. Chan SM, Wu JC, Teoh AY, Yip HC, Ng EK, et al. Comparison of early outcomes and quality of life after laparoscopic Heller's cardiomyotomy to peroral endoscopic myotomy for treatment of achalasia. Dig Endosc. 2016;28(1):27–32.
67. Hungness ES, Teitelbaum EN, Santos BF, Arafat FO, Pandolfino JE, et al. Comparison of perioperative outcomes between peroral esophageal myotomy (POEM) and laparoscopic Heller myotomy. J Gastrointest Surg. 2013;17(2):228–35.
68. Zhang Y, Wang H, Chen X, Liu L, Wang H, et al. Per-Oral endoscopic myotomy versus Laparoscopic Heller Mytomy for achalasia: a meta-analysis of nonrandomized comparative studies. Medicine (Baltimore). 2016;95(6):e2736.
69. Marano L, Pallabazzer G, Solito B, Santi S, Pigazzi A, et al. Surgery or peroral esophageal myotomy for achalasia: a systematic review and meta-analysis. Medicine (Baltimore). 2016;95(10):e3001.
70. Kumbhari V, Tieu AH, Onimaru M, El Zein MH, Teitelbaum EN, et al. Peroral endoscopic myotomy (POEM) vs laparoscopic Heller myotomy (LHM) for the treatment of Type III achalasia in 75 patients: a multicenter comparative study. Endosc Int Open. 2015;3(3):e195–201.
71. Teitelbaum EN, Soper NJ, Arafat FO, Santos BF, Kahrilas PJ, et al. Analysis of a learning curve and predictors of intraoperative difficulty for peroral esophageal myotomy (POEM). J Gastrointest Surg. 2014;18(1):92–8; discussion 98-9.
72. Hernández Mondragón OV, Rascón Martínez DM, Muñoz Bautista A, Altamirano Castañeda ML, Blanco-Velasco G, et al. The per oral endoscopic myotomy (POEM) technique: how many preclinical procedures are needed to master it? Endosc Int Open. 2015;3(6):E559–65.
73. Bechara R, Inoue H. POEM, the prototypical "new NOTES" procedure and first successful NOTES procedure. Gastrointest Endosc Clin N Am. 2016;26(2):237–55.
74. Desilets DJ, Romanelli JR, Earle DB. Starting a peroral endoscopic myotomy program at your institution. Tech Gastrointest Endosc. 2013;15:157–9.
75. Modayil R, Stavropoulos SN. A western perspective on "new NOTES" from POEM to full-thickness resection and beyond. Gastrointest Endosc Clin N Am. 2016;26(2):413–32.
76. Inoue H, Ikeda H, Hosoya T, Onimaru M, Yoshida A, et al. Submucosal endoscopic tumor resection for subepithelial tumors in the esophagus and cardia. Endoscopy. 2012;44(3):225–30.
77. Xu MD, Cai MY, Zhou PH, Qin XY, Zhong YS, et al. Submucosal tunneling endoscopic resection: a new technique for treating upper GI submucosal tumors originating from the muscularis propria layer (with videos). Gastrointest Endosc. 2012;75(1):195–9.
78. Gong W, Xiong Y, Zhi F, Liu S, Wang A, et al. Preliminary experience of endoscopic submucosal tunnel dissection for upper gastrointestinal submucosal tumors. Endoscopy. 2012;44(3):231–5.
79. Swanstrom LL, Lebaras C. Per-Oral Pyloromyotomy (POP): An Emerging Application of Submucosal Tunneling for the Treatment of Refractory Gastroparesis. Gastrointest Endosc Clin N Am. 2016;26 (2):257–70.

Per-oral Endoscopic Myotomy (POEM) for Non-achalasia Disorders

7

Majidah A. Bukhari, Payal Saxena
and Mouen A. Khashab

Abstract

Per-oral endoscopic myotomy (POEM) is a novel endoscopic procedure, which has been performed to treat achalasia with favorable outcomes. Emerging data suggest that POEM may also have a role in the treatment of patients with spastic esophageal disorders (SEDs). SEDs include spastic or type III achalasia, distal esophageal spasm (DES), and hypercontractile (Jackhammer) esophagus. Despite the difference in pathophysiology, these disorders share many similarities, including their clinical manifestations. Patients may present with one or all of the following symptoms: dysphagia, non-cardiac chest pain, regurgitation, and refractory gastroesophageal reflux symptoms. The gold standard to diagnose these disorders is high-resolution esophageal manometry. While medical therapy fails in the majority of these patients, surgical myotomy is invasive and associated with suboptimal results due to the need for long esophageal myotomy. POEM provides an ideal therapy for SEDs, as it allows for long esophageal myotomy in addition to myotomy of the lower esophageal sphincter (LES). Emerging data suggest POEM is both effective and safe for treating patients with SEDs. Similarly, gastric POEM (G-POEM) or endoscopic pyloromyotomy is a novel procedure for the treatment of patients with gastroparesis refractory to medical therapy. Emerging data

M.A. Bukhari · P. Saxena · M.A. Khashab
Department of Medicine and Division of Gastroenterology and Hepatology, The Johns Hopkins Medical Institutions, Baltimore, MD, USA
e-mail: mbukhar4@jhmi.edu

P. Saxena
e-mail: psaxena1@jhmi.edu

P. Saxena
Department of Medicine and Division of Gastroenterology and Hepatology, Royal Prince Alfred Hospital, Missenden Rd, Camperdown, NSW 2050, Australia

M.A. Bukhari
Department of Gastroenterology, Sheikh Zayed Tower, Suite M2058, 1800 Orleans Street, Baltimore, MD 21287, USA

M.A. Khashab (✉)
Division of Gastroenterology and Hepatology, Johns Hopkins Hospital, Sheikh Zayed Building, 1800 Orleans Street, Suite 7125B, Baltimore, MD 21287, USA
e-mail: mkhashab@jhmi.edu

J.R. Romanelli et al. (eds.), *NOTES and Endoluminal Surgery*, Clinical Gastroenterology, DOI 10.1007/978-3-319-50610-4_7

suggest promising outcomes. Prospective multicenter data on POEM for SEDs and G-POEM for gastroparesis are awaited.

Keywords
Spastic esophageal disorders · Refractory gastroparesis · Per-oral endoscopic myotomy · Endoscopic myotomy · Nutcracker esophagus · Jackhammer esophagus

Abbreviations

CI	Contractile integral
DCI	Distal contractile integral
DES	Distal esophageal spasm
DL	Distal latency
DM	Distal esophageal segments with myotomy
EGJOO	Esophagogastric junction outflow obstruction
EPT	Esophageal pressure topography
EUS	Endoscopic ultrasonography
GERD	Gastroesophageal reflux disease
GES	Gastric electrical stimulation
G-POEM	Gastric per-oral endoscopic myotomy
HREM	High-resolution esophageal manometry
IRP	Integrated relaxation pressure
LES	Lower esophageal sphincter
LHM	Laparoscopic Heller myotomy
PNM	Proximal esophageal segments with no myotomy
POEM	Per-oral endoscopic myotomy
SED	Spastic esophageal disorder
TPS	Trans-pyloric stenting
UES	Upper esophageal sphincter

Introduction

Esophageal motility disorders are a broad class of diseases that are characterized by abnormal or absent contractions of the esophageal body and abnormal function of the upper and/or lower esophageal sphincters (LESs). The Chicago classification categorized esophageal motility disorders utilizing high-resolution esophageal manometry (HREM) imaged with pressure topography plots, and it is considered the gold standard for the diagnosis and classification of esophageal motility disorders [1]. Spastic esophageal disorders (SEDs) are characterized by hyperactive esophageal contractions of either abnormal propagation (premature contraction) or extreme vigorous contractions [2]. SEDs include spastic or type III achalasia, distal esophageal spasm (DES), and hypercontractile (Jackhammer) esophagus. Esophagogastric junction outflow obstruction (EGJOO) is considered a fourth potential subtype of achalasia [3]. Hypertensive peristalsis, also known as nutcracker esophagus, has been eliminated from the updated 2015 Chicago classifications, because it has no apparent clinical significance [1].

Per-oral endoscopic myotomy (POEM) is a novel endoscopic procedure, which has been performed to treat achalasia with favorable outcomes [4–6]. Emerging data suggest that POEM techniques may also have a role in the treatment of patients with gastroesophageal motility disorders such as SEDs and refractory gastroparesis. The aim of this chapter is to discuss the diagnosis, clinical management, utility, and the outcomes of POEM in non-achalasia conditions, including SEDs and refractory gastroparesis.

Spastic Esophageal Disorders (SEDs)

Spastic Achalasia and Esophagogastric Junction Outflow Obstruction (EGJOO)

The first assessment of esophageal motility as per the Chicago classification is to assess for the presence of EGJOO, which is defined by integrated relaxation pressure (IRP) >15 mmHg [1]. Disorders of GEJ outflow obstruction are further subdivided into achalasia and EGJ outflow obstruction. According to the updated 2015 Chicago classification version 3.0, achalasia is then divided into three subtypes (Types I, II, and III), which are differentiated by the patterns of non-peristaltic esophageal pressurization that accompany the elevated IRP. Type III achalasia, (also known as spastic achalasia and formerly known as vigorous achalasia) is defined by elevated median IRP >15 mmHg, absence of normal peristalsis, and premature (spastic) contractions with a distal contractile integral (DCI) >450 mmHg.s.cm, involving ≥20% of swallows. These swallows associated with spastic contractions may be mixed with panesophageal pressurization (Fig. 7.1). Type III achalasia is the least common type of achalasia and accounts for only 10% of cases [7]. EGJOO is defined by an elevated median IRP >15 mmHg, with some intact or weak peristalsis such that the criteria of achalasia are not met. Some consider this a fourth potential achalasia phenotype [3]. EGJOO is present in 1.8–9.5% of patients referred for manometric evaluation [8].

Distal Esophageal Spasm (DES)

DES is an uncommon disorder characterized by impairment of ganglionic inhibition in the distal esophagus [2, 9]. DES is now considered a major disorder of peristalsis based upon the updated Chicago classification. DES is characterized by a normal median IRP, ≥20% premature contractions (contraction occurring within a phase when esophageal contractile activity is normally inhibited), and with a DCI >450 mmHg.s.cm. Normal peristalsis may also be present. It is important to note that DES is intermittent, and so the typical manometric findings may not be seen with all test swallows. Although most patients with DES usually have normal relaxation of the LES, approximately 30% may have high resting pressure or incomplete relaxation. The prevalence of DES is low and accounts for only 2% of patients evaluated for dysphagia by HRE manometry [9].

Hypercontractile (Jackhammer) Esophagus

Hypercontractile or Jackhammer esophagus is characterized by at least two swallows with DCI >8000 mmHg.s.cm (Fig. 7.2). Hypercontractility may involve, or even only be localized to, the LES [1]. Jackhammer esophagus is likely due to an excess of cholinergic drive causing asynchronous contraction of the circular and longitudinal muscle layers of the esophagus [10]. Jackhammer esophagus is a rare disorder that is present in 4.1% of patients referred for manometric evaluation in a tertiary center [9].

Clinical Manifestations of SEDs

Despite differences in pathophysiology, these disorders share many similarities, including their clinical manifestations. Patients with SEDs may present with one or all of the following symptoms: dysphagia (for solids or both solids and liquids), non-cardiac chest pain, regurgitation, and refractory gastroesophageal reflux disease (GERD) symptoms. Dysphagia is the predominant symptom and occurs because of impairment of bolus transit through the esophagus. Chest pain is another frequent symptom and is often severe in nature.

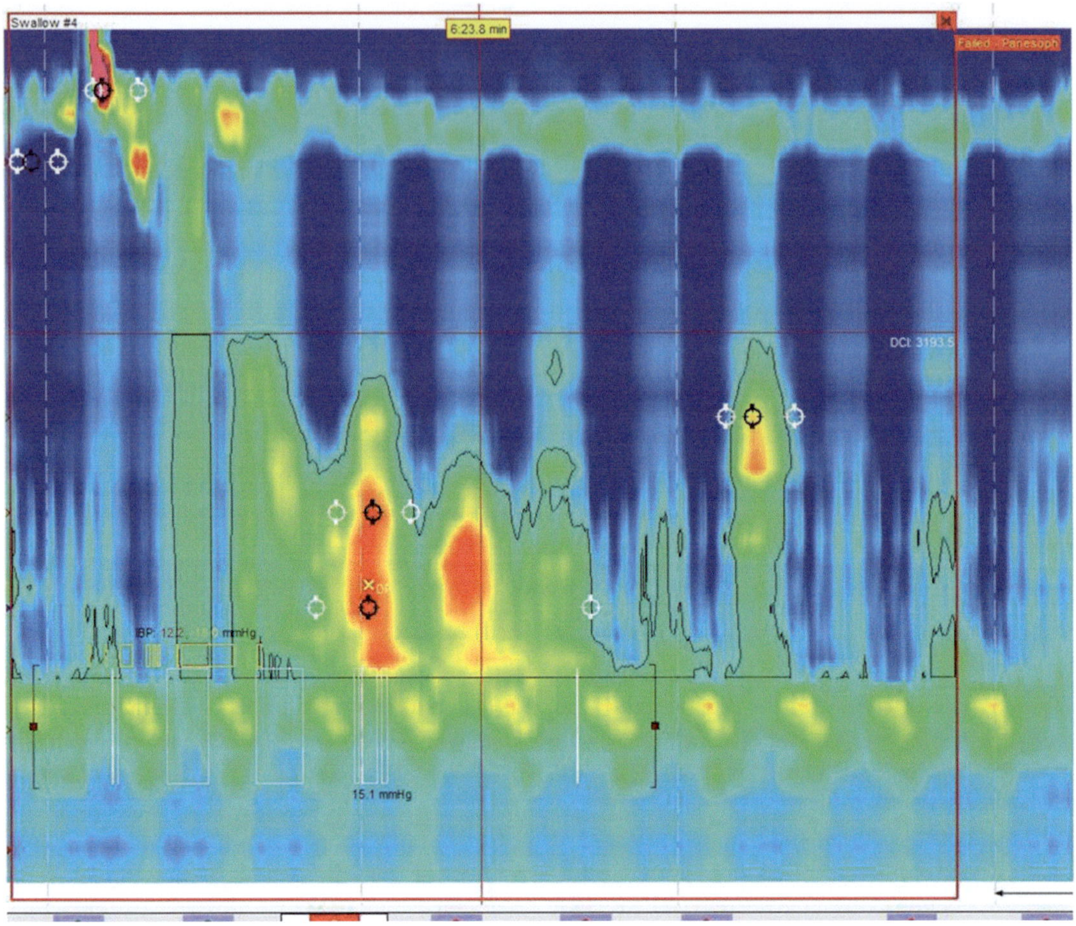

Fig. 7.1 Type III achalasia: defined as elevated median IRP >15 mmHg, no normal peristalsis, and premature (spastic) contractions with a distal contractile integral (DCI) >450 mmHg.s.cm, and with ≥20% of swallows which may be mixed with panesophageal pressurization

Diagnostic Work-Up for SEDs

Identification of SEDs is based on the contractile patterns observed during HRE manometry with esophageal pressure topography (EPT). Other diagnostic tests are required to rule out structural abnormalities or other causes of dysphagia.

- ***Upper endoscopy***

Upper endoscopy is required during the initial evaluation of SEDs to exclude mechanical causes of dysphagia such as malignancy, stenosis, peptic strictures, or eosinophilic esophagitis. Endoscopic findings of esophageal dilation and/or resistance to passage of endoscope at the GEJ may suggest a motility disorder. However, none of these endoscopic findings is specific.

- ***Barium swallow***

In patients with DES severe, non-peristaltic contractions may result in the classic corkscrew appearance of the esophagus. In patients with

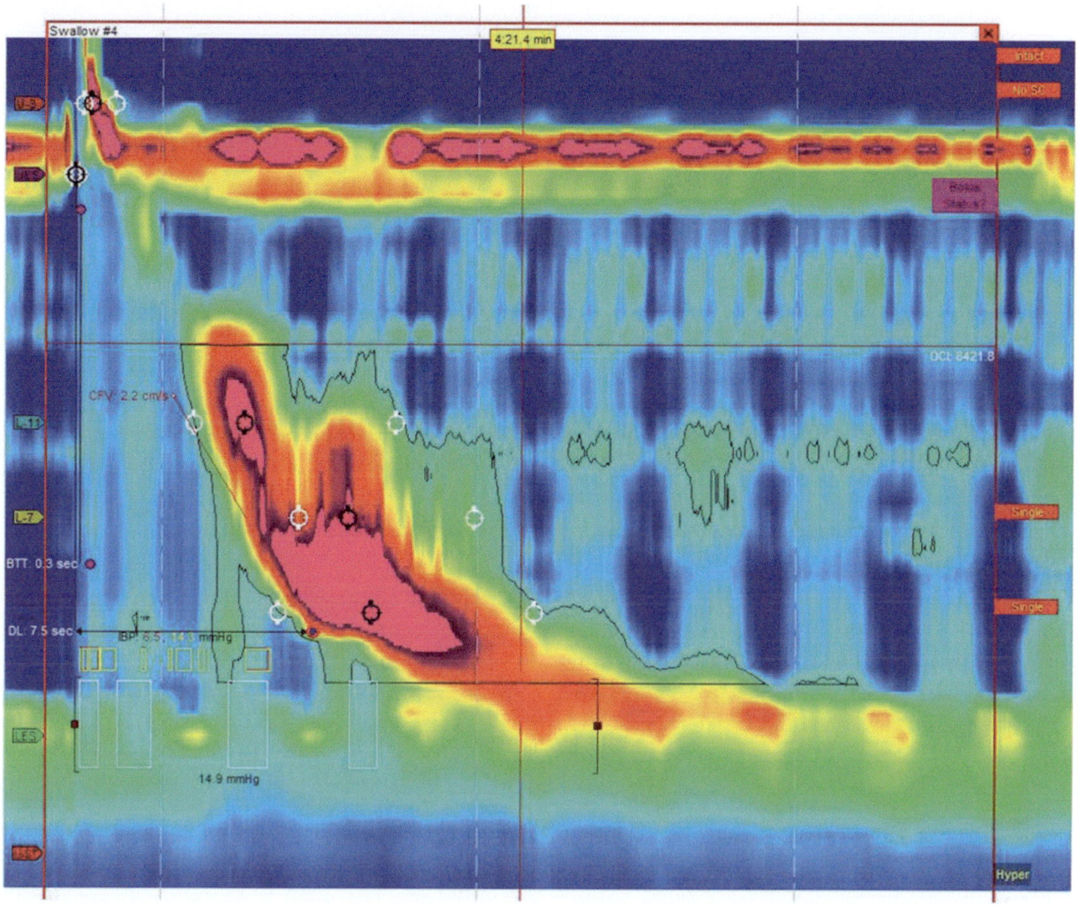

Fig. 7.2 Hypercontractile or Jackhammer esophagus, which is characterized by at least two swallows with DCI >8000 mmHg.s.cm

hypercontractile esophagus barium swallow usually shows normal sequential peristalsis [11].

- ***24-h pH monitoring***

There is a potential overlap of symptoms in DES and GERD. Therefore, 24-h pH monitoring should be considered in patients with chest pain, regurgitation, and/or heartburn [2].

- ***High-resolution esophageal manometry (HREM) with esophageal pressure topography (EPT)***

HRE manometry with EPT is the gold standard for diagnosis of esophageal motility disorders. HRE manometry with EPT is superior to conventional manometry, as EGJ relaxation is more reliably seen with HRE manometry in comparison to conventional manometry. EGJ relaxation is essential for distinguishing DES from spastic achalasia [2]. Furthermore, the use of IRP, the DCI, and the distal latency (DL) measurements in HRE manometry are more accurate than the metrics used in conventional manometry [1, 2]. Identification of these spastic disorders is based on the esophageal contractile pattern and IRP observed in HRE manometry with EPT (Table 7.1).

- ***Other investigations including CT scan and endoscopic ultrasound (EUS)***

Cross-sectional imaging can detect esophageal muscle thickening in patients with SEDs.

Table 7.1 High-resolution patterns of spastic esophageal disorders (SEDs)

Spastic disorders	EGJ relaxation	Esophageal contraction
1. Spastic achalasia (type III)	Impaired (elevated median IRP >15 mmHg)	• No normal peristalsis • ≥20% of swallow with premature (spastic contraction with DCI >450 mmHg.s.cm)
2. EGJ outflow obstruction	Impaired (elevated median IRP >15 mmHg)	• Sufficient evidence of peristalsis which does not meet the achalasia I–III
3. Distal esophageal spasm	Normal median IRP <15 mmHg	• ≥20% of swallow with premature (spastic contraction with DCI >450 mmHg.s.cm)
4. Jackhammer esophagus	Normal (IRP <15 mmHg) or impaired (IRP >15 mmHg)	• At least two swallow with DCI >8000 mmHg.s.cm

CT scan revealed marked esophageal wall thickening at the lower esophagus in 21% of patients with DES ($p < 0.01$), which corresponded to non-propulsive contractions detected on barium study [12]. A CT scan is not routinely indicated in patients with spastic disorders unless there is a suspicion of extrinsic esophageal compression. Alternatively, endoscopic ultrasonography (EUS) can quantify esophageal thickening and reveal mediastinal, infiltrative/malignant extramural, or intramural abnormalities that may mimic achalasia (pseudoachalasia). A retrospective study of 62 patients with esophageal motility disorders evaluated the clinical utility of a radial endoscopic ultrasound examination [3]. EUS identified 15% clinically relevant findings that altered patients' management and explained the etiology of the esophageal outflow obstruction. These included aortic compression, intramural mass, leiomyoma, congenital muscular ring, and sarcoidosis. There were no pathological EUS findings in patients with DES or hypercontractility [3].

Treatment of Spastic Esophageal Disorders

Although multiple medical, endoscopic, and surgical therapeutic modalities have been used to treat SEDs, the treatment success rates have been less than ideal. In order to meet the treatment objective of alleviating patients' symptoms, we believe the anatomic and physiologic goal is to reduce the vigorous abnormal esophageal contraction and to alleviate the EGJ obstruction.

- **Pharmacological therapy**

Medical therapies include calcium channel blockers, nitrates, or tricyclic antidepressants. One small, randomized, crossover study compared the effect of nifedipine (10 mg three times daily) versus placebo for 4 weeks in 20 patients with primary esophageal disorders (hypertensive LES $n = 10$, DES $n = 4$, spastic achalasia $n = 3$, nutcracker $n = 2$, and achalasia $n = 1$). Patients who received nifedipine had significantly higher rates of relief of chest pain ($p < 0.01$) and dysphagia ($p < 0.05$) within 1–6 weeks of treatment [13].

Visceral analgesic agents such as tricyclic antidepressants have also been proposed as therapy for these disorders. A low dose of clomipramine (25 mg daily for 4 weeks) was shown to be effective in a small case-control study of nine patients with DES compared with 26 healthy volunteers. Patients with DES received initial isosorbide dinitrate (15 mg daily) for 1 month, followed by clomipramine (25 mg daily) for an additional month. Patients with DES had greater improvement of chest pain ($n = 88\%$, $p < 0.05$), but only 40% of those patients had slight manometric improvement after treatment [14].

- **Endoscopic therapy**

Endoscopic therapies include botulinum toxin injection and esophageal dilation. Botulinum toxin reduces smooth muscle tone in the gastrointestinal tract by blocking the release of acetylcholine in the excitatory motor neurons. Botulinum toxin injection results unlimited degeneration of the nerve endings. However, after a few months nerves regenerate, which leads to the loss of toxin effect [15]. A recent retrospective study evaluated the effect of botulinum toxin injection in 45 patients with SEDs (Type III achalasia $n = 22$, Jackhammer esophagus $n = 8$, DES $n = 7$, EGJOO $n = 5$, nutcracker $n = 1$, unclassified $n = 2$) [16]. After Botulinum toxin injection, 71% had significant improvement of symptoms at 2 months, and 57% remained in remission for more than 6 months. The clinical response rates were apparently worse (although not significantly, $p = 0.13$) in patients with normal EGJ relaxation (Jackhammer esophagus, DES, nutcracker esophagus, and type III achalasia with IRP <15 mmHg; 10/22, 45%) compared to those patients with abnormal EGJ relaxation (achalasia with IRP >15 mmHg, EGJOO; 14/20, 70%).

Pneumatic balloon dilation has been proposed for treating SEDs. In a study of 61 patients with DES, pneumatic balloon dilation was performed in 20 patients who were refractory to medical therapy. Seventy percent of those patients had significant improvement of dysphagia [17]. However, Pandolfino et al. [18] observed that pneumatic balloon dilation was ineffective in patients with spastic achalasia compared with other types of achalasia. A total of 1000 HRE manometry studies were reviewed, and 213 with impaired EGJ relaxation were identified. Ninety-nine patients were newly diagnosed with achalasia (21 Type I, 49 Type II, and 29 Type III). All patients underwent therapeutic interventions including botulinum toxin injection, pneumatic balloon dilation, or Heller myotomy. Patients with Type III achalasia had the worst response to therapy, despite having a significant number of therapeutic interventions during a mean follow-up of 20 months (success rate was 22% with botulinum toxin injection, 0% with pneumatic balloon dilation, and 0% with Heller myotomy) [18].

- **Surgical therapy**

Heller myotomy is an established treatment for achalasia; however, a lower response rate has been observed in patients with spastic achalasia [2, 18, 19]. In SEDs, the disease process involves the proximal esophageal body in addition to the LES. Hence, a longer surgical myotomy is likely needed to target the proximal esophageal body [2]. Patti and colleagues compared the outcomes in patients with DES and nutcracker esophagus treated by surgical myotomy with the outcomes in those treated medically. Thirty patients with nutcracker and DES were treated with dilation and/or medication (a calcium channel blocker), and ten patients underwent a thoracoscopic myotomy. A higher response rate was seen in the surgical myotomy group compared to the medical group (80% vs. 26%, $p = 0.001$) [20].

Per-oral Endoscopic Myotomy (POEM) for Spastic Esophageal Disorders

The literature suggests that the management of SEDs is challenging. Efficacy of pharmacological therapies is disappointing, and botulinum toxin injection achieves only short-term relief in a subset of patients. Surgical myotomy is more effective than medical therapies; however, the results are less than optimal. One reason is that the disease process in SED is primarily in the proximal esophagus. Access to the thoracic esophagus via a surgical approach is technically challenging, and myotomy of the esophageal segments with spastic contractions may not be possible. POEM permits access and therapy to the entire esophagus, thereby alleviating the challenges faced during other surgical approaches.

Why Is POEM Potentially the Ideal Therapy for Spastic Esophageal Disorders?

POEM is an effective procedure that has been performed to treat achalasia with clinical success rates of 82–100% [21]. Data suggest that a long

Table 7.2 Published data on POEM for spastic esophageal disorders

Reference	Type of study	SEDs	Clinical success rate	Adverse events
1. Shiwaku et al. [22]	Case report	DES	Yes	None
2. Minami et al. [23]	Case series	2 DES	Yes	None
3. Louis et al. [24]	Case report	DES	Yes	None
4. Khashab et al. [25]	Case report	Jackhammer esophagus	Yes	None
5. Kandulski et al. [26]	Case report	Jackhammer esophagus	No	Mild emphysema and pneumothorax
6. Kristensen et al. [31]	Case series	3 nutcracker esophagus	Yes	None
7. Ko et al. [28]	Case report	Jackhammer esophagus	yes	None
8. Takahashi et al. [29]	Case report	DES	100%	None
9. Sharata et al. [30]	Retrospective cohort study	2 spastic achalasia 12 nutcracker esophagus 5 DES	70.8%	6%
10. Khashab et al. [34]	Retrospective cohort study	9 DES 10 Jackhammer esophagus 54 spastic achalasia	93%	11%
11. Kumbhari et al. [27]	Retrospective cohort study	49 spastic achalasia	98%	6%

surgical myotomy may be effective in treating patients with SEDs [22–26]. Surgical myotomy of the upper thoracic esophagus is technically challenging via transabdominal approach [20]. However, during POEM, the endoscopist is able to access the entire length of the esophagus, which renders POEM an attractive, minimally invasive therapeutic modality for the treatment of SEDs. POEM facilitates myotomy of the LES as well as the esophageal body, where hypertensive contractions occur. There have been multiple case reports and case series demonstrating excellent clinical efficacy of POEM for various SEDs including Jackhammer esophagus, DES, spastic achalasia, and Nutcracker esophagus (Table 7.2) [22–31]. A retrospective trial comparing 49 patients who underwent POEM for spastic achalasia (Type III achalasia) with 26 patients who underwent laparoscopic Heller myotomy (LHM) showed a higher rate of clinical success in the POEM group (98% vs. 80.8%, $p = 0.01$). Furthermore, procedure duration was significantly shorter in the POEM group (102 min vs. 264 min, $p < 0.01$) despite longer myotomy (16 cm vs. 8 cm, $p < 0.01$). The rate of adverse events was also significantly lower in the POEM group (6% vs. 27%, $p < 0.01$) [27].

POEM may have additional benefits even in the setting of prior therapies such as balloon dilation, botulinum toxin injection, or surgical myotomy. Surgical re-do myotomy is known to be difficult due to fibrosis and scaring [32]. A retrospective analysis of 40 POEM procedures, including treatment-naïve patients ($n = 28$) and patients with previous endoscopic intervention (2 with nutcracker and 1 with DES; 10 with previous botulinum toxin injection and 2 with previous pneumatic balloon dilation) ($n = 12$), demonstrated no significant difference in the mean procedure duration (131 ± 41 min vs. 134 ± 43 min, $p = 0.8$) or the incidence of intraoperative complications (3% vs. 17%, $p = 0.2$) between the two groups [33].

Modification of POEM Technique for Spastic Esophageal Disorders

During standard POEM procedures, a submucosal tunnel is initially created prior to performance of endoscopic myotomy of the LES and esophageal body. Performance of POEM occurs in four consecutive steps: (1) mucosal incision, (2) formation of submucosal tunnel, (3) myotomy, and (4) closure of mucosal incision. The myotomy is started 2–5 cm distal to the mucosal incision and continued to the end of the submucosal tunnel (2–3 cm distal to the GEJ). The length of the esophageal myotomy in patients with achalasia types I and II is typically 6–8 cm but varies based on patient symptoms (such as amount of chest pain), manometry results, and even operator preference [21]. However, the length of myotomy in SEDs should be based on the proximal extent of hypertensive contractions seen on HRE manometry and has been reported to be 14–16 cm on average [34]. Patients with spastic achalasia and DES are believed to have a higher response rate than those with Jackhammer esophagus (96.3, 100, and 70%, respectively) [34]. The reason is not well known, but it may be due to extreme hypercontractility of the esophageal body in jackhammer patients [34]. Therefore, concomitant bilateral (anterior and posterior) myotomy in patients with Jackhammer esophagus may be considered as possible alternative for such patients, although this approach remains to be studied. Insufficient myotomy or remnant of esophageal body contraction may lead to residual symptoms in those patients [26].

Do We Have to Perform LES Myotomy in Patients with Jackhammer or DES?

Patients with Jackhammer esophagus may or may not have EGJ outflow obstruction, and some patients with DES do not have this abnormal manometric finding [2]. It is arguable whether patients without outflow obstruction will require myotomy of the LES. Myotomy of the esophageal body induces aperistalsis, and this may result in dysphagia in patients who do not undergo LES myotomy. The inclusion of the LES seems warranted by the potential after effects of myotomy, even in the setting of normal LES pressure, since preserving the LES pressure may result in postoperative dysphagia caused by induced aperistalsis [25]. After POEM, there are several esophageal motility changes such as a decrease in the LES resting pressure, as well a dramatic decrease in LES relaxation pressure [4, 35, 36].

A recent retrospective study by Ren et al. [37] reported the therapeutic effect of POEM on the proximal esophagus in all types of achalasia. Thirty-two patients with achalasia (Type I $n = 6$, Type II $n = 17$, Type III $n = 9$) who underwent POEM and follow-up high-resolution esophageal manometry were included in the analysis. The LES resting pressure and IRP were significantly decreased post POEM (38.12 ± 13.48 mmHg vs. 14.53 ± 4.92 mmHg, $P < 0.001$ and 31.28 ± 10.03 mmHg vs. 8.80 ± 4.22 mmHg, $P < 0.001$). POEM also resulted in a significant reduction in the contractile integral (CI) in both the distal esophageal segments with myotomy (DM) and the proximal segments with no myotomy (PNM) (CI-DM: 43.95 mmHg.s.cm vs. 3.79 mmHg.s.cm, $p < 0.001$, and CI-PNM, 1337.73 mmHg.s.cm vs. 480.85 mmHg.s.cm, $p < 0.001$). The upper esophageal sphincter relaxing pressure (UES) was also reduced after POEM (12.74 ± 7.14 mmHg vs. 5.79 ± 6.11 mmHg, $p < 0.001$). Nevertheless, the UES resting pressure and relaxation duration were unchanged [37]. After POEM, there was a positive linear correlation of CI changes between the distal esophageal body segment with myotomy and the proximal esophageal body without myotomy (correlation coefficient = 0.901, $p < 0.001$). The changes in the UES relaxing pressure were positively correlated with CI of the distal segment of esophageal body with myotomy and the proximal segment of esophageal body without myotomy (CI-DM: correlation coefficient = 0.705, $p < 0.001$, and CI-PNM: correlation coefficient = 0.755, $p < 0.001$). In type II achalasia, the positive correlation of changes of CI was significant between the distal esophageal body with myotomy and the proximal esophageal body without myotomy (correlation coefficient = 0.917, $p = 0.001$). These findings suggested that myotomy of the distal esophagus could influence contraction of the proximal esophagus and UES relaxation pressure [37]. Ren et al. [38] hypothesized that simultaneous contraction or pressurization of esophageal body would provide a "viscous resistance" to food bolus during swallow. Therefore, myotomy of the distal esophagus was found to significantly inhibit the pressurization of the whole esophageal body and lead to less "viscous resistance" [37, 38].

The Outcomes of POEM in Patients with Spastic Esophageal Disorders

There have been multiple case reports and case series reporting the efficacy of POEM for SEDs (Table 7.2) [22–31]. The clinical efficacy of POEM is assessed based on symptomatic improvement as measured by Eckardt score. The Eckardt score is the sum of the symptom scores for dysphagia, regurgitation, chest pain, and weight loss. Clinical success is defined as decrease in Eckardt score to ≤3.

Sharata et al. [30] reported a series of 100 patients with primary esophageal disorders, 75 patients with achalasia, and 25 patients with non-achalasia spastic disorders (nutcracker $n = 12$, DES $n = 5$, and isolated, hypertensive, non-relaxing LES $n = 8$). Complete resolution of dysphagia post POEM was seen in 70.8% of patients with non-achalasia disorders compared to 97.8% with achalasia at an average of 21.5 months after POEM [30]. Furthermore, improvement of chest pain was seen in 75% of patients with non-achalasia compared to 100% resolution in patients with achalasia [30].

Khashab et al. [34] reported an international multicenter study of 73 patients who underwent POEM for SEDs (DES $n = 9$, Jackhammer esophagus $n = 10$, and spastic achalasia $n = 54$). Selective inner circular myotomy was performed in 64 patients (87.7%), whereas full thickness myotomy was performed in nine patients (12.3%). The mean length of the submucosal tunnel was 19 cm, and the mean myotomy length was 16 cm [34]. Overall, clinical success was observed in 93% of patients after an average of 8 months follow-up. There was a significant decrease in the mean Eckardt score after POEM (6.73 vs. 1.13, $p < 0.001$) [34]. Mean post-POEM Eckardt score was significantly lower in patients with spastic achalasia and DES as compared to patients with Jackhammer esophagus (1 vs. 2.6, $p = 0.01$). A repeat HRE manometry after POEM was performed in 60% of patients, showing 100% resolution of the initial manometric abnormalities [34]. There were eight adverse events (11%), the majority of which were mild according to the American Society for Gastrointestinal Endoscopy lexicon severity grading system [39]. Two patients had mucosotomy, which was managed with endoscopic clips. Infectious esophagitis was seen in one patient and was treated with antibiotics. Subcutaneous emphysema was found in two patients and resolved spontaneously with conservative management. Epigastric pain requiring hospitalization occurred in two patients, and one patient had pulmonary embolism treated with anticoagulation [34].

Another retrospective, cross-sectional study of 35 patients with spastic esophageal motility disorders ($n = 10$) and achalasia ($n = 25$) who underwent POEM demonstrated significant improvement of dysphagia in 75% of patients with SEDs at average follow-up of 7 months. The overall rate of complications requiring intervention was 5.7% ($n = 2$). One patient developed a pleural sterile effusion and required placement of a pigtail catheter for drainage, and the other developed mucosotomy closure dehiscence that was treated conservatively with proton pump inhibitor. However, this patient developed recurrent dysphagia secondary to a stricture at the site of the mucosal defect and eventually required LHM with partial fundoplication [40].

GERD is one of the most frequent complications after any treatment of achalasia [41]. GERD occurs if there is incompetence of antireflux barriers at the gastroesophageal junction. The antireflux mechanisms include the LES, the diaphragmatic crura (which function as an external sphincter), and the phrenoesophageal ligament. The phrenoesophageal ligament helps maintain the anatomic integrity of the GEJ. This ligament is commonly divided in Heller myotomy, which can lead to anatomical displacement of the esophagus and reflux of gastric contents (20–100%) [42–44]. Hence, a concomitant Dor or Toupet fundoplication is often performed with Heller myotomy.

On the other hand, the incidence of GERD after POEM appears to be lower than previously seen with Heller myotomy. A recent prospective study by Shiwaku et al. [45] reported the association of POEM with reflux esophagitis. There were 105 patients who underwent POEM, and 70 of these were followed up to 3 months after POEM [45]. Endoscopic evidence of esophagitis was found in 42 patients (60%). The majority was LA grade A esophagitis (73.8%), and none of the patients had grade D esophagitis. Symptomatic GERD occurred in only five patients (7%) [45]. Treatment with PPI in patients with reflux esophagitis and symptomatic GERD resulted in clinical improvement.

During POEM, myotomy is limited to the esophageal body and LES, thereby preserving the surrounding structures of the distal esophagus such as the phrenoesophageal ligament and the angle of His. Therefore, the risk of post-POEM GERD is likely to be lower than is seen in surgical Heller myotomy [46]. Although not yet the standard of care, we propose that routine 24-hour pH testing should be considered in all patients following POEM to prevent complications of chronic esophageal acid exposure in symptomatic and asymptomatic patients.

Refractory Gastroparesis

Gastroparesis is a common chronic disorder characterized by objective delayed gastric emptying in the absence of mechanical obstruction. The incidence of gastroparesis in the general population is 0.2–4% [47, 48]. The cardinal symptoms of gastroparesis are early satiety, postprandial fullness, nausea and vomiting, bloating, and upper abdominal pain. These symptoms are often debilitating to the patient [47]. The three most common causes of gastroparesis are idiopathic, diabetes mellitus, and postsurgical. Other causes include Parkinson's disease, hypothyroidism, collagen vascular disease, and iatrogenic secondary to certain medications. Refractory gastroparesis is defined as persistent symptoms despite dietary modifications, prokinetic, and antiemetic therapy. Patients with refractory gastroparesis are unable to maintain oral nutrition and require frequent emergency room visits. Recent limited data suggest that surgical pyloroplasty might lead to sustained improvement in patients with refractory symptoms [49].

Diagnosis of Gastroparesis

A scintigraphic gastric emptying study is the gold standard for evaluation of gastric emptying. Delayed gastric emptying is defined variably depending on the center where the study is performed and on how it is performed (liquid, solid, or mixed). One common definition of delayed gastric emptying is a gastric retention of >10% of contents at 4 h and/or >60% at 2 h when using a standard low-fat meal [50]. Alternatives to scintigraphy include wireless motility capsule and ^{13}C breath testing using octanoate or spirulina incorporated into the solid meal [50]. Upper endoscopy is required to rule out mechanical obstruction as the cause of delayed gastric emptying.

Therapies for Gastroparesis

Despite a large number of patients suffering from the disease, few effective treatments exist. The treatment of gastroparesis is challenging and can be frustrating for the patient and the physician. First-line treatment includes dietary modification with or without prokinetic and antiemetic therapy. The response to metoclopramide varies between 29 and 60% based on clinical trials [50]. Injection of botulinum toxin into the pylorus may improve gastric emptying but does not result in symptom improvement in comparison with saline solution injections based on two randomized, double-blind clinical trials [51, 52].

Gastric electrical stimulation (GES) delivers high-frequency lower-energy electrical stimulation to the stomach. GES improves nausea and vomiting, oral tolerance, and the quality of life in subset of patients with refractory gastroparesis. A meta-analysis by Chu et al. [53] in 2012 confirmed significant improvement in symptom severity and gastric emptying with GES ($p < 0.00001$). This technique seems to be effective in patients with diabetic gastroparesis [50, 54]. However, placement of the GES requires surgical implantation.

Khashab et al. [54, 55] described the effect of trans-pyloric stenting (TPS) using a fully covered, self-expandable metallic stent in 30 patients with refractory gastroparesis (idiopathic gastroparesis $n = 16$, diabetic gastroparesis $n = 8$, postsurgical gastroparesis $n = 6$). A clinical response was observed in 75% of patients with an average weight gain of 5 kg. Clinical success in patients with predominant symptoms of nausea and vomiting was higher than those with abdominal pain alone (79% vs. 21%, $p = 0.12$). A repeat gastric emptying study was performed in 16 patients at a mean of 49 days after stent placement. The mean 4-h gastric emptying normalized in six patients (gastric emptying pre-stent of 75% vs. 98% post stent, $p = 0.2$), and significantly improved in five others (54% vs. 73%, $p = 0.02$). TPS may be considered as salvage therapy for inpatients with intractable symptoms, or potentially as a method to select patients who may respond to more permanent directed therapies to the pylorus. These include surgical pyloroplasty and endoscopic pyloromyotomy via gastric per-oral endoscopic myotomy (G-POEM) [55].

G-POEM

Hibbard et al. [49] suggested that surgical pyloroplasty might lead to sustained improvement of symptoms in patients with refractory gastroparesis. Kawai et al. [56] performed endoscopic pyloromyotomy in eight pigs with successful result. Given these data, Khashab et al. [57] performed the first human case of G-POEM in a patient with severe refractory diabetic gastroparesis.

Efficacy and the Outcomes of Gastric POEM

G-POEM is performed by complete dissection of the pylorus using principles of submucosal endoscopy [57]. After the initial report by Khashab, multiple case reports showed that G-POEM had excellent clinical efficacy in patients with gastroparesis (Table 7.3) [58–62]. A retrospective study demonstrated the safety and feasibility of G-POEM in seven patients with gastroparesis (idiopathic $n = 4$, postsurgical gastroparesis $n = 2$, severe clinical gastroparesis and negative gastric emptying study $n = 1$) who underwent endoscopic pyloromyotomy with 100% technical success, and without immediate complications [63].

Symptomatic improvement occurred in 85% of patients. Significant symptomatic improvement was observed for nausea and epigastric burning ($p < 0.05$). However, symptomatic improvement of vomiting, early satiety, postprandial fullness, and epigastric pain was not statically significant ($p > 0.05$). During follow-up, normalization of gastric emptying was seen in 85% of patients at mean follow-up of 6.5 months. One patient had bleeding 2 weeks post procedure requiring blood transfusion and endoscopic clipping of a pyloric channel ulcer. One patient who underwent concomitant Nissen fundoplication developed temporary dysphagia [63].

Technique of G-POEM

The G-POEM endoscopic pyloromyotomy is similar in principle to submucosal dissection and myotomy performed for the treatment of achalasia. The procedure consists of four steps similar to those described for esophageal POEM. The tunnel is typically created 5 cm proximal to the pylorus, along the greater curvature or anterior gastric wall. A short, 2-cm antral myotomy in addition to pyloromyotomy is then performed. Further technical details on this procedure can be found in the per-oral pyloromyotomy chapter.

Table 7.3 Summary of published data on G-POEM

Reference	Study	Cause of gastroparesis	Clinical success	Adverse event	Follow-up
Khashab et al. [57]	1 case report	Diabetic	Yes	No	12 weeks
Chaves et al. [59]	1 case report	Postsurgical gastroparesis	Yes	No	12 weeks
Bapaye et al. [60]	2 case reports	Postsurgical gastroparesis	Yes	No	10 weeks
Chung et al. [61]	1 case report	Postsurgical gastroparesis	Yes	No	4 weeks
Shlomovitz et al. [63]	Retrospective study (7 patients)	4 idiopathic 2 postsurgical gastroparesis 1 severe clinical gastroparesis and negative gastric emptying study	85%	1 GI bleed	26 weeks
Gonzalez et al. [58]	1 case report	Diabetic	Yes	No	4 weeks

Post-procedural Care

Patients should be admitted to the hospital for observation and kept nil per os. Intravenous prophylactic antiemetics and broad-spectrum antibiotics should be prescribed. An upper GI series is typically obtained on the following day, and if there is no evidence of leakage, a liquid diet is commenced and advanced to a soft diet the following day for two weeks. A gastric scintigraphy study is recommended during follow-up to assess the effect of the myotomy on gastric emptying.

Conclusion

There are limited data to guide the management of SEDs and refractory gastroparesis. The most effective treatment has yet to be defined. However, POEM is an elegant, minimally invasive, endoscopic procedure used worldwide to treat a variety of gastroesophageal disorders with excellent short-term clinical response rates and low rates of adverse events. POEM and G-POEM are promising procedures for SEDs and refractory gastroparesis, respectively.

Conflicts of Interest Dr. Khashab is a consultant for Boston Scientific. All other authors have no relevant disclosures.

References

1. Kahrilas PJ, Bredenoord AJ, Fox M, Gyawali CP, Roman S, Smout AJ, et al. The Chicago classification of esophageal motility disorders, v3.0. Neurogastroenterol Motil (The Official Journal of the European Gastrointestinal Motility Society). 2015;27(2):160–74. Epub 4 Dec 2014.
2. Roman S, Kahrilas PJ. Management of spastic disorders of the esophagus. Gastroenterol Clin N Am. 2013;42(1):27–43. Epub 5 Mar 2013.
3. Krishnan K, Lin CY, Keswani R, Pandolfino JE, Kahrilas PJ, Komanduri S. Endoscopic ultrasound as an adjunctive evaluation in patients with esophageal motor disorders subtyped by high-resolution manometry. Neurogastroenterol Motil (The Official Journal of the European Gastrointestinal Motility Society). 2014;26(8):1172–8. Epub 22 July 2014.
4. Inoue H, Minami H, Kobayashi Y, Sato Y, Kaga M, Suzuki M, et al. Peroral endoscopic myotomy (POEM) for esophageal achalasia. Endoscopy. 2010;42(4):265–71. Epub 1 Apr 2010.
5. Costamagna G, Marchese M, Familiari P, Tringali A, Inoue H, Perri V. Peroral endoscopic myotomy (POEM) for oesophageal achalasia: preliminary results in humans. Dig Liver Dis (Official Journal of the Italian Society of Gastroenterology and the Italian Association for the Study of the Liver). 2012;44(10):827–32. Epub 23 May 2012.
6. Lee BH, Shim KY, Hong SJ, Bok GH, Cho JH, Lee TH, et al. Peroral endoscopic myotomy for treatment of achalasia: initial results of a Korean study. Clin Endosc. 2013;46(2):161–7. Epub 25 Apr 2013.
7. Boeckxstaens G, Zaninotto G. Achalasia and esophago-gastric junction outflow obstruction: focus

on the subtypes. Neurogastroenterol Motil (The Official Journal of the European Gastrointestinal Motility Society). 2012;24 Suppl 1:27–31. Epub 25 Jan 2012.

8. Pandolfino JE, Ghosh SK, Rice J, Clarke JO, Kwiatek MA, Kahrilas PJ. Classifying esophageal motility by pressure topography characteristics: a study of 400 patients and 75 controls. Am J Gastroenterol. 2008;103(1):27–37. Epub 29 Sep 2007.
9. Valdovinos MA, Zavala-Solares MR, Coss-Adame E. Esophageal hypomotility and spastic motor disorders: current diagnosis and treatment. Curr Gastroenterol Rep. 2014;16(11):421. Epub 8 Nov 2014.
10. Roman S, Pandolfino JE, Chen J, Boris L, Luger D, Kahrilas PJ. Phenotypes and clinical context of hypercontractility in high-resolution esophageal pressure topography (EPT). Am J Gastroenterol. 2012;107(1):37–45. Epub 21 Sept 2011.
11. Ott DJ, Richter JE, Wu WC, Chen YM, Gelfand DW, Castell DO. Radiologic and manometric correlation in "nutcracker esophagus". AJR Am J Roentgenol. 1986;147(4):692–5. Epub 1 Oct 1986.
12. Goldberg MF, Levine MS, Torigian DA. Diffuse esophageal spasm: CT findings in seven patients. AJR Am J Roentgenol. 2008;191(3):758–63. Epub 22 Aug 2008.
13. Nasrallah SM, Tommaso CL, Singleton RT, Backhaus EA. Primary esophageal motor disorders: clinical response to nifedipine. South Med J. 1985;78(3):312–5. Epub 1 Mar 1985.
14. Handa M, Mine K, Yamamoto H, Hayashi H, Tsuchida O, Kanazawa F, et al. Antidepressant treatment of patients with diffuse esophageal spasm: a psychosomatic approach. J Clin Gastroenterol. 1999;28(3):228–32. Epub 7 Apr 1999.
15. Boeckxstaens GE. Achalasia. Best Pract Res Clin Gastroenterol. 2007;21(4):595–608. Epub 24 July 2007.
16. Marjoux S, Brochard C, Roman S, Gincul R, Pagenault M, Ponchon T, et al. Botulinum toxin injection for hypercontractile or spastic esophageal motility disorders: may high-resolution manometry help to select cases? Dis Esophagus (Official Journal of the International Society for Diseases of the Esophagus/ISDE). 2015;28(8):735–41. Epub 13 Sept 2014.
17. Irving JD, Owen WJ, Linsell J, McCullagh M, Keightley A, Anggiansah A. Management of diffuse esophageal spasm with balloon dilatation. Gastrointest Radiol. 1992;17(3):189–92. Epub 1 Jan 1992.
18. Pandolfino JE, Kwiatek MA, Nealis T, Bulsiewicz W, Post J, Kahrilas PJ. Achalasia: a new clinically relevant classification by high-resolution manometry. Gastroenterology. 2008;135(5):1526–33. Epub 30 Aug 2008.
19. Rohof WO, Salvador R, Annese V, des Varannes SB, Chaussade S, Costantini M, et al. Outcomes of treatment for achalasia depend on manometric subtype. Gastroenterology. 2013;144(4):718–25; quiz e13–4. Epub 2 Jan 2013.
20. Patti MG, Pellegrini CA, Arcerito M, Tong J, Mulvihill SJ, Way LW. Comparison of medical and minimally invasive surgical therapy for primary esophageal motility disorders. Arch Surg. 1995;130(6):609–15; discussion 15–6. Epub 1 June 1995.
21. Stavropoulos SN, Desilets DJ, Fuchs KH, Gostout CJ, Haber G, Inoue H, et al. Per-oral endoscopic myotomy white paper summary. Gastrointest Endosc. 2014;80(1):1–15. Epub 22 June 2014.
22. Shiwaku H, Inoue H, Beppu R, Nakashima R, Minami H, Shiroshita T, et al. Successful treatment of diffuse esophageal spasm by peroral endoscopic myotomy. Gastrointest Endosc. 2013;77(1):149–50. Epub 10 Apr 2012.
23. Minami H, Isomoto H, Yamaguchi N, Ohnita K, Takeshima F, Inoue H, et al. Peroral endoscopic myotomy (POEM) for diffuse esophageal spasm. Endoscopy. 2014;46 Suppl 1 UCTN:E79–81. Epub 29 Mar 2014.
24. Louis H, Covas A, Coppens E, Deviere J. Distal esophageal spasm treated by peroral endoscopic myotomy. Am J Gastroenterol. 2012;107(12):1926–7. Epub 6 Dec 2012.
25. Khashab MA, Saxena P, Kumbhari V, Nandwani M, Roland BC, Stein E, et al. Peroral endoscopic myotomy as a platform for the treatment of spastic esophageal disorders refractory to medical therapy (with video). Gastrointest Endosc. 2014;79(1):136–9. Epub 18 Dec 2013.
26. Kandulski A, Fuchs KH, Weigt J, Malfertheiner P. Jackhammer esophagus: high-resolution manometry and therapeutic approach using peroral endoscopic myotomy (POEM). Dis Esophagus (Official Journal of the International Society for Diseases of the Esophagus/ISDE). 2014. Epub 28 Jan 2014.
27. Kumbhari V, Tieu AH, Onimaru M, El Zein MH, Teitelbaum EN, Ujiki MB, et al. Peroral endoscopic myotomy (POEM) vs. laparoscopic Heller myotomy (LHM) for the treatment of Type III achalasia in 75 patients: a multicenter comparative study. Endosc Int Open. 2015;3(3):E195–201. Epub 15 July 2015.
28. Ko WJ, Lee BM, Park WY, Kim JN, Cho JH, Lee TH, et al. Jackhammer esophagus treated by a peroral endoscopic myotomy. Korean J Gastroenterol = Taehan Sohwagi Hakhoe chi. 2014;64(6):370–4. Epub 23 Dec 2014.
29. Takahashi K, Sato H, Sato Y, Takeuchi M, Takeda SR, Mizuno K, et al. Education and imaging. Gastroenterology: histopathological investigation of distal esophageal spasm (DES) using per-oral endoscopic myotomy (POEM). J Gastroenterol Hepatol. 2015;30(7):1113. Epub 23 June 2015.
30. Sharata AM, Dunst CM, Pescarus R, Shlomovitz E, Wille AJ, Reavis KM, et al. Peroral endoscopic myotomy (POEM) for esophageal primary motility disorders: analysis of 100 consecutive patients. J Gastrointest Surg (Official Journal of the Society for Surgery of the Alimentary Tract). 2015;19(1):161–70; discussion 70. Epub 4 Sept 2014.
31. Kristensen HO, Bjerregaard NC, Rask P, Mortensen FV, Kunda R. Peroral endoscopic myotomy (POEM) for nutcracker esophagus. Three cases

with 12 months follow-up. Scand J Gastroenterol. 2014;49(11):1285–9. Epub 17 Sept 2014.
32. Youn YH, Minami H, Chiu PW, Park H. Peroral endoscopic myotomy for treating achalasia and esophageal motility disorders. J Neurogastroenterol Motil. 2016;22(1):14–24. Epub 1 Jan 2016.
33. Sharata A, Kurian AA, Dunst CM, Bhayani NH, Reavis KM, Swanstrom LL. Peroral endoscopic myotomy (POEM) is safe and effective in the setting of prior endoscopic intervention. J Gastrointest Surg (Official Journal of the Society for Surgery of the Alimentary Tract). 2013;17(7):1188–92. Epub 24 Apr 2013.
34. Khashab MA, Messallam AA, Onimaru M, Teitelbaum EN, Ujiki MB, Gitelis ME, et al. International multicenter experience with peroral endoscopic myotomy for the treatment of spastic esophageal disorders refractory to medical therapy (with video). Gastrointest Endosc. 2015;81(5):1170–7. Epub 31 Jan 2015.
35. Chiu PW, Wu JC, Teoh AY, Chan Y, Wong SK, Liu SY, et al. Peroral endoscopic myotomy for treatment of achalasia: from bench to bedside (with video). Gastrointest Endosc. 2013;77(1):29–38. Epub 10 Oct 2012.
36. Swanstrom LL, Kurian A, Dunst CM, Sharata A, Bhayani N, Rieder E. Long-term outcomes of an endoscopic myotomy for achalasia: the POEM procedure. Ann Surg. 2012;256(4):659–67. Epub 18 Sept 2012.
37. Ren Y, Tang X, Chen F, Deng Z, Wu J, Nei S, et al. Myotomy of distal esophagus influences proximal esophageal contraction and upper esophageal sphincter relaxation in patients with achalasia after peroral endoscopic myotomy. J Neurogastroenterol Motil. 2016;22(1):78–85. Epub 16 Oct 2015.
38. Ren Y, Ke M, Fang X, Zhu L, Sun X, Wang Z, et al. Response of esophagus to high and low temperatures in patients with achalasia. J Neurogastroenterol Motil. 2012;18(4):391–8. Epub 30 Oct 2012.
39. Berzosa M, Villa N, El-Serag HB, Sejpal DV, Patel KK. Comparison of endoscopic ultrasound guided 22-gauge core needle with standard 25-gauge fine-needle aspiration for diagnosing solid pancreatic lesions. Endosc Ultrasound. 2015;4(1):28–33. Epub 20 Mar 2015.
40. Hoppo T, Thakkar SJ, Schumacher LY, Komatsu Y, Choe S, Shetty A, et al. A utility of peroral endoscopic myotomy (POEM) across the spectrum of esophageal motility disorders. Surg Endosc. 2016;30(1):233–44. Epub 8 Apr 2015.
41. Familiari P, Greco S, Gigante G, Cali A, Boskoski I, Onder G, et al. Gastroesophageal reflux disease after peroral endoscopic myotomy: analysis of clinical, procedural and functional factors, associated with gastroesophageal reflux disease and esophagitis. Dig Endosc (Official Journal of the Japan Gastroenterological Endoscopy Society). 2016;28(1):33–41. Epub 16 July 2015.
42. Campos GM, Vittinghoff E, Rabl C, Takata M, Gadenstatter M, Lin F, et al. Endoscopic and surgical treatments for achalasia: a systematic review and meta-analysis. Ann Surg. 2009;249(1):45–57. Epub 25 Dec 2008.
43. Richards WO, Torquati A, Holzman MD, Khaitan L, Byrne D, Lutfi R, et al. Heller myotomy versus Heller myotomy with Dor fundoplication for achalasia: a prospective randomized double-blind clinical trial. Ann Surg. 2004;240(3):405–12; discussion 12–5. Epub 21 Aug 2004.
44. Boeckxstaens GE, Zaninotto G, Richter JE. Achalasia. Lancet. 2014;383(9911):83–93. Epub 23 July 2013.
45. Shiwaku H, Inoue H, Sasaki T, Yamashita K, Ohmiya T, Takeno S, et al. A prospective analysis of GERD after POEM on anterior myotomy. Surg Endosc. 2015. Epub 30 Sept 2015.
46. Simic AP, Radovanovic NS, Skrobic OM, Raznatovic ZJ, Pesko PM. Significance of limited hiatal dissection in surgery for achalasia. J Gastrointest Surg (Official Journal of the Society for Surgery of the Alimentary Tract). 2010;14(4):587–93. Epub 25 Dec 2009.
47. Camilleri M, Bharucha AE, Farrugia G. Epidemiology, mechanisms, and management of diabetic gastroparesis. Clin Gastroenterol Hepatol (The Official Clinical Practice Journal of the American Gastroenterological Association). 2011;9(1):5–12; quiz e7. Epub 19 Oct 2010.
48. Hasler WL. Gastroparesis: symptoms, evaluation, and treatment. Gastroenterol Clin N Am. 2007;36 (3):619–47, ix. Epub 24 Oct 2007.
49. Hibbard ML, Dunst CM, Swanstrom LL. Laparoscopic and endoscopic pyloroplasty for gastroparesis results in sustained symptom improvement. J Gastrointest Surg (Official Journal of the Society for Surgery of the Alimentary Tract). 2011;15(9):1513–9. Epub 2 July 2011.
50. Camilleri M, Parkman HP, Shafi MA, Abell TL, Gerson L. Clinical guideline: management of gastroparesis. Am J Gastroenterol. 2013;108(1):18–37; quiz 8. Epub 14 Nov 2012.
51. Friedenberg FK, Palit A, Parkman HP, Hanlon A, Nelson DB. Botulinum toxin A for the treatment of delayed gastric emptying. Am J Gastroenterol. 2008;103(2):416–23. Epub 12 Dec 2007.
52. Arts J, Holvoet L, Caenepeel P, Bisschops R, Sifrim D, Verbeke K, et al. Clinical trial: a randomized-controlled crossover study of intrapyloric injection of botulinum toxin in gastroparesis. Aliment Pharmacol Ther. 2007;26(9):1251–8. Epub 20 Oct 2007.
53. Chu H, Lin Z, Zhong L, McCallum RW, Hou X. Treatment of high-frequency gastric electrical stimulation for gastroparesis. J Gastroenterol Hepatol. 2012;27(6):1017–26. Epub 2 Dec 2011.
54. Khashab MA, Besharati S, Ngamruengphong S, Kumbhari V, El Zein M, Stein EM, et al. Refractory gastroparesis can be successfully managed with

endoscopic transpyloric stent placement and fixation (with video). Gastrointest Endosc. 2015;82(6):1106–9. Epub 9 Aug 2015.

55. Clarke JO, Sharaiha RZ, Kord Valeshabad A, Lee LA, Kalloo AN, Khashab MA. Through-the-scope transpyloric stent placement improves symptoms and gastric emptying in patients with gastroparesis. Endoscopy. 2013;45 Suppl 2 UCTN:E189–90. Epub 5 July 2013.
56. Kawai M, Peretta S, Burckhardt O, Dallemagne B, Marescaux J, Tanigawa N. Endoscopic pyloromyotomy: a new concept of minimally invasive surgery for pyloric stenosis. Endoscopy. 2012;44(2):169–73. Epub 25 Jan 2012.
57. Khashab MA, Stein E, Clarke JO, Saxena P, Kumbhari V, Chander Roland B, et al. Gastric peroral endoscopic myotomy for refractory gastroparesis: first human endoscopic pyloromyotomy (with video). Gastrointest Endosc. 2013;78(5):764–8. Epub 15 Oct 2013.
58. Gonzalez JM, Vanbiervliet G, Vitton V, Benezech A, Lestelle V, Grimaud JC, et al. First European human gastric peroral endoscopic myotomy, for treatment of refractory gastroparesis. Endoscopy. 2015;47 Suppl 1 UCTN:E135–6. Epub 11 Apr 2015.
59. Chaves DM, de Moura EG, Mestieri LH, Artifon EL, Sakai P. Endoscopic pyloromyotomy via a gastric submucosal tunnel dissection for the treatment of gastroparesis after surgical vagal lesion. Gastrointest Endosc. 2014;80(1):164. Epub 20 May 2014.
60. Bapaye A, Dubale N, Pujari R, Kulkarni A, Jajoo Naval R, Vyas V, et al. Peroral endoscopic pyloromyotomy for delayed postoperative gastroparesis. Endoscopy. 2015;47(S 01):E581–2. Epub 10 Dec 2015.
61. Chung H, Dallemagne B, Perretta S, Lee SK, Shin SK, Park JC, et al. Endoscopic pyloromyotomy for postesophagectomy gastric outlet obstruction. Endoscopy. 2014;46 Suppl 1 UCTN:E345–6. Epub 5 Aug 2014.
62. Jung Y, Lee J, Gromski MA, Kato M, Rodriguez S, Chuttani R, et al. Assessment of the length of myotomy in peroral endoscopic pyloromyotomy (G-POEM) using a submucosal tunnel technique (video). Surg Endosc. 2015;29(8):2377–84. Epub 27 Nov 2014.
63. Shlomovitz E, Pescarus R, Cassera MA, Sharata AM, Reavis KM, Dunst CM, et al. Early human experience with per-oral endoscopic pyloromyotomy (POP). Surg Endosc. 2015;29(3):543–51. Epub 12 Aug 2014.

Flexible Endoscopic Zenker's Diverticulotomy

8

Vikram Budhraja and David J. Desilets

Abstract

Zenker's diverticulum (ZD) often presents with symptoms of dysphagia, regurgitation, choking, and coughing. Opcn approaches to repairing the diverticulum have been plagued by high morbidity, leaving surgeons to search for other alternatives. Rigid endoscopic approaches are typically safe and produce good results, although they require the use of a diverticuloscope and the need for the patient to extend their neck. Using lessons learned from per-oral endoscopic myotomy (POEM), flexible endoscopic approaches have begun to be described. Although highly operator dependent, the flexible approach may have the highest success rate and the lowest morbidity rate.

Keywords

Zenker's diverticulum · Surgery · Myotomy · Endoscopy

Abbreviations

APC	Argon plasma coagulator
CP	Cricopharyngeal
ENT	Otorhinolaryngology ("ear, nose, and throat")
ESD	Endoscopic submucosal dissection
NG	Nasogastric
NPO	Nil per os
NOTES	Natural orifice, translumenal, endoscopic surgery
POEM	Per-oral endoscopic myotomy
ZD	Zenker's diverticulum

V. Budhraja · D.J. Desilets (✉)
Gastroenterology Division, Department of Medicine, Baystate Health, 759 Chestnut Street, Springfield, MA 01199, USA
e-mail: david.desilets@baystatehealth.org

V. Budhraja
e-mail: vikram.budhrajaMD@baystatehealth.org

J.R. Romanelli et al. (eds.), *NOTES and Endoluminal Surgery*, Clinical Gastroenterology, DOI 10.1007/978-3-319-50610-4_8

Background, Anatomy, Definition of Zenker's Diverticulum

Zenker's diverticulum (ZD) was first described in 1769 by Abraham Ludlow, but was subsequently named by German pathologist Freidrich Albert von Zenker after he published a series of 28 patients with the disorder in 1877 [1, 2].

A ZD is a pouch that may form in the posterior hypopharynx through a relative weakness in the area known as Killian's triangle. Autopsy studies show that the presence and size of Killian's triangle is correlated with male gender and anthropomorphic measurements [3]. Although often thought of as an esophageal diverticulum, it is neither esophageal, nor a true diverticulum. The pouch is thought to form through pulsion forces in the hypopharynx coupled with decreased compliance of the cricopharyngeus muscle, as fibrosis of the muscle increases with age [4]. Decreased cricopharyngeal (CP) compliance results in increased pressure during swallowing in the hypopharynx which, over time, can lead to a protrusion or herniation of the pharyngeal wall above the cricopharyngeus muscle (and therefore, above the esophagus) and below the inferior pharyngeal constrictor muscles (within Killian's triangle) (Fig. 8.1). A true diverticulum contains all layers of the parent organ, typically also involving serosa for intestinal diverticula. ZD is composed of only mucosa and submucosa and, therefore, is not a true diverticulum.

Clinical Manifestations

Zenker's diverticula are relatively rare, with an incidence of symptomatic disease estimated at 2 per 100,000, and seem to have a higher incidence in populations from northern European decent [5, 6]. Most symptomatic patients are men over the age of 60. It generally presents with transient oropharyngeal dysphagia, but as the pouch

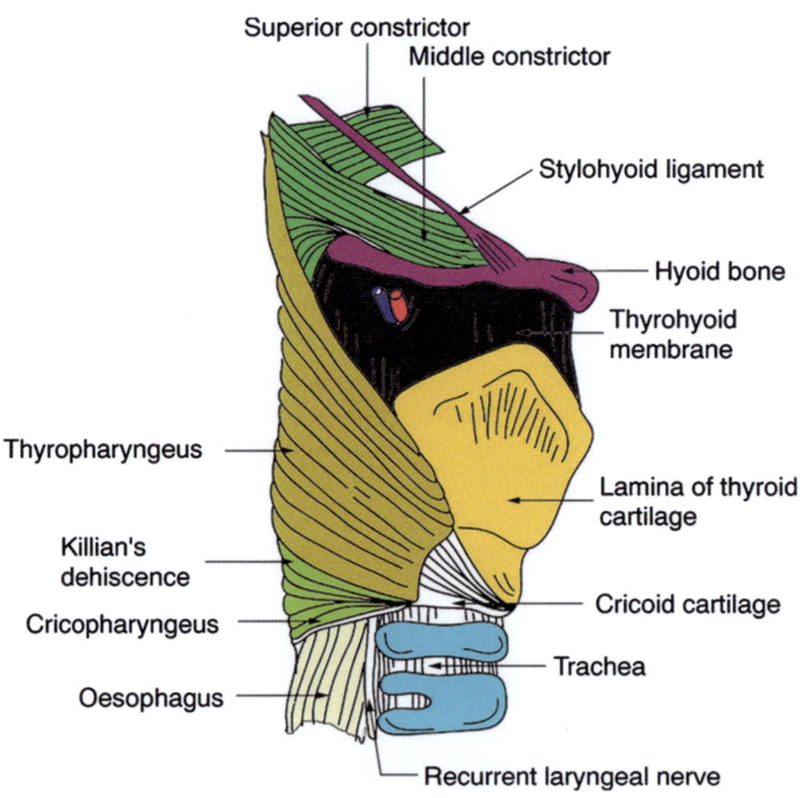

Fig. 8.1 Schematic of Killian's triangle

enlarges and becomes the preferential route of ingested food, symptoms generally become more regular and severe. While dysphagia is the most common symptom, 60% will have regurgitation, 30–40% cough, and 20% choking, hoarseness, weight loss, or a globus sensation [7]. Large diverticula can be palpated on neck examination (more often on the left) and may even show Boyce's sign (a splashing sound from fluid within the diverticulum). Bleeding or localized pain is less common and should alert the clinician to the possibility of ulceration or malignant transition, with squamous cell carcinoma having an incidence of approximately 1% in ZD [8, 9].

Approach to Management

Open Surgical

Historically, treatment of ZD has evolved from surgical to rigid endoscopic and now to flexible endoscopic approaches. Early treatment was often diverticulectomy through a neck incision. As understanding of pathophysiology evolved, it became apparent that increased hypopharyngeal bolus pressures were a result of decreased compliance of the cricopharyngeus muscle and that disruption of the muscle was necessary to prevent recurrence [10]. With the open approach, pouches >5 cm in length are often excised with stapled closure of the defect. Pouches 25–50 mm are often treated with diverticulopexy and CP myotomy. Smaller diverticula may be treated with diverticulopexy or just CP myotomy alone. The open approach is associated with a 10.5% rate of morbidity, but good success rates, with resolution of symptoms in about 95% of patients [11].

Rigid Endoscopic

The rigid transoral approach utilizes a diverticuloscope, which acts as a speculum with its long blade in the esophagus and its short blade in the diverticulum, exposing the common wall. Division of the common wall (including the cricopharyngeus) is then performed using anything from electrocautery, carbon dioxide laser, ultrasonic dissection, or stapling [11]. The idea is to incise the common wall (formed at the top by the cricopharyngeus muscle and perpetuated by the adhesion of the posterior esophageal wall to the anterior aspect of the diverticular sac) (Fig. 8.2). The diverticulum thus becomes contiguous with the posterior wall of the esophagus. Comprehensive reviews of this approach confirmed similar rates of clinical success compared to the open approach (90%), but with slightly lower morbidity (7%), and so this methodology has become the current standard [11].

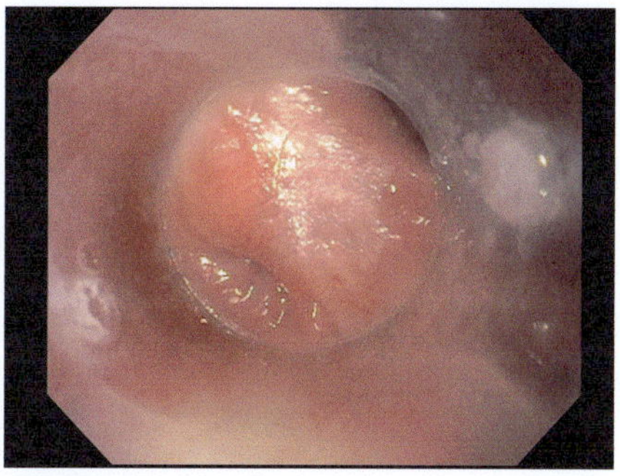

Fig. 8.2 Endoscopic view of the septum between the true and false lumen

Flexible Endoscopic

Some patients may not be candidates for the rigid transoral approach for anatomic reasons such as inadequate neck mobility, upper teeth protrusion, or inadequate jaw opening. Flexible endoscopic techniques have emerged, especially over the last decade, utilizing a variety of technologies. The first case was performed in 1982, but recently there has been a resurgence of interest as an exploding array of endoscopic tools has become available [12, 13]. Prophylactic antibiotics are frequently used, and patients are kept nil per os (NPO) prior to the procedure. The use of a soft diverticuloscope improves maneuverability and is associated with a lower risk of perforation and a higher likelihood of technical success on the first procedure [14] (Fig. 8.3). Another option

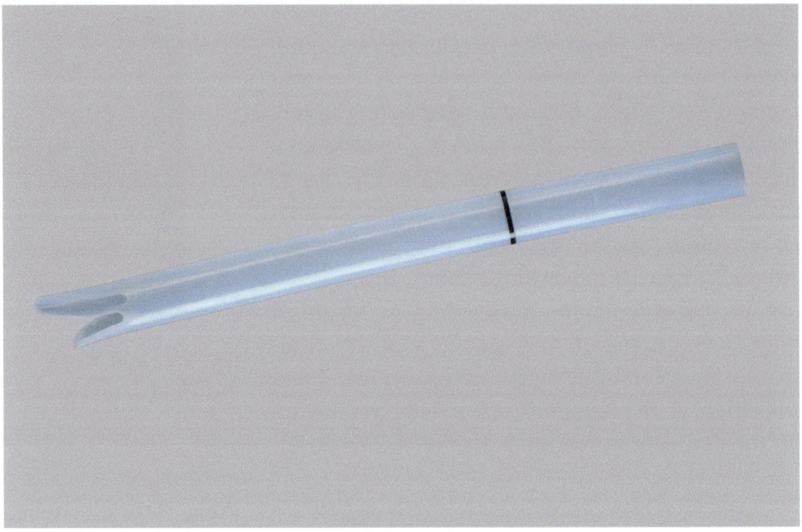

Fig. 8.3 Flexible diverticuloscope (photograph courtesy of Cook Medical, Winston-Salem, NC)

would be to utilize a transparent cap that can be attached to the tip of the endoscope, as is often done in endoscopic submucosal dissection (ESD). A guidewire or nasogastric tube may be placed in the stomach, which also serves to guide the incision from the diverticulum to the esophageal lumen, although we find it is typically not necessary. A variety of endoscopic tools can be used to incise the common wall, including a needle knife (multiple manufacturers), the Hybrid Knife® (Erbe USA, Marietta, GA), Hook Knife™ (Olympus America, Center Valley, PA), hot biopsy forceps, or argon plasma coagulator (APC™) (Erbe USA). No particular incisional device was found to be superior, but most studies have been relatively small and underpowered to detect these differences [15]. The most important landmark to identify is the muscular septum between the true lumen and false lumen. The incision is begun with a mucosotomy performed over the cricopharyngeus muscle (Fig. 8.4). This exposes the underlying muscle (Fig. 8.5). All muscle fibers are then divided to complete the myotomy (Fig. 8.6). The incision is then carried down further until the septum is completely incised. An endoscopic clip is typically placed at the vertex of the incision and is thought to decrease the risk of subsequent perforation, or the incision is closed on both sides with multiple clips (Fig. 8.7). Patients are either NPO or

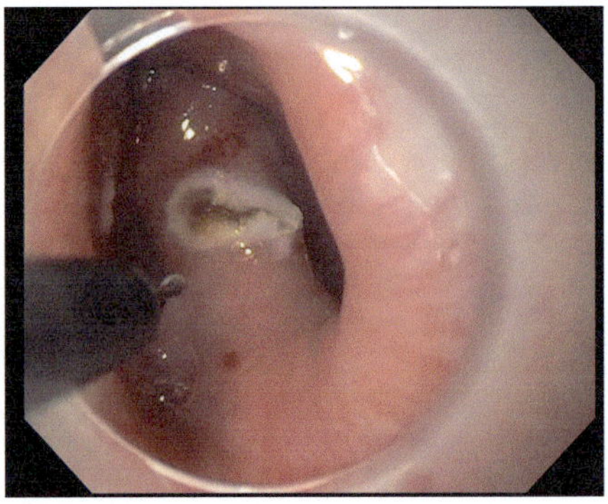

Fig. 8.4 Endoscopic view of the mucosal opening over the cricopharyngeal septum

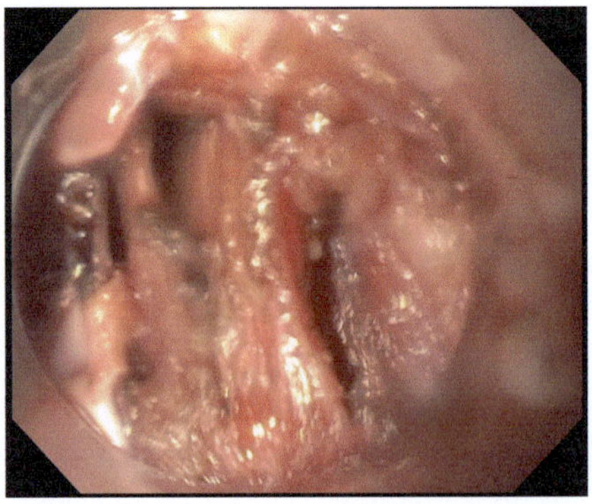

Fig. 8.5 Endoscopic view of the exposed cricopharyngeal muscle fibers

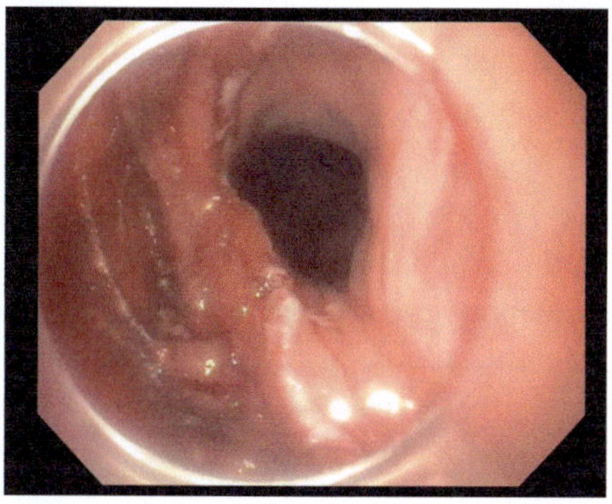

Fig. 8.6 Endoscopic view of the completed division of the muscular septum

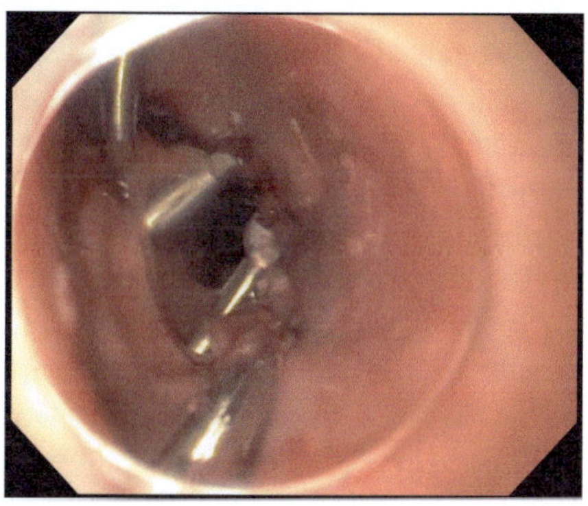

Fig. 8.7 Endoscopic view of the completed diverticulotomy, with mucosal clips closing the mucosa

allowed to have liquids post-procedure, and the diet is generally advanced that evening or the next day. Barium swallow evaluations were historically obtained after septotomy, but findings generally did not correlate well with clinical outcomes [16]. Therefore, some surgeons are abandoning this practice.

Great technological variety has lead to significant heterogeneity in the published literature regarding flexible endoscopic therapy, but overwhelmingly results are at least comparable to other modalities. A recent publication found that septotomy length ≤ 25 mm and diverticulum size ≥ 50 mm were associated with clinical failure at 6 months [17]. Post-procedural radiographic appearance does not correlate well with symptoms as noted above, but the presence of a post-treatment diverticulum ≥ 10 mm was associated with clinical failure at 48 months. Success rates were best for diverticula measuring 30–49 mm and a septotomy >25 mm with 100% clinical success at 6 months.

A recent meta-analysis identified 20 studies of flexible endoscopic treatment of ZD, including 813 total patients [15]. Pooled success rates were 91%, recurrence rates were 11%, and the adverse events rate was 11.6%. All of these parameters showed heterogeneity. Lower rates of adverse events were seen in larger studies. Clinical success rates correlated with the year of publication, with publications since 2006 having a pooled success rate of 97%. These data support the conclusion that flexible endoscopic treatment is rapidly evolving and highly operator dependent with success and complication rates that rival other modalities.

Discussion

Treatment results appear to be acceptable with any method of treatment, and absolute differences in complication rates are small. As treatment modalities evolved from open surgical, to rigid endoscopic, to flexible endoscopic approaches, so too did the operator from surgeon, to ENT specialist, to endoscopist. Experts continue to be divided in their opinion, mostly advocating for the modality with which they are most familiar [7, 13]. This is understandable, as the procedure appears to be highly operator dependent, and the most important factor in achieving good treatment results may be the operator rather than the modality.

Some of the purported advantages of a flexible endoscopic approach include decreased costs and shorter postoperative length of stay. Since studies of endoscopic therapy are highly variable, it seems likely that further experience will result in better outcomes. The use of the diverticuloscope in the flexible endoscopic approach is associated with improved completion rates and reduced perforation rates [17]. It enhances visibility but may also limit septotomy to the cricopharyngeus, which is readily visible. The needle knife has been used for most large series; this is used with a downward cutting action and can make it harder to control the extent of dissection. A Hook Knife or similar device can be used to identify and lift muscle fibers away from the septum, resulting in a more controlled dissection, as is often done in per-oral endoscopic myotomy (POEM). Suturing devices may offer better closure of the severed septum, but the apparatus can be unwieldy and difficult to maneuver in the tight spaces of the hypopharynx [18].

The incision should be carried out to the bottom extent of the pouch to eliminate the diverticulum completely. Some authors favor a more conservative approach and leave a small "residual pouch" so as to avoid extending the dissection too deep [17]. These authors report low perforation rates, but also reported lower clinical success rates than other series utilizing flexible endoscopic therapy. Though not yet specifically studied, the use of clips to close the cut edges and/or vertex of the incision is thought to be a significant advance in the prevention of leakage resulting in mediastinitis.

Not all endoscopists will be technically equipped with the tools and expertise necessary to perform this advanced procedure. Those who incorporate it will likely have familiarity with other advanced endoscopic techniques such as ESD or POEM, as these techniques utilize similar instruments and involve similar dissection techniques. The porcine model offers an excellent opportunity for interested endoscopists to practice the technique, as pigs have a normal anatomical pharyngeal pouch similar to a Zenker's diverticulum that also permits an analogous septotomy [19]. Once a particular team has developed an optimized technique, results generally continue to improve, reflecting the learning curve of the procedure. As such, there may be little incentive to change techniques. Great thought and care should be invested in preparing to offer this procedure so as to find techniques that work well for the providers, assistants, and institution involved.

True mastery of flexible endoscopic Zenker's treatment will hinge not just on achieving an adequate septotomy with low rates of complications, but also on appropriate management of complications, both common and rare. The two potentially life-threatening adverse events that may occur with flexible endoscopic treatment of ZD are bleeding and perforation. Bleeding can virtually always be managed endoscopically. Perforation can usually be managed conservatively (keeping the patient NPO and giving prophylactic antibiotics) [15].

Although the majority of patients with a Zenker's diverticulum may be candidates for flexible endoscopic therapy, determining the optimal treatment modality remains a subject of debate. The diverticulum is usually located below the cricopharyngeus and adheres to the posterior wall of the esophagus, but rarely, it may protrude caudally [20]. If it is not located in the typical anatomic position, endoscopic therapy should not be attempted. Small diverticula (<30 mm) may be difficult to visualize especially without the use of a diverticuloscope. Additionally, if the diverticulum is too small, the septotomy may be carried to the end of the diverticulum while still not having completely transected the CP muscle. This may lead to continued elevation of hypopharyngeal pressures and recurrence of the diverticulum. Indeed, a septotomy <25 mm was identified as a poor prognostic factor for flexible endoscopic therapy [17].

Therapy for small diverticula might best remain surgical so as to allow complete myotomy. This limitation could potentially be overcome utilizing ESD techniques to complete the myotomy even below the extent of the diverticulum. Finally, with small diverticula, careful clinical assessment is needed to ensure that symptoms are in fact related to the diverticulum, as it can be an incidental finding in patients with dysphagia from other etiologies.

In large diverticula (>50 mm), even a longer septotomy may not result in complete obliteration of the pouch and may leave a residual pouch. The pouch, having become the new posterior wall of the esophagus, is aperistaltic and may itself result in similar symptoms of dysphagia with incomplete clinical resolution. Therefore, some favor surgical myotomy with diverticulectomy or diverticulopexy for these patients, which preserves the integrity of proximal esophageal body. Flexible endoscopic therapy may have found its niche in the 30–50 mm range, with the best-reported clinical outcomes for patients with these sized diverticula [17].

Tips and Tricks

We now prefer to use the Hook Knife™ rather than fashioning a homemade hook cautery or using the Hybrid Knife®. We have found that using a cap-fitted endoscope provides the best results when ease of performance of the procedure is the goal. The upper esophageal sphincter area and the proximal esophagus are already anatomically tight areas in which to work, with little space to maneuver the endoscope. Having a transparent cap allows redundant or constricting tissue to be pushed aside while still maintaining a good endoscopic view. The cap also provides assistance with mucosal clipping. The endoscopic clip can be positioned half way out of the cap and in proper orientation to appose the mucosal edges. Then, suction can be applied, prolapsing the mucosa into the cap and making it easier for the clip to grab the edges. Occasionally, a nasogastric tube or guidewire in the true esophageal lumen can assist with the procedure, acting variably as a landmark or as a backstop against which to cut the septum. It is useful to have coagulation forceps or hot biopsy forceps on hand, unopened, so that they can be quickly employed in the case of significant bleeding.

Conclusion

Treatment of ZD has made dramatic advances over the years, and we are poised to be able to offer most patients therapy with a flexible endoscopic approach. The two main goals of therapy—severing the septum between esophagus and diverticulum and performing myotomy of the cricopharyngeus muscle—can be obtained in most patients with ZD. Early experience with this technique seems to support comparable success rates and similar or lower adverse event rates as compared to an open surgical approach. Flexible endoscopic approaches will likely become the new standard, leaving little advantage to performing rigid endoscopic septotomy. Surgical intervention will remain relevant, as it may still be the preferred modality to manage the both very small and very large diverticula. Flexible endoscopic techniques will continue to evolve, and the addition of dissection techniques may allow for even better technical and clinical success.

References

1. Ludlow A. A case of obstructed deglutition from a preternatural dilatation of, and bag formed in, the pharynx. Med Observ Inq 1769;3:85–101.
2. von Zenker FA, von Ziemssen H. Krankheiten des Oesophagus. In: von Ziemssen H, editor. Handbuch der Speciellen Pathologie und Therapie. Leipzig: FC Vogel; 1877. p. 1–87.
3. Anagiotos A, Preuss SF, Koebke J. Morphometric and anthropometric analysis of Killian's triangle. Laryngoscope. 2010;120:1082–8.
4. Cook IJ, Gabb M, Panagopoulos V, Jamieson GG, Dodds WJ, et al. Pharyngeal (Zenker's) diverticulum is a disorder of upper esophageal sphincter opening. Gastroenterology. 1992;103:1229–35.
5. Laing MR, Murthy P, Ah-See KW, Cockburn JS. Surgery for pharyngeal pouch: audit of management with short- and long-term followup. J R Coll Surg Edinb. 1995;40:315–8.
6. van Overbeek JJ. Meditation on the pathogenesis of hypopharyngeal (Zenker's) diverticulum and a report of endoscopic treatment in 545 patients. Ann Otol Rhinol Laryngol. 1994;103:178–85.
7. Lerut T, Coosemans W, Decaluwe H, Decker G, De Leyn P, et al. Zenker's diverticulum. Multimedia Manual of Cardiothoracic Surgery. 2009;224:2881.
8. Odemis B, Ataseven H, Basar O, Ertugrul I, Yüksel O, et al. Ulcer in the basis of Zenker's diverticulum mimicking esophageal malignancy. J Natl Med Assoc. 2006;98:1177–80.
9. Bradley PJ, Kochaar A, Quraishi MS. Pharyngeal pouch carcinoma: real or imaginary risks? Ann OtolRhinolLaryngol. 1999;108:1027–32.
10. Ellis FH Jr, Sclegel JF, Lynch VP, Payne WS. Cricopharyngeal myotomy for pharyngo-esophageal diverticulum. Ann Surg. 1969;170:340–9.
11. Yuan Y, Zhao YF, Hu Y, Chen LQ. Surgical treatment of Zenker's diverticulum. Dig Surg. 2013;30:214–25.
12. Ishioka S, Sakai P, Maluf-Filho F, Melo JM. Endoscopic incision of Zenker's diverticulum: a new approach. Endoscopy. 1995;27:438–42.

13. Law R, Katzka DA, Baron TH. Zenker's diverticulum. Clin Gastro Hep. 2014;12:1773–82; quiz 1773–82.
14. Costamagna G, Iacopini F, Tringali A, Marchese M, Spada C, et al. Flexible endoscopic Zenker's diverticulotomy: cap-assisted technique vs. diverticuloscope-assisted technique. Endoscopy. 2007;39:146–52.
15. Ishaq S, Hassan C, Antonello A, Tanner K, Bellisario C, et al. Flexible endoscopic treatment for Zenker's diverticulum: a systematic review and meta-analysis. Gastrointest Endosc. 2016 Jan 21; Epub ahead of print.
16. Mantsopoulos K, Psychogios G, Karatzanis A, Künzel J, Lell M, et al. Clinical relevance and prognostic value of radiographic findings in Zenker's diverticulum. Eur Arch Otorhinolaryngol. 2014;271: 583–8.
17. Costamagna G, Iacopini F, Bizzotto A, Familiari P, Tringali A, et al. Prognostic variables for the clinical success of flexible endoscopic septotomy of Zenker's diverticulum. Gastrointest Endosc. 2016;83:765–73.
18. Sakai Paulo. Endoscopic myotomy of Zenker's diverticulum: lessons from 3 decades of experience. Gastrointest Endosc. 2016;83(4):774.
19. Seaman DL, de la Mora Levy J, Gostout CJ, Rajan E, Herman L, et al. An animal training model for endoscopic treatment of Zenker's diverticulum. Gastrointest Endosc. 2007;65:1050–3.
20. Nehring P, Ireneusz W. Krasnodębski. Zenker's diverticulum: aetiopathogenesis, symptoms and diagnosis. Comparison of operative methods. Przeglad Gastroenterologiczny 8.5 (2013):284–289. PMC. Web. 1 Apr 2016.

Per-oral Endoscopic Pyloromyotomy

9

Eran Shlomovitz, Kristel Lobo Prabhu
and Kevin M. Reavis

Abstract

Given the initial enthusiasm for per-oral endoscopic myotomy (POEM), surgeons and endoscopists began to search for other applications for the technique. Gastroparesis is a motility disorder of the stomach which is often refractory to medical therapy. Other options for treatment include endoscopic options such as botox injection or transpyloric stenting, gastric electrical stimulation, and surgical therapy such as laparoscopic pyloroplasty. Recently, surgeons have begun to apply POEM inspired techniques to the pylorus in an attempt to perform a transluminal pyloromyotomy. Although early series are small and limited largely to case reports, the early data is encouraging for this nascent procedure.

Keywords

Per-oral pyloromyotomy (POP) · Gastroparesis · Per-oral endoscopic myotomy (POEM) · Natural orifice translumenal endoscopic surgery (NOTES) · Surgical endoscopy · Motility

Abbreviations

GES	Gastric emptying study
GCSI	Gastroparesis cardinal symptom index
NSAIDs	Nonsteroidal anti-inflammatory drugs
PAGI-SYM	Patient assessment of upper gastrointestinal disorders–symptom severity index
POEM	Per-oral endoscopic myotomy

E. Shlomovitz (✉)
Toronto General Hospital, PMB 1-298, 585 University Avenue, Toronto, ON, Canada
e-mail: eran.shlomovitz@uhn.ca

K.L. Prabhu
Department of Surgery, University Health Network, Toronto, ON M5V 4A1, Canada
e-mail: kristelprabhu@gmail.com

K.M. Reavis
Division of Gastrointestinal and Minimally Invasive Surgery, Foregut and Bariatric Surgery, The Oregon Clinic, 4805 NE Glisan Street, Ste 6N60, Portland, OR 97213, USA
e-mail: kreavis@orclinic.com

J.R. Romanelli et al. (eds.), *NOTES and Endoluminal Surgery*,
Clinical Gastroenterology, DOI 10.1007/978-3-319-50610-4_9

POP	Per-oral pyloromyotomy
PPI	Proton pump inhibitor
PSG	Postsurgical gastroparesis
WMC	Wireless motility capsules

Introduction

Gastroparesis is a motility disorder of the stomach characterized by objectively delayed gastric emptying in the absence of mechanical obstruction [1]. The most common symptoms associated with this condition include nausea, vomiting, and early satiety [1]. Postprandial fullness and abdominal pain have also been reported [2]. The magnitude of delay in gastric emptying does not, however, correlate well with symptom severity [3]. Symptoms may be chronic or manifest as episodic flares [2]. In severe cases of gastroparesis, these symptoms can be debilitating and result in weight loss, malnutrition, and dehydration [2]. The gastroparesis cardinal symptom index (GCSI) is a validated patient-rated symptom assessment tool used in the assessment of disease severity and for monitoring treatment outcomes [4]. GCSI scores are based on the combined results of the nausea/vomiting, postprandial fullness/early satiety, and bloating subscales of the patient assessment of upper gastrointestinal disorders–symptom severity index (PAGI-SYM) [4]. This tool does not, however, take into account the impact of pain on disease severity.

The incidence of gastroparesis is estimated at 2.4 per 100,000 person-years for men and 9.8 for women [5]. The age-adjusted prevalence of gastroparesis per 10,000 persons is estimated at 9.6 for men and 37.8 for women [5].

The underlying etiology of gastroparesis remains unknown in the majority of patients. Known contributing etiologies for gastroparesis include diabetes and postsurgical gastroparesis [6]. When gastroparesis occurs as a result of diabetes mellitus, the cumulative incidence of the condition is 4.8% in type 1 and 1% in type 2 diabetics [7]. Diabetic gastroparesis is typically late in onset and develops more than 10 years after disease onset [7]. Diabetic patients with gastroparesis are also more likely to have cardiovascular disease, hypertension, and retinopathy, indicating that the underlying pathology may be due to micro- and macroangiopathy [8].

Postsurgical gastroparesis (PSG) is typically seen in the setting of prior foregut gastrointestinal or thoracic surgery and is thought to result from the disruption of the vagus nerve resulting in impaired gastric emptying [9]. The surgical management of peptic ulcer disease has been associated with the development of gastroparesis. This, however, has declined significantly with the introduction of proton pump inhibitors (PPI) and is now largely of historical significance. Currently, Nissen fundoplication is the surgical procedure most commonly linked to the development of gastroparesis [2]. This underlines the need for careful dissection, identification, and preservation of the vagus nerves in any procedure involving the dissection of the hiatus and esophagus.

Post-viral gastroparesis is also thought to occur, with some patients describing the onset of gastroparesis following a viral prodrome. Viral or post-viral, immune-related injury to the innervation of the stomach or the interstitial cells of Cajal has been proposed as a possible mechanism for this etiology of gastroparesis [2]. These cases of gastroparesis that follow an infectious prodrome may gradually improve over time [1].

Multiple medications have also been implicated in delayed gastric emptying. These include narcotics, tricyclic antidepressants, anticholinergics, and calcium channel blockers [10].

Finally, a multitude of medical conditions can result or contribute to gastroparesis including, thyroid dysfunction, neurologic disease, and autoimmune disorders [1].

The pathophysiology of gastroparesis has not been well elucidated. Gastric emptying occurs via a complex interaction between smooth muscle, enteric and extrinsic autonomic nerves, and the interstitial cell of Cajal [11]. The two most important currently accepted mechanisms for the development of gastroparesis include the loss of expression of neuronal nitric oxide synthase (the function of which is control of the muscle tone of the lower esophageal sphincter, the pylorus, the sphincter of Oddi, and the anus) and loss of the interstitial cells of Cajal [11]. In diabetic patients, hyperglycemia-related stimulation of pyloric contraction may be an additional mechanism resulting in delayed gastric emptying [12].

Diagnostic Workup

A thorough history and physical examination are the first steps in the diagnostic workup of gastroparesis. History taking will help identify the nature and severity of symptoms as well as elucidate reversible causes such as medications, rumination syndromes, and eating disorders that may mimic gastroparesis [3]. Orthostatic hypotension (related to autonomic neuropathy and severe dehydration) and a succussion splash may occasionally be demonstrated on physical examination [3]. Upper gastrointestinal endoscopy is an essential part of the workup and is used to rule out the presence of an obstructive lesion or any other gastric or proximal small bowel abnormalities [13]. The results of endoscopy may be supplemented with the use of cross-sectional imaging in the form of computed tomography or magnetic resonance enterography [3]. Electrolyte abnormalities such as hypokalemia, hypercalcemia, and hypomagnesemia may cause acute, reversible gastroparesis. Thus, serum electrolyte levels should be monitored as a part of the diagnostic evaluation [3].

Once mechanical obstruction has been excluded, the next step in the diagnostic assessment is the investigation of gastric motility. Four-hour gastric emptying scintigraphy of a solid-phase meal is the gold standard test used to objectively demonstrate delayed gastric emptying and to make the diagnosis of gastroparesis. A technetium 99-m sulfur colloid-labeled test meal is used by most centers for scintigraphy studies. Delayed gastric emptying is defined as retention greater than 60% at two hours, or greater than 10% at 4 h postprandially [14]. Medications that affect gastric emptying must be stopped 48 h prior to testing. Since hyperglycemia delays gastric emptying in diabetics, testing should be delayed until relative euglycemia has been achieved [1].

^{13}C breath testing has been proposed as an alternative to scintigraphy. In this test, the patient ingests a test meal containing ^{13}C substrates. Gastric emptying is the rate-limiting step in the absorption of the ^{13}C isotopes from the small intestine and therefore affects the rate of detection of expired ^{13}C [3]. This carbon breath test has been found to have a sensitivity of 86% and a specificity of 80% [15]. Breath testing also has the advantage of being less expensive and technically complex than scintigraphy and does not expose the patient to ionizing radiation [3]. This test, however, has not been validated in patients with impaired respiratory function and small intestinal disease [3].

Wireless motility capsules (WMC) have also been developed which measure intraluminal pH and determine the timing of gastric emptying through the rapid rise in pH that occurs during the transfer from the acidic environment of the stomach to the alkaline duodenum [1]. The overall correlation between WMC and the gold standard 4-h gastric emptying scintigraphy has been demonstrated to be about 0.73 [16].

Once the diagnosis of gastroparesis has been established using the diagnostic approach outlined above, investigation into the etiology must begin. This involves biochemical screening tests for diabetes mellitus, thyroid dysfunction, and autoimmune disease. In cases where the etiology remains unclear, gastroduodenal manometry may be used to distinguish between neuropathic (antral hypomotility, abnormal propagation of the migrating motor complex, and hypercontractility) and myopathic (low-amplitude contractions) disease processes [17].

Overview of Available Treatment Options for Gastroparesis

Medical Treatment

The first step in treatment is the correction of any fluid or metabolic abnormality resulting from ongoing emesis and poor oral intake. Oral hydration and vitamin supplementation are preferred; however, parenteral support may be needed in those with severe symptoms. Due to the risk of refeeding syndrome, close monitoring of electrolytes is recommended during this period [18]. Patients should receive counseling regarding dietary modification. Small, frequent meals low in fat and insoluble fiber are recommended [19]. Oral nutrition is the preferred route of feeding in this patient group. If oral nutrition is not tolerated, then post-pyloric feeding via a jejunostomy or gastrojejunostomy tube is recommended [1]. Parenteral nutrition is only used in cases where enteral nutrition cannot be maintained [1]. Glycemic control should be optimized in diabetic patients [7].

Medications that target the dopamine D_2 receptors are the first-line therapy in the treatment of gastroparesis. Metoclopramide is currently the only FDA-approved medication for the treatment of gastroparesis, with a recommendation that it not be used for a period exceeding 12 weeks due to the risk of irreversible tardive dyskinesia [20]. Metoclopramide has been shown to improve gastric motility and emptying as well as the symptoms of gastroparesis [18]. Domperidone, also a D_2 receptor antagonist, may be used in cases where metoclopramide is contraindicated. Domperidone should be avoided in patients with QT prolongation and is associated with a risk of sudden cardiac death [13]. Antiemetic medications may also be used in combination with prokinetic agents for the treatment of nausea and vomiting [3].

Macrolide antibiotics such as erythromycin and azithromycin exert their prokinetic effects through action on motilin receptors as well as cholinergic agonism of gastric smooth muscle [13]. The macrolides improve gastric emptying but are associated with tachyphylaxis, which may present 2 weeks after the onset of treatment [20]. Clonidine, an α_2-receptor agonist, has also shown some benefit in treating symptoms of bloating and early satiety in diabetic gastroparesis [3]. If pain is a major associated symptom, the use of nonsteroidal anti-inflammatory drugs (NSAIDs), such as indomethacin or ketorolac, may be considered [3], although one must consider the risk of ulcers and bleeding.

Tricyclic antidepressants have been observed to result in symptom reduction when used for the treatment of functional vomiting and diabetic gastroparesis. Other novel medical therapies such as ghrelin agonists and 5-HT_4 receptor agonists are currently being evaluated for the treatment of gastroparesis [20].

Endoscopic Treatment

Botulinum toxin blocks neurotransmitter release at peripheral cholinergic skeletal and smooth muscle nerve terminals [13]. Given this inhibitory effect on neuromuscular transmission, endoscopic botulinum injection was previously used in the treatment of gastroparesis with pylorospasm. However, randomized, controlled trials have failed to demonstrate the efficacy of this procedure, and it is no longer routinely recommended for the treatment of gastroparesis [21]. In patients with refractory gastroparesis, endoscopic placement of a transpyloric stent has been also been evaluated in small, open-label studies [20]. The stent is deployed over a guidewire under endoscopic visualization with the proximal flared end of the stent located in the antrum and the distal end in the duodenum proximal to the ampulla [20]. Stent migration remains one of the main challenges with this technique. Despite various anchoring techniques including clips or endoscopic suturing, stent migration remains a frequent occurrence.

Gastric electrical stimulation is also used for the compassionate treatment of gastroparesis in those who experience persistent symptoms and have failed prokinetic therapy [22]. Temporary gastric stimulators may be placed endoscopically to determine the response to electric stimulation prior to permanent surgical stimulator implantation [20].

Surgical Treatment

Laparoscopic pyloroplasty involves the horizontal division of the pylorus followed by vertical closure in a Heineke–Mikulicz fashion. Laparoscopic pyloroplasty was found to result in reduction in symptom severity, improved quality of life, and acceleration of gastric emptying in a retrospective study of 42 patients with refractory gastroparesis [23]. Toro et al. were also able to demonstrate an improvement in gastric emptying time following laparoscopic pyloroplasty in their study, which included 50 patients with refractory gastroparesis. This was accomplished with low morbidity associated with the procedure [24].

In patients with significant upper gastrointestinal symptoms, a venting gastrostomy may be placed with or without a feeding jejunostomy [1]. The jejunostomy serves as a conduit to maintain nutrition, hydration, and blood glucose. Its use should be considered in patients suffering from ongoing weight loss [25]. Wound breakdown and infection are the most common complications of this procedure [3]. In patients with refractory postsurgical gastroparesis, extensive subtotal or completion gastrectomy is the preferred surgical management [25]. While gastrectomy can offer symptom relief, this must be weighed against the risk of major surgery and malnutrition in this patient population [26].

Per-oral Pyloromyotomy

Despite the early excitement and research regarding natural orifice surgery in the early 2000s, most of the procedures have failed to catch on or gain mainstream acceptance. The technical difficulties in performing such procedures and the limited tools available have largely dampened the early enthusiasm. However, this was changed in 2007 with the introduction of the per-oral endoscopic myotomy (POEM) technique by Pasricha and colleagues. Their experimental work in 4 pig models demonstrated that a true esophageal myotomy, equivalent to what could be achieved surgically, can be safely performed endoscopically [27]. Esophageal manometry performed on the fifth postoperative day demonstrated a significant decrease in average lower esophageal sphincter pressures from 16.4 to 6.7 mmHg. This technique of endoscopically developing a submucosal tunnel followed by division of the circular muscles of the esophagus and lower esophageal sphincter using electrocautery was adapted shortly thereafter by Inoue et al. for use in humans. The description of the successful application of this technique in achalasia has revolutionized the surgical management of this condition [28]. Since the first four cases were described, thousands of patients around the world have successfully undergone the procedure. This newfound comfort with operating in the submucosal space sets off a search for new applications for this novel endoscopic technique. Endoscopic myotomy of the pylorus can therefore be thought of as a natural extension of the success of the POEM technique for achalasia.

Pyloric disruption by means of a surgical pyloroplasty has been previously well documented for the treatment of benign gastric outlet obstruction and gastroparesis. Although this technique has shown efficacy in the improvement of gastric emptying, it is associated with a risk of leakage and potential further narrowing of the gastric outlet through "frame shifting." Furthermore, as a surgical procedure, it carries all the risks of general anesthesia and requires advanced laparoscopic suturing skills. Therefore, the development of a less invasive yet reliable method of improving gastric emptying is highly desirable. The feasibility of per-oral endoscopic pyloromyotomy (POP) was demonstrated by Kawai and colleagues in animals [29]. Reduced pyloric pressure following the per-oral pyloromyotomy (POP) was demonstrated after the procedure, thus supporting the potential effectiveness of this concept whereby complete ablation of the pylorus may result in improved gastric emptying.

Technique

The per-oral pyloromyotomy technique is similar in its basic principles to the endoscopic submucosal dissection and myotomy techniques performed during a POEM procedure for achalasia. Routine preoperative antibiotics and steroids (8 mg IV Decadron) are given prior to the start of the procedure. The procedure is performed under general anesthesia with the patient in the supine position. Upper endoscopy is performed using a high-definition, forward-viewing gastroscope. Insufflation is obtained using low-flow carbon dioxide throughout the procedure. The stomach and proximal duodenum are carefully inspected and thoroughly lavaged of any retained gastric contents. A transparent dissection cap is then fitted onto the gastroscope, and an overtube is placed down the esophagus. A mucosotomy site is selected approximately 2–3 cm proximal to the pylorus on the posterior aspect of the greater curvature of the stomach. Mucosotomy is facilitated by a submucosal injection of a 5–10 cc lift solution (500 cc of normal saline mixed with 0.5 cc of 1:1000 epinephrine and 0.5 cc of methylene blue), creating a submucosal lift. A 1–2 cm longitudinal mucosal incision 1–2 cm in length is then performed with an endoscopic dissection knife using dry cut mode at 180 W, effect 4 (ERBE, Tubingen, Germany). To facilitate entry into the submucosal tunnel, the scope can be inserted over a 15-mm inflated biliary extraction balloon. Upon entry into the submucosal space, a submucosal tunnel is created using a submucosal dissection technique by dividing the loose submucosal areolar tissue with spray or forced coagulation. Tunneling can be made easier by repeated injections of the lifting solution using the distal injection port of the biliary extraction balloon to improve distention of the submucosal space and delineation of the layers. Dissection knives which incorporate an injection port are also available and may decrease the number of instrument exchanges required. Care must be taken not to injure the overlying mucosal layer. Therefore, the dissection proceeds along the deep submucosal level adjacent to the muscularis layer of the gastric wall (Fig. 9.1). Tunneling continues just past the pylorus and into the most proximal duodenal bulb. Scope orientation and the position of the pylorus can also be estimated by exiting the tunnel and observing the length dissected from the gastric lumen (Fig. 9.2).

Once the submucosal tunnel has been completed, the endoscopic myotomy is initiated roughly 2 cm proximal to the pylorus. No attempt is made to selectively divide a certain muscle layer (as in POEM) and a full-thickness myotomy of all muscle layers, and the pylorus is performed down to the serosa. The myotomy continues until the visible pyloric bar is fully divided as confirmed by its thinning into the duodenal musculature. Considerable care must

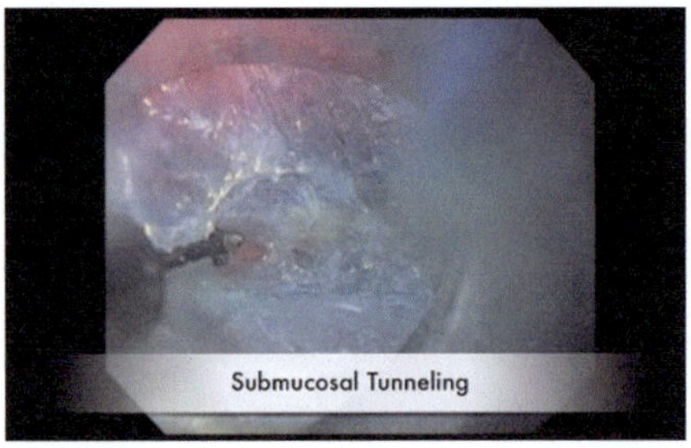

Fig. 9.1 Image of the submucosal tunnel during dissection

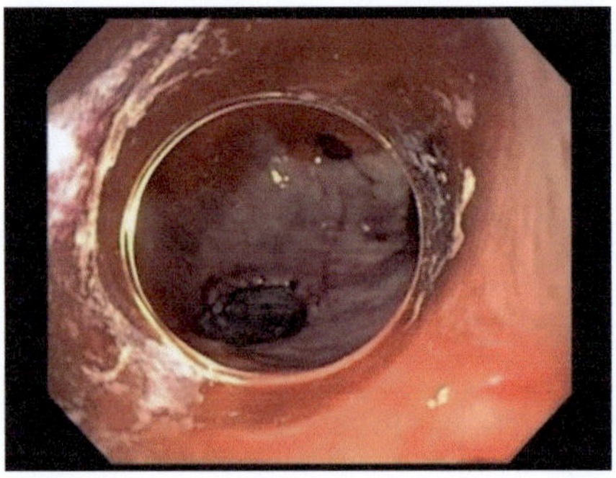

Fig. 9.2 Image of the view from the gastric lumen after the submucosal tunnel is completed

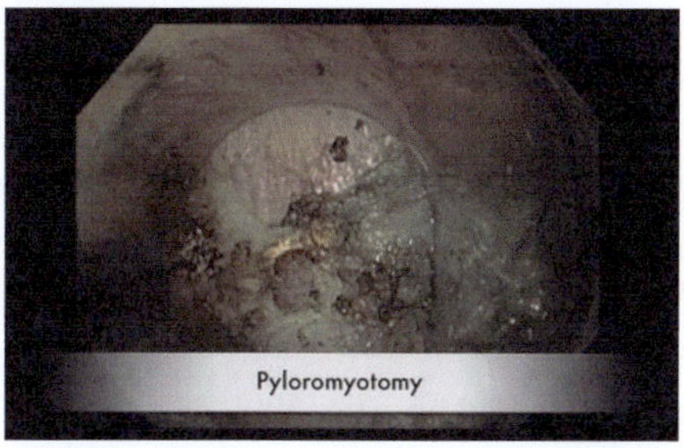

Fig. 9.3 Image of the pyloromyotomy, with duodenal mucosa visible

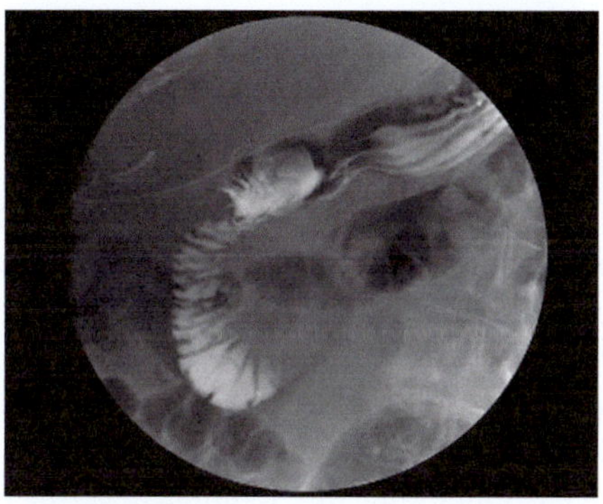

Fig. 9.4 UGI taken postoperative day #1, showing an open lumen and no leak

be taken when dividing the distal edge of the pylorus, as the duodenal mucosa drapes over in a perpendicular fashion (Fig. 9.3), thus increasing the risk of an inadvertent perforation of the duodenal mucosa. At the completion of the dissection, the tunnel is inspected for hemostasis, and the mucosotomy is closed using clips or an endoscopic suturing device.

Following the procedure, the patient is admitted for overnight observation. Diet is held until an upper GI series is performed the next day confirming adequate pyloric opening and absence of a leak (Fig. 9.4). If no complications are demonstrated, the patient is started on a clear liquid diet. A puree/soft diet is started the following day which the patient is asked to continue for a two-week period to avoid inadvertent clip dislodgement. A high-dose PPI is started following the procedure and continued for a period of 6 weeks. The patient then returns at 3 months postoperatively for follow-up endoscopy (Fig. 9.5) and a gastric emptying study.

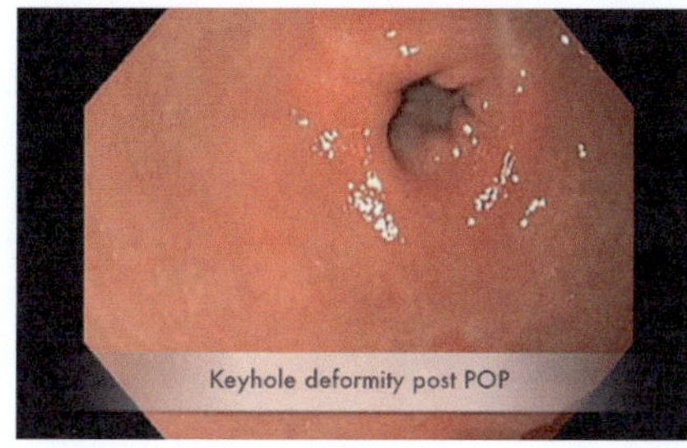

Fig. 9.5 Three-month postoperative endoscopy demonstrating a keyhole deformity of the pylorus in keeping with a recent pyloromyotomy

The first human experience with POP was reported by Khashab et al. [30]. A 27-year-old female with diabetic gastroparesis, daily symptoms of nausea and vomiting, and multiple admissions for refractory symptoms and dehydration was treated with POP. No complications were reported and objective and subjective results confirmed the success of treatment.

A subsequent early case series was reported by Shlomovitz et al. [31], documenting seven non-diabetic patients with refractory gastroparesis treated with the POP procedure. In this series, the most common cause of gastroparesis was idiopathic (n = 5). Two patients had PSG based on a history of prior foregut surgery. Six procedures were performed under laparoscopic guidance, given that patients required other concurrent laparoscopic procedures. A purely endoscopic procedure was performed in one patient who did not require additional laparoscopic procedures.

POP was technically successful in all seven cases, and there were no intraoperative adverse events. A delayed complication related to the procedure consisted of an upper GI bleed two weeks post-procedure, necessitating a blood transfusion. This occurred in a patient who did not comply with the usual regimen of postoperative, high-dose PPI. Upper endoscopy demonstrated a 1-cm ulcer in the pyloric channel, with an exposed vessel that was clipped. This resulted in complete resolution of the bleeding. In this patient series, six of the seven patients reported symptom improvement or resolution at 6-month follow-up. Objective nuclear medicine gastric emptying studies (GES) were available in five of the patients. In 4 out of these 5 patients, follow-up GES documented successful normalization of gastric emptying [31].

A recent multicenter trial was published with 30 patients with refractory gastroparesis (11 diabetic, 12 postsurgical, and 7 idiopathic) [32]. Twenty-six out of 30 patients (86%) responded to POP with a median follow-up of 5.5 months. There were two adverse events in the series: one case of capnoperitoneum, and one prepyloric ulcer.

POP has also been shown to be effective in the treatment of gastroparesis caused by vagal injury after esophagectomy and after fundoplication.

Technical Differences

Some technical differences do exist between the POP and the POEM techniques. Unlike in a POEM, we prefer to keep a fairly short submucosal tunnel with the mucosal incision that is performed only about 2–3 cm proximal to the pylorus. Also, the myotomy itself is fairly restricted to the pylorus and only extends proximally by about 1 cm. During the pyloromyotomy, no specific attempt is made to selectively divide only the circular muscular layer, and it is typically divided in a full-thickness fashion down to the serosal layer. Special attention must be paid when performing the distal portion of the pyloromyotomy since the duodenal mucosa will drape over it in a perpendicular direction and could easily be perforated during this portion of the dissection. Finally, there is still some disagreement as to the optimal location to perform the myotomy. We prefer to perform the pyloromyotomy on the posterior aspect of the greater curvature to benefit from the natural positioning of the endoscope. An argument, however, can be made to perform the myotomy along the anterior aspect so that the procedure can more easily be converted to a laparoscopic pyloroplasty in case of an endoscopic full-thickness perforation.

Future Perspectives

The success of POEM expanded the indications and the acceptance of endoscopic submucosal dissection techniques. This is evident by the increasing numbers of gastroenterologists and surgeons in the Western world performing advanced endoscopic techniques such as endoscopic pyloromyotomies. Further studies with larger number of patients are of course required to determine the long-term outcomes, indications, and optimal patient selection for per-oral pyloromyotomy.

An important limitation to widespread acceptance is that significant challenges remain with respect to adequate physician training to perform these advanced procedures. Only a few centers have evaluated the learning curve for POEM. Estimated numbers of procedures required to reach mastery of the POEM procedure vary between 20 and 60 cases [33, 34]. Per-oral pyloromyotomy may in fact be even more challenging than a myotomy of the lower esophageal sphincter. Obtaining this required level of experience can be quite challenging, especially in the setting of these relatively rare disorders. Future research must therefore also focus on the improvement in the training and simulation of these procedures. With time, the available endoscopic surgical platforms will continue to improve and evolve, perhaps making these techniques accessible to an increasing group of practitioners.

References

1. Camilleri M, Parkman HP, Shafi MA, Abell TL, Gerson L. Clinical Guideline: Management of Gastroparesis. Am J Gastroenterol. 2013;108(1):18–37.
2. Pasricha PJ, Parkman HP. Gastroparesis: definitions and diagnosis. Gastroenterol Clin North Am. 2015;44(1):1–7.
3. Khoo J, Rayner CK, Jones KL, Horowitz M. Pathophysiology and management of gastroparesis. Expert Rev Gastroenterol Hepatol. 2009;3(2):167–81.
4. Revicki DA, Rentz AM, Dubois D, et al. Gastroparesis cardinal symptom index (GCSI): development and validation of a patient reported assessment of severity of gastroparesis symptoms. Qual Life Res. 2004;13(4):833–44.

5. Jung H-K, Choung RS, Locke GR, et al. The incidence, prevalence, and outcomes of patients with gastroparesis in Olmsted County, Minnesota, from 1996 to 2006. Gastroenterology. 2009;136(4):1225–33.
6. Soykan I, Sivri B, Sarosiek I. Demography, clinical characteristics, psychological and abuse profiles, treatment, and long-term follow-up of patients with gastroparesis. Dig Dis Sci. 1998;43(11):2398–404.
7. Camilleri M, Bharucha AE, Farrugia G. Epidemiology, mechanisms, and management of diabetic gastroparesis. Clin Gastroenterol Hepatol. 2011;9(1):5–12.
8. Hyett B, Martinez FJ, Gill BM, et al. Delayed radionucleotide gastric emptying studies predict morbidity in diabetics with symptoms of gastroparesis. Gastroenterology. 2009;137(2):445–52.
9. Fich A, Neri M, Camilleri M, Kelly KA, Phillips SF. Stasis syndromes following gastric surgery: clinical and motility features of 60 symptomatic patients. J Clin Gastroenterol. 1990;12(5):505–12.
10. Parkman HP, Hasler WL, Fisher RS. American Gastroenterological Association technical review on the diagnosis and treatment of gastroparesis. Gastroenterology. 2004;127(5):1592–622.
11. Oh JH, Pasricha PJ. Recent advances in the pathophysiology and treatment of gastroparesis. J Neurogastroenterol Motil. 2013;19(1):18–24.
12. Fraser R, Horowitz M, Dent J. Hyperglycaemia stimulates pyloric motility in normal subjects. Gut. 1991;32(5):475–8.
13. Langworthy J, Parkman HP, Schey R. Emerging strategies for the treatment of gastroparesis. Expert Rev Gastroenterol Hepatol. 2016.
14. Tougas G, Eaker EY, Abell TL, et al. Assessment of gastric emptying using a low fat meal: establishment of international control values. Am J Gastroenterol. 2000;95(6):1456–62.
15. Viramontes BE, Kim DY, Camilleri M, et al. Validation of a stable isotope gastric emptying test for normal, accelerated or delayed gastric emptying. Neurogastroenterol Motil. 2001;13(6):567–74.
16. Kuo B, McCallum RW, Koch KL, Sitrin MD, Wo JM, et al. Comparison of gastric emptying of a nondigestible capsule to a radio-labelled meal in healthy and gastroparetic subjects. Aliment Pharmacol Ther. 2008;27(2):186–96.
17. Camilleri M, Hasler WL, Parkman HP, Quigley EMM, Soffer E. Measurement of gastrointestinal motility in the GI laboratory. Gastroenterology. 1998;115(3):747–62.
18. Bharadwaj S, Meka K, Tandon P, Rathur A, Rivas JM, Vallabh H, Jevenn A, Guirguis J, Sunesara I, Nischnick A, Ukleja A. The management of gastroparesis associated malnutrition. J Dig Dis. 2016 Apr 25 (Epub ahead of print).
19. Parkman HP, Yates KP, Hasler WL, et al. Dietary intake and nutritional deficiencies in patients with diabetic or idiopathic gastroparesis. Gastroenterology. 2011;141(2):486–98.
20. Camilleri M. Novel diet, drugs, and gastric interventions for gastroparesis. Clin Gastroenterol Hepatol. 2016;(February):1–10.
21. Ukleja A, Tandon K, Shah K, Alvarez A. Endoscopic botox injections in therapy of refractory gastroparesis. World J Gastrointest Endosc. 2015;7(8):790–8.
22. Heckert J, Sankineni A, Hughes WB, Harbison S, Parkman H. Gastric electric stimulation for refractory gastroparesis: a prospective analysis of 151 patients at a single center. Dig Dis Sci. 2016;61(1):168–75.
23. Mancini SA, Angelo JL, Peckler Z, Philp FH, Farah KF. Pyloroplasty for refractory gastroparesis. Am Surg. 2015;81(7):738–46.
24. Toro JP, Lytle NW, Patel AD, et al. Efficacy of laparoscopic pyloroplasty for the treatment of gastroparesis. J Am Coll Surg. 2014;218(4):652–60.
25. Jones MP, Maganti K. Clinical reviews a systematic review of surgical therapy for gastroparesis. 2003;98(10).
26. Speicher JE, Thirlby RC, Burggraaf J, Kelly C, Levasseur S. Results of completion gastrectomies in 44 patients with postsurgical gastric atony. J Gastrointest Surg. 2009;13(5):874–80.
27. Pasricha PJ, Hawari R, Ahmed I, Chen J, Cotton PB, et al. Submucosal endoscopic esophageal myotomy: a novel experimental approach for the treatment of achalasia. Endoscopy. 2007;39(9):761–4.
28. Inoue H, Minami H, Kobayashi Y, Sato Y, Kaga M, et al. Peroral endoscopic myotomy (POEM) for esophageal achalasia. Endoscopy. 2010;42(4):265–71.
29. Kawai M, Perretta S, Burckhardt O, Dallemagne B, Marescaux J, Tanigawa N. Endoscopic pyloromyotomy: a new concept of minimally invasive surgery for pyloric stenosis. Endoscopy. 2012;44(2):169–73.
30. Khashab MA, Stein E, Clarke JO, Saxena P, Kumbhari V, et al. Gastric peroral endoscopic myotomy for refractory gastroparesis: first human endoscopic pyloromyotomy (with video). Gastrointest Endosc. 2013;78(5):764–8.
31. Shlomowitz E, Pescarus R, Cassera MA, Sharata AM, Reavis KM, et al. Early human experience with per-oral endoscopic pyloromyotomy (POP). Surg Endosc. 2015;29(3):543–51.
32. Khashab MA, Ngamruengphong S, Carr-Locke D, Bapaye A, Benais PC, et al. Gastric peroral endoscopic myotomy for refractory gastroparesis: results from the first multicenter study on endoscopic pyloromyotomy (with video). Gastrointest Endosc. 2016 Jun 25 (Epub ahead of print).
33. Kurian AA, Dunst CM, Sharata A, Bhayani NH, REavis KM, et al. Peroral endoscopic esophageal myotomy: defining the learning curve. Gastrointest Endosc. 2013;77(5):719–25.
34. Patel KS, Calixte R, Modayil RJ, Friedel D, Brathwaite CE, et al. The light at the end of the tunnel: a single-operator learning curve analysis for per oral endoscopic myotomy. Gastrointest Endosc. 2015;81(5):1181–7.

10 Endoluminal Bariatric Procedures

Jonah Cohen and Ram Chuttani

Abstract

Obesity is a disease that is growing in burden. It is estimated that over 1.4 billion people worldwide suffer from obesity, and 68% of Americans are considered overweight or obese. While bariatric surgery has also increased in popularity over the last two decades, the morbidity of these procedures has led investigators to develop less invasive therapies that may cause weight loss and resolution of comorbid conditions associated with obesity. There are two intragastric balloons on the market in the USA, which have been widely available in Europe and other countries, and three more remain under investigation but should be available soon. These balloons are typically placed endoscopically and are removed after a duration of months. Other novel technologies to treat obesity that are under investigation include endoscopic suturing devices to create anatomic simulations of bariatric procedures, endoluminal sleeves that create malabsorptive states, aspiration therapy to reduce caloric intake, duodenal mucosal resurfacing to induce malabsorption, and endoscopic magnetic anastomotic devices to create intestinal bypasses. These new devices may eventually become part of a growing toolbox for surgeons and endoscopists to offer therapy to morbidly obese patients in a much less invasive manner than bariatric surgery, although more data are needed.

Keywords

Obesity · Bariatric surgery · Intragastric balloons · Endoluminal surgery · Endoluminal suturing · Aspiration therapy · Duodenal mucosal resurfacing

J. Cohen · R. Chuttani (✉)
Department of Medicine and Division of Gastroenterology, Center for Advanced Endoscopy, Beth Israel Deaconess Medical Center, Harvard Medical School, 330 Brookline Avenue, Stoneman 458, Boston, MA, USA
e-mail: rchuttan@bidmc.harvard.edu

J. Cohen
e-mail: jmcohen@bidmc.harvard.edu

J.R. Romanelli et al. (eds.), *NOTES and Endoluminal Surgery*, Clinical Gastroenterology, DOI 10.1007/978-3-319-50610-4_10

Abbreviations

ASGE/ASMBS	American Society of Gastrointestinal Endoscopy/ American Society for Metabolic and Bariatric Surgery
BIB	Bioenterics Intragastric Balloon, now known as Orbera™
BMI	Body mass index
CC	Completed cases
CVD	Cardiovascular disease
DJBS	Duodenojejunal bypass sleeve
DMR	Duodenal mucosal resurfacing
EBT	Endoscopic bariatric therapy
EBW	Excess BMI weight loss
ESG	Endoscopic sleeve gastroplasty
EWL	Excess weight loss
FDA	Food and Drug Administration
HDL	High-density lipoprotein
IGB	Intragastric balloon
IOP	Incisionless operating platform
POSE	Primary obesity surgery endoluminal
ITT	Intent to treat
LDL	Low-density lipoprotein
NHANES	National Health and Nutrition Examination Survey
NIH	National Institutes of Health
PEG	Percutaneous endoscopic gastrostomy
TWL	Total weight loss
WHO	World Health Organization

Obesity: Growing Burden of Disease

Obesity is a chronic disease increasing in prevalence in adults and children on a global scale. Worldwide, more than 1.4 billion adults are overweight or obese, and in the USA, 68% of adults are overweight or obese [1–4]. Furthermore, the morbidity and mortality associated with being overweight (body mass index (BMI) defined as the weight in kilograms (kg) divided by height in meters squared of 25–29.9 kg/m^2) or obese (BMI of ≥30 kg/m^2) have been known for many years, and mounting evidence increasingly implicates obesity as an independent risk factor for various medical conditions, with enormous economic costs as well [5]. The USA spent $190 billion on obesity-related healthcare expenses in 2005, and obesity-attributable medical problems accounted for 21% of healthcare expenditures [4, 6]. Based upon data collected for the National Health and Nutrition Education Survey (NHANES) between 2011 and 2012, the measured prevalence of obesity in adults in the USA is 34.9% [7]. Notably, BMI classifications of obesity as per the National Institutes of Health (NIH) and World Health Organization (WHO) for Caucasian, Hispanic, and Black individuals refer to Class I as BMI of 30.0–34.9 kg/m^2, Class II as BMI of 35.0–39.9 kg/m^2, and Class III (or severe) as BMI ≥ 40 kg/m^2 [8]. Morbid obesity is defined as a BMI > 40, or ≥35 in the presence of comorbidities. The age-adjusted prevalence of class III obesity (BMI ≥ 40) in the USA has been estimated to be around 6% [3]. BMI is increasing worldwide, with 36.9% of men and 38% of women estimated to have a BMI ≥ 25 kg/m^2 [9, 10]. It is important to note that obesity is ultimately a complex, multi-factorial, metabolic, and psychoneuroendocrine disease, and not simply an imbalance between energy intake and energy expenditure. While many elements have contributed to this increase in obesity, sedentary lifestyle and diet are among the most important etiologies.

Obesity is associated with myriad complications including increased rate of death from all causes and from cardiovascular disease (CVD) [11]. Obesity and central adiposity are also associated with increased morbidity in addition to mortality [1]. Compared with normal weight individuals, overweight and obese individuals have a higher relative risk of diabetes mellitus, hypertension, hypercholesterolemia, nonalcoholic fatty liver disease, gout, stroke, venous thrombosis, cholelithiasis, depression, symptomatic osteoarthritis, gastroesophageal reflux disease, infertility, and obstructive sleep apnea, as well as CVD including heart failure, atrial fibrillation, and coronary disease [12]. Obesity is also an independent risk factor for many different cancers including breast, pancreatic, endometrial, gallbladder, kidney, liver, colon, and cervical cancer as well as leukemia [13]. Additionally, multiple studies have showed impaired quality of life among obese individuals including negative social and economic consequences [14].

Endoscopic Bariatric Therapies: A New Paradigm

Decreasing total body weight by only 5–10% has been shown to slow and even prevent the onset of obesity-related comorbidities, and has historically been recommended as the initial goal for weight-loss therapy [15, 16]. A reasonable time period for a 10% reduction in total body weight is 6 months [17]. While this amount of weight loss may appear modest, it is associated with a decrease in systolic blood pressure of 10 mmHg and in diastolic blood pressure of 20 mmHg; a reduction in total cholesterol by 10% and low-density lipoprotein (LDL) by 15%; and an increase of 7% in high-density lipoprotein (HDL) [18]. Interestingly, ovarian function is improved by only 5% weight loss. Furthermore, weight loss of 10–20% has been shown to improve glycemic control, while 15–20% of weight loss may reverse the elevated mortality risk of diabetes mellitus [18]. While to date first-line therapy, behavioral modification, including physical activity and dietary programs, thus far has yielded only modest long-term outcomes for treating obesity and metabolic disease [19–23]. Current pharmacologic therapies for obesity, including orlistat and lorcaserin, increase weight loss by 3–9% compared with lifestyle modification therapy alone, but are associated with significant side effects [24]. Unfortunately, both lifestyle and pharmacologic therapies are subject to significant rates of weight-loss recidivism [25]. While bariatric surgery has shown to be the most effective alternative for achieving durable weight loss as well as remission of diabetes in many obese patients, it is limited for use only in patients with a BMI > 40 or ≥35 with comorbidities. In addition, it is expensive, difficult to reverse, and associated with significant short- and long-term complications and even risk of death [26–32]. Some of the complications of bariatric surgery include cardiopulmonary events, anastomotic leak, stomal stenosis, marginal ulceration, incisional hernias, internal hernias, and formation of fistulae, as well as nutritional deficiencies, risk of reoperation, and chronic abdominal pain [30]. Current bariatric surgical procedures include open and laparoscopic Roux-en-Y gastric bypass, laparoscopic adjustable gastric banding, laparoscopic sleeve gastrectomy, and open or laparoscopic biliopancreatic diversion with duodenal switch. Evidence indicates that less than 1% of morbidly obese patients who qualify for bariatric surgery actually undergo operative management which has been attributed to cost, access, and patient concerns regarding morbidity and mortality of surgery [33]. Thus, the majority of overweight and obese patients are left without significant options aside from surgery once diet, lifestyle modifications, and weight-loss medications are unsuccessful. This provides a significant opportunity for novel therapeutic alternatives [17]. Indeed, as previously mentioned, the relatively low reduction in total body weight leading to significant improvements in comorbidities creates an exciting opportunity for these novel therapeutic options.

Recent technological advances have led to the emergence of endoscopic bariatric therapies (EBTs) for obesity and metabolic disease. Endoscopic procedures in development and in clinical trials, as well as those already used in practice, have the opportunity to bridge a significant gap between medical therapies and bariatric surgery and may serve as an alternative or an adjunct to medical treatment [34, 35]. Notably, endoscopic therapies for weight loss are potentially less invasive, lower cost, and reversible, with the option for repeat procedures as necessary [17, 36]. These include a variety of devices that work via different mechanisms of action including intragastric balloons, implantable sleeves, neuromodulatory, and gastric restriction devices, as well as endoscopic suturing and stapling platforms [34, 35]. Endoluminal bariatric procedures can be also organized into six main categories defined by their potential role as follows: (1) *early-intervention procedures* to treat patients that are overweight and obese but whom do not meet criteria for conventional weight-loss surgery; (2) *primary obesity or metabolic procedures* that may provide durable weight-loss similar to traditional bariatric surgeries or focus on obesity-related comorbid metabolic conditions such as diabetes; (3) *bridge procedures* that offer short-term weight reduction to decrease the operative risks associated with morbid obesity; (4) *revisional procedures* that repair failed traditional bariatric operations where patients have not lost or re-gained weight; (5) *postsurgical complication procedures* that endoscopically manage entities such as anastomotic leaks, bleeding, strictures, and fistulae; and (6) *routine endoscopy in postsurgical patients* which includes procedures to access the biliopancreatic limb and endoscopic retrograde cholangiopancreatography (ERCP) in patients who have previously underwent bariatric surgery (Table 10.1) [37, 38]. Finally, current *primary obesity or metabolic* endoscopic therapies can be classified as follows: (1) space-occupying; (2) restrictive; (3) bypass; (4) aspiration; or (5) other novel therapies. This chapter will focus on recent advances in the field of EBTs as primary management to treat obesity or metabolic

Table 10.1 Endoluminal bariatric procedures

Categories of endoluminal bariatric procedures	Examples
1. Early-intervention procedures	Treat patients that are overweight and obese but whom do not meet criteria for conventional weight-loss surgery
2. Primary obesity or metabolic procedures	Provide durable weight-loss similar to traditional bariatric surgeries or focus on obesity-related comorbid metabolic conditions such as diabetes
3. Bridge procedures	Offer short-term weight reduction to decrease the operative risks associated with morbid obesity prior to bariatric surgery
4. Revisional procedures	Repair failed traditional bariatric operations
5. Postsurgical complication procedures	Manage entities such as anastomotic leaks, bleeding, strictures, and fistulae
6. Routine endoscopy in postsurgical patients	Includes procedures to access the biliopancreatic limb and endoscopic retrograde cholangiopancreatography (ERCP) in patients who have previously underwent bariatric surgery

disease via devices or procedures in clinical practice or in advanced stages of development; however, many of these interventions may overlap as *early-intervention* or *bridge procedures*.

Challenge of Weight-Loss Reporting and Goals of Endobariatric Therapy

Of note, challenges exist in interpreting the available clinical data on primary endoscopic therapies for weight loss given that studies often differ in endpoints and have variable follow-up. Additionally, many factors other than weight loss play an important role in post-procedural quality of life, and such data are often not clearly reported [39]. Finally, central adiposity data *vis a vis* the metabolic syndrome are measured by waist circumference, and these data are not captured by relative weight-loss measures commonly used and may not be reported.

Weight-loss results are expressed in absolute terms such as kg or BMI, as well as relative terms such as percentage excess weight loss (%EWL), percentage excess BMI loss (%EBL), or percentage total weight loss (%TWL). The %EWL and %EBL are compared to reference points of ideal body weight and BMI of 25, respectively. Interestingly, one of the strongest links between obesity and health risks including mortality has been reported via BMI specifically in an almost 1-million-subject study [40]. Furthermore, there are limitations of relative measures such as %EWL and %TWL as they depend on a patient's initial status, and thus, percentage change may correspond with a variety of possible BMI results in different patients. Thus, %EWL and %TWL are unable to express health risk reduction unequivocally among different patients [41]. As lighter patients show higher %EWL and %TWL, studies and physicians may improve "their power" paradoxically by enrolling patients on the safer and lower end of the scale. Therefore, absolute terms are often favored by investigators in nonsurgical studies on weight loss, while relative measures tend to be used by proceduralists [42, 43].

Given this bias, it has been advocated by some that weight and BMI at all time points should be provided as a minimum by all journals reporting on intentional weight loss [42]. However, one recent report carefully showed that %TWL is less affected by the variation caused by initial BMI than %EWL, and thus, %TWL may be better suited for comparing weight loss among different patients or studies than %EWL if only relative measures are used [41]. Nevertheless, in most endobariatric studies, %EWL is the most commonly used endpoint.

Finally, other confounding variables such as dietary compliance, as well as nutritional and exercise interventions, affect the outcomes of weight-loss studies, introducing heterogeneity and limiting comparisons between studies. Such limitations are relevant and should be considered when interpreting data in the field of bariatric surgery and endobariatric procedures. A recent white paper by the ASGE/ASMBS Task Force on Endoscopic Bariatric Therapy delineated requirements of EBTs with respect to targets of safety, weight-loss efficacy, durability, reversibility, repeatability, costs, and the alteration of anatomy [44]. Therein, they advocate defining successful weight loss in primary interventions as %EWL $\geq$ 25% at 12 months or 15% greater %EWL compared to a control group. They also recommended a minimum threshold of total weight loss of 5% for early, bridge-to-surgery, and metabolic interventions, based on the aforementioned health benefits of 5% weight loss. The threshold for incidence of serious adverse events associated with a particular EBT was set at 5% or less. Hence, the expected lower complication rates with EBTs allow the efficacy bar to be lower compared to surgical therapies.

Importance of Patient Selection, Follow-Up, and Multidisciplinary Teams

Like any medical intervention, contraindications exist and correct patient selection is essential. Aside from the aforementioned indication categories for EBT patient selection (i.e., early intervention, primary intervention, bridge, metabolic), other factors also play a role in successful management. For example, extensive preprocedural counseling and prophylactic symptom management is important in the case of intragastric balloons. These help minimize early device removal by managing expectations and reducing nausea and vomiting. This deters patients with a high likelihood of attrition from proceeding [45]. Contraindications for primary EBTs include the following: endocrine cause for obesity, alcoholism or drug abuse, desire of pregnancy or lactation, lack of patient compliance with previous lifestyle or medical therapies, inadequately treated psychiatric disease or eating disorders, malignancy in previous 5 years, and previous gastric surgery [44, 46]. Other procedure-specific contraindications also exist and will be discussed when applicable. One of the most critical aspects of creating a successful EBT program is the formation of a team of providers that can assist with patient selection as well as frequent and durable follow-up [47]. Recent work has highlighted that the number of nutritional and psychological contacts predicted successful weight loss [48]. Internists, endocrinologists, gastroenterologists, bariatric surgeons, dietitians, psychologists/psychiatrists, and exercise physiologists each play an important role and ideally are integrated via weight-loss centers or programs [49].

Space-Occupying Devices

Space-occupying devices most often take the form of temporarily placed prostheses such as endoscopically placed intragastric balloons (IGBs). However, space-occupying devices other than balloons are also in clinical trials. Such space-occupying devices induce gastric distention and displace volume but likely also work via alterations in gastrointestinal motility such as delaying gastric emptying, as well as neurohormonal shifts [50]. IGBs were first described in 1982 and approved for use in the USA in 1985 with the air-filled Garren-Edwards Gastric Bubble [51]. These balloons unfortunately had limited efficacy and were associated with multiple adverse events including gastric ulceration and small-bowel obstructions related to spontaneous balloon deflation and migration [52, 53]. Since that time, IGBs have demonstrated decades of improved safety and efficacy internationally. As of 2015 two devices, the Orbera™ and ReShape Duo® intragastric balloons were approved for use by the US Food and Drug Administration (FDA) [54, 55]. Other space-occupying devices in development which will not be discussed in this chapter include IGBs such as the Heliosphere BAG, satiety-inducing devices such as Full Sense™, and transpyloric devices designed to impair gastric emptying such as Transpyloric Shuttle® and SatiSphere™.

Orbera™ Intragastric Balloon

The Orbera™ (formerly Bioenterics) intragastric balloon (Apollo Endosurgery, Austin, Texas) is an elastic spherical balloon made of silicone (Fig. 10.1). It is placed blindly into the stomach and then under endoscopic visualization is filled with approximately 500–700 mL of saline solution and often 10 mL of methylene blue which acts as an indicator of inadvertent balloon deflation via urine discoloration. It is indicated for intragastric residence up to 6 months at which time it is punctured and retrieved endoscopically. The Orbera™ balloon has been used worldwide for several decades with extensive experience and data supporting its efficacy and safety. While a Cochrane Systematic Review in 2007 lacked sufficient evidence to clearly recommend benefit on weight loss via the Orbera™ balloon, a subsequent meta-analysis from 2008 showed clear safety and efficacy data for short-term weight loss [53, 56]. This 2008 meta-analysis evaluated 3608 patients and 15 studies with estimates for weight lost at time of balloon removal after 6 months of implantation was 14.7 kg in total weight, 12.2% TWL, 5.7 kg/m^2 BMI, and 32.1% EWL.

However, it is important to note that there were limited data following patients post balloon

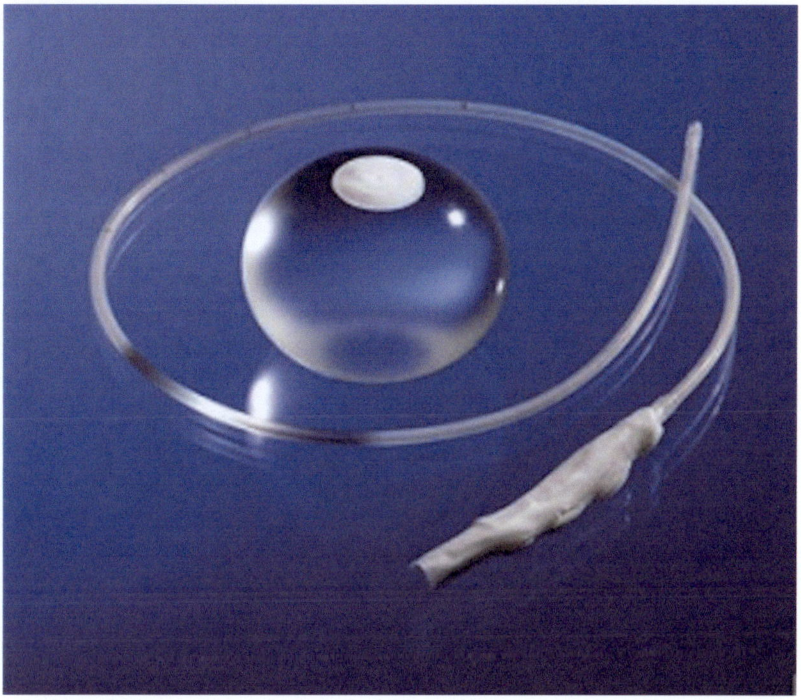

Fig. 10.1 Orbera™ intragastric balloon

removal. Regarding safety, the majority of complications were mild, and the early removal rate was 4.2%. The largest study from the meta-analysis evaluating 2515 patients from Italy included dietary counseling recommending approximately 1000 kcal/day. The reported overall complication rate was 2.8% [49]. They reported gastric perforation occurring in 5 patients (0.19%), 4 of whom had undergone previous gastric surgery. Two died and 2 were successfully treated by laparoscopic repair after balloon removal. Thus, the authors of this study concluded that the previous gastric surgery is a contraindication to BIB placement.

Of note, 19 gastric obstructions (0.76%) presented in the first week after positioning and were successfully treated by balloon removal. Balloon rupture occurred in 9 patients (0.36%) and was treated by removal. Finally, esophagitis ($n = 32$; 1.27%) and gastric ulcer ($n = 5$; 0.2%) presented in patients without a history of peptic disease and were treated conservatively with medical therapy. After 6 months, %EWL was 33.9 and BMI loss was 4.9 kg/m^2. Of note, there was statistically significant improvement in fasting glucose, blood pressure, and lipid markers, while hemoglobin A1c decrease or normalization was reported in 87.2% of thc 488 patients with diabetes in the study.

A recent ASGE Technology Review aggregated much of the available evidence on Orbera™ in over 18 studies and cited a median %TWL of 12% at 6 months when the device was removed [57]. With respect to longer-term weight loss, they reported %EWL ranging from 11 to 51% at 12 months (6 months after balloon removal) based on 10 prospective trials with 1161 patients. Two trials reported long-term data with approximately 6% TWL maintained 36 months after implantation, and mean %EWL was 55.6% at 6 months and 29.1% at 3 years [58, 59]. One study followed patients out to 5 years after balloon placement and found that about 40% of patients presented weight loss of 7 kg, BMI reduction of 2.5 kg/m^2, and %EWL of 13 [60]. In another meta-analysis of 17 studies including 1638 patients, Abu Dayyeh et al. [46] reported that %EWL with the Orbera™ IGB at 12 months was 25.44 (95% CI, 21.47–29.4). Three RCTs compared %EWL in patients who received the Orbera™ IGB with a control group, with the mean difference in %EWL in patients who received the Orbera™ IGB over controls being 26.9% (95% CI, 15.6–38.2; $P \leq 0.001$) [47–49]. Finally, a recent systematic review evaluating weight loss in 547 patients and 9 trials after Orbera™ removal showed that at removal patients lost on average 16.7 kg, 6 months post-removal, had a net loss of 15.9 kg (sustaining 95% weight loss), and 12 months post-removal had a net loss of 8.7 kg (sustaining 52% of the initial weight lost) [50].

Importantly, sequential placement of IGBs after an IGB-free time interval has been suggested as a mechanism for resetting the stomach's normal motility prior to repeating therapy to provide additional weight loss. Lopez-Nava et al. [61] and Genco et al. [62] reported that a second Orbera™ IGB after a 1-month balloon-free period led to an additional average decrease in BMI of 2.6 and 4.2 kg/m^2, respectively, and to an increase in the percentage of EWL from 25.1 to 51.9% compared to patients who underwent a single 6-month Orbera™ balloon placement followed by 7 months of dietary counseling [62]. Finally, Dumonceau et al. [63] found that obese patients who repeat Orbera™ IGB therapy after a balloon-free period lost approximately 9.0 kg during their second Orbera™ balloon placement in addition to the 14.6 kg lost from the first balloon.

In a meta-analysis evaluating Orbera™ safety in 68 studies [46], the most frequent side effects were pain and nausea occurring in over one-third of subjects. The pooled early removal rate was approximately 7%, and serious adverse events from Orbera™ were uncommon with an incidence of migration and gastric perforation of 1.4 and 0.1%, respectively. Notably 4 of 8 gastric perforations occurred in patients with previous gastric surgeries, and the four reported deaths were related to gastric perforation or aspiration events. While delayed gastric emptying is felt to be induced by the IGB, once removed, it is felt the there is no long-term risk of gastroparesis based on current available evidence.

Reshape Duo® Intragastric Balloon

The ReShape Duo® (ReShape Medical, San Clemente, California) is an endoscopically inserted and retrieved, saline-filled, dual intragastric balloon system with 2 balloons attached to each other by a flexible tube which helps prevents migration if one balloon inadvertently deflates (Fig. 10.2). Filling volume is recommended at 900 mL of saline solution with methylene blue via a power pump delivering 450 mL to each balloon. The device is recommended for removal after 6 months similar to Orbera™. Again similar to Orbera™, ReShape Duo® was officially FDA-approved in 2015 for adult obese patients who have a BMI of 30–40 kg/m^2 and who have been unable to lose weight through diet and exercise. Furthermore, patients must also have one or more obesity-related conditions such as diabetes, high blood pressure, or high cholesterol, and they must also participate in a supervised diet and exercise plan. FDA approval was based on of the REDUCE Pivotal Trial which was a prospective, sham-controlled, double-blinded, randomized, Multicenter, clinical study that enrolled 326 subjects [55]. The results showed that ReShape Duo® patients lost over twice the amount of weight of those patients who underwent sham endoscopy with diet and exercise alone. Duo patients had significantly greater %EWL at 24 weeks (25.1% intent to treat (ITT), 27.9% completed cases (CC, $n = 167$) compared with control group patients (11.3% ITT, $P = 0.004$, 12.3% CC, $n = 126$). Notably, the secondary endpoint evaluating weight maintenance was not met as more than 50% of treatment subjects who lost weight with the device did not maintain greater than 40% of their %EWL for the 24 weeks after the device was removed. Regarding total weight loss, the average number of pounds in the ReShape® group was 14.4 (6.8% TWL) versus 7.2 (3.3% TWL) in the control group at 24 weeks via ITT analysis, and 9.9 lb in ReShape® group at 48 weeks. Balloon deflation occurred in 6% but without migrations,

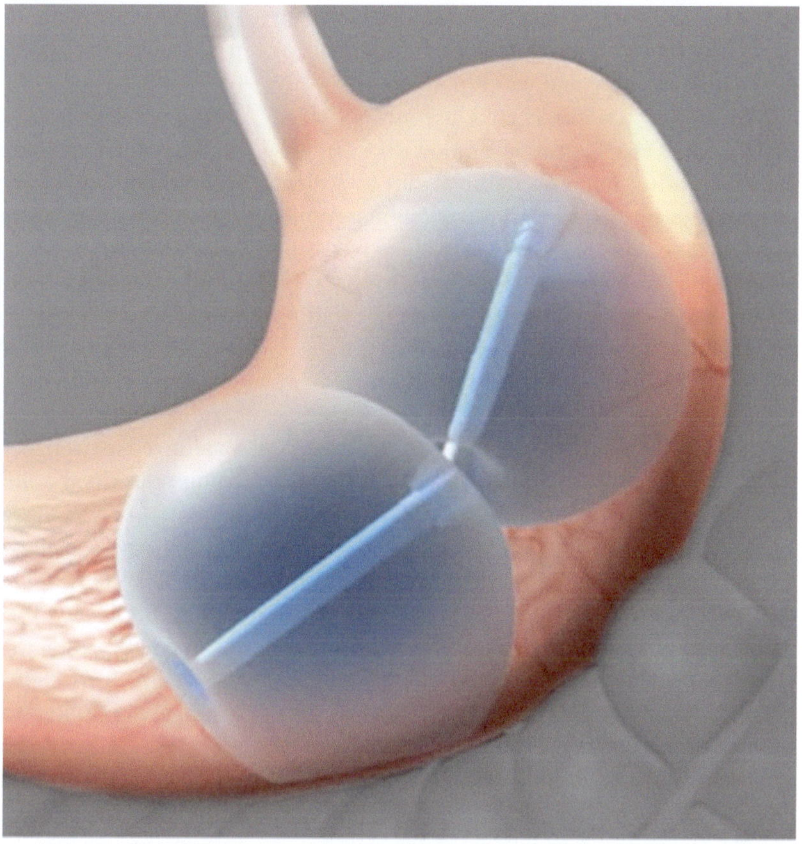

Fig. 10.2 Reshape Duo™ intragastric balloon

and early retrieval for nonulcer intolerance occurred in 9% of subjects. Gastric ulcers were observed, and a minor device change led to significantly reduced ulcer size and frequency (10%). Based on these data, the FDA felt the risk–benefit profile was favorable enough to grant approval.

Obalon Intragastric Balloon

The Obalon Gastric Balloon (Obalon Therapeutics Inc., Carlsbad, California) is a 250-mL gas-filled balloon that is packaged within a large dissolvable gelatin capsule. It is swallowed under fluoroscopic visualization but does not require endoscopic placement. A catheter, which extends through the esophagus and outside the mouth, is used to fill the balloon by using a gas-filled canister. The Obalon balloon requires endoscopic removal via puncture and forceps extraction. Up to 3 balloons can be swallowed during the same or sequential sessions, and balloons are removed endoscopically after 12–24 weeks. The target population is patients with BMI 27 or greater who have failed previous conservative measures for weight loss. Initial feasibility data demonstrated proof of concept for preliminary safety and efficacy in 17 patients [64]. Based on data from the European Union Limited Market Release (unpublished data from Obalon) from eleven centers throughout Belgium, Germany, Italy, and Spain studying 119 subjects in the absence of a control group, they found a 50.2% EWL, 8.3% %TWL, 2.8-point reduction in BMI, and mean weight loss of 8.0 ± 5.8 kg over the 3-month period. In this study, most commonly reported adverse events were nausea (10.1%), vomiting (6.7%), and 9 patients (7.6%) requested early removal of balloons mainly due to a lack of commitment to the full 3-month therapy period. One (0.8%) small

(<1 cm), nonbleeding ulcer was observed during the endoscopy to remove balloons at the end of the treatment period and was reported as possibly related to the contraindicated use of NSAIDs. Finally, one esophageal laceration (0.8%) was observed after balloon removal in a patient diagnosed with eosinophilic esophagitis. While the device is currently not FDA-approved, the US Pivotal Trial for the Obalon IGB has been under way with published results awaiting release.

Elipse Gastric Balloon

The Elipse™ balloon (Allurion Technologies, Wellesley, MA) is another example of an intragastric balloon. While an IGB is technically not an EBT, as novel technology is utilized eliminating endoscopy and sedation for both implantation and removal, these devices should be included under nonsurgical approaches to procedural management of obesity. The Elipse is enclosed inside a capsule and is attached to a thin, flexible catheter long enough to remain outside the patient's mouth once the capsule is swallowed (Fig. 10.3). Once in the stomach the capsule quickly dissolves, the balloon is filled with 550 mL of fluid. When filling is complete, the detachable catheter is removed. The Elipse balloon is designed to remain within the stomach for a predetermined period of several months, at which point a valve opens based on timed-release technology, allowing the balloon to empty automatically from the stomach and be excreted spontaneously from the GI tract. In a proof-of-concept pilot study, 8 patients swallowed a smaller prototype Elipse balloon intended to remain in the stomach for 6 weeks, self-empty, and then pass [65]. There were no serious adverse events, and all balloons were swallowed as well as excreted safely. Despite not being prescribed a diet or exercise plan, all eight patients lost weight, and after 6 weeks of Elipse therapy, the mean weight loss was 2.4 kg and mean %EWL was 12.4%. In results presented at the 2015 Obesity Week conference and submitted for publication, a larger study of 34 individuals with BMI between 27 and 40 found an average weight loss of 10 kg (22 lb), 39% EWL, 10% TWL, and 8 cm off their waist circumference over the 4-month treatment period, with improvements in triglycerides, hemoglobin A1c, and quality of life. All balloons were safely and naturally excreted. In 2015, the device received European Marketing Approval and is in the

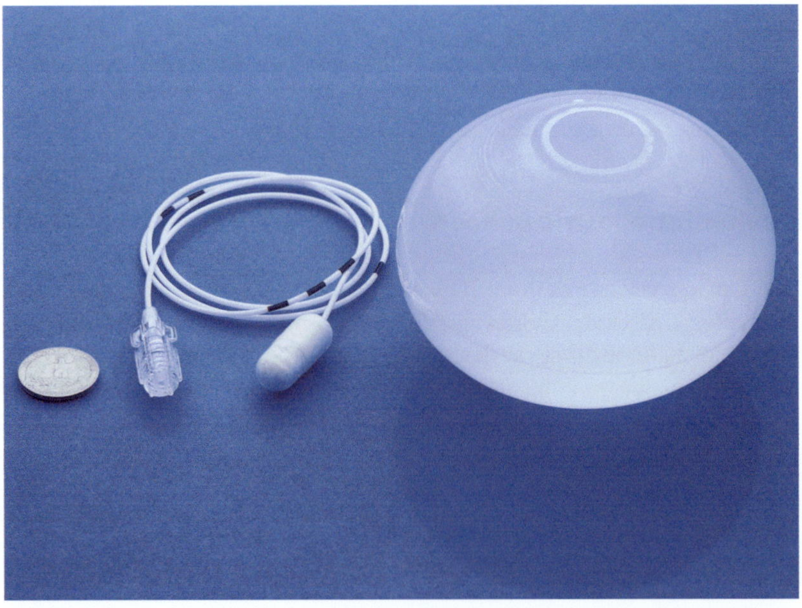

Fig. 10.3 Elipse™ intragastric balloon (Courtesy of Allurion Technologies)

planning phases for a US Pivotal Trial-seeking FDA approval.

Spatz3 Adjustable Balloon System®

The Spatz3 Adjustable Balloon System® (Spatz Medical, Great Neck, NY) is an endoscopically placed IGB that is filled with saline. It has an extractable inflation tube allowing for variable volume adjustment while the balloon remains in the stomach. Balloon volume may be increased to enhance the efficacy or decreased to improve the patient tolerance and is approved for 12-month implantation outside of the USA. Regarding efficacy data, two small observational studies evaluated weight-loss outcomes after Spatz3 Adjustable Balloon® deployment in 94 obese patients. At 12 months, when the balloon was removed, % EWL was 46% [66, 67]. Finally, a case–control study comparing Spatz3® to Orbera™ balloons found no difference in weight-loss outcomes at 12 months. The study evaluated 80 patients who had sequential placement of two Orbera balloons (6 months each) to 40 patients with the Spatz3 adjustable balloon for 12 months; however, 15% of the Spatz devices were removed due to complications related to device hardware and migration [68]. Newer versions of the Spatz3 balloon are addressing these engineering challenges.

Restrictive Procedures and Devices

Restrictive procedures remodel the stomach via stapling, suturing, or tissue anchor placement to reduce gastric volume and achieve effects analogous to gastric pouch formation as in the Roux-en-Y gastric bypass or sleeve gastrectomy.

OverStitch™ for Endoscopic Sleeve Gastroplasty

Endoscopic sleeve gastroplasty (ESG) is a transoral endoscopic gastric volume reduction procedure that reduces gastric capacity in a similar fashion to sleeve gastrectomy without the need for gastric surgery. The Apollo OverStitch™ device (Apollo Endosurgery, Austin, TX), which is FDA-approved, allows placement of full-thickness sutures in a variety of interrupted or running patterns using a double-channel therapeutic gastroscope (Fig. 10.4a). ESG is accomplished by placing these full-thickness sutures through the gastric wall utilizing a tissue helix device to capture tissue extending from the prepyloric antrum to the gastroesophageal junction reducing the entire stomach along the greater curvature (Fig. 10.4b). Increasing data have been published showing the safety and efficacy of ESG. A 20-subject trial from Spain, in subjects with a mean baseline BMI of 38.5 kg/m^2, demonstrated a mean body weight reduction of 19.3 ± 8.9 kg at 6 months (17.8% TWL). In a New York study, ESG was performed on 10 subjects with a mean BMI of 45.2 kg/m^2 and reported no significant adverse events [69]. After 1 month, 3 months, and 6 months, excess weight loss of 18, 26, and 30% and mean weight loss of 11.5, 19.4, and 33.0 kg, respectively, were observed. In a 1-year follow-up study from Spain with 25 patients, there were no major intraprocedural, early, or delayed adverse events from ESG, and mean %TWL was 18.7 ± 10.7 at 1 year. In regression analysis, predictors of successful weight loss were the number of nutritional and psychological contacts each patient had. Notably, at 1-year follow-up, only one patient underwent a revision partial gastroplasty because of loosened applications, demonstrating significant durability of ESG suture lines. Finally, a Mayo Clinic series of 25 patients with mean BMI of 35.5 ± 2.6 kg/m^2 has been released [70]. After 6, 9, 12, and 20 months, subjects had lost 53 ± 17%, 56 ± 23%, 54 ± 40%, and 45 ± 41% of excess body weight, respectively, after the procedure. Endoscopy at 3 months showed intact gastroplasty in all subjects. Physiological analyses of 4 patients showed that ESG delays gastric emptying and induces early satiety. Finally, 3 subjects had serious adverse events (a perigastric inflammatory collection, a pulmonary embolism, and a small pneumothorax) but made full recoveries without surgical intervention.

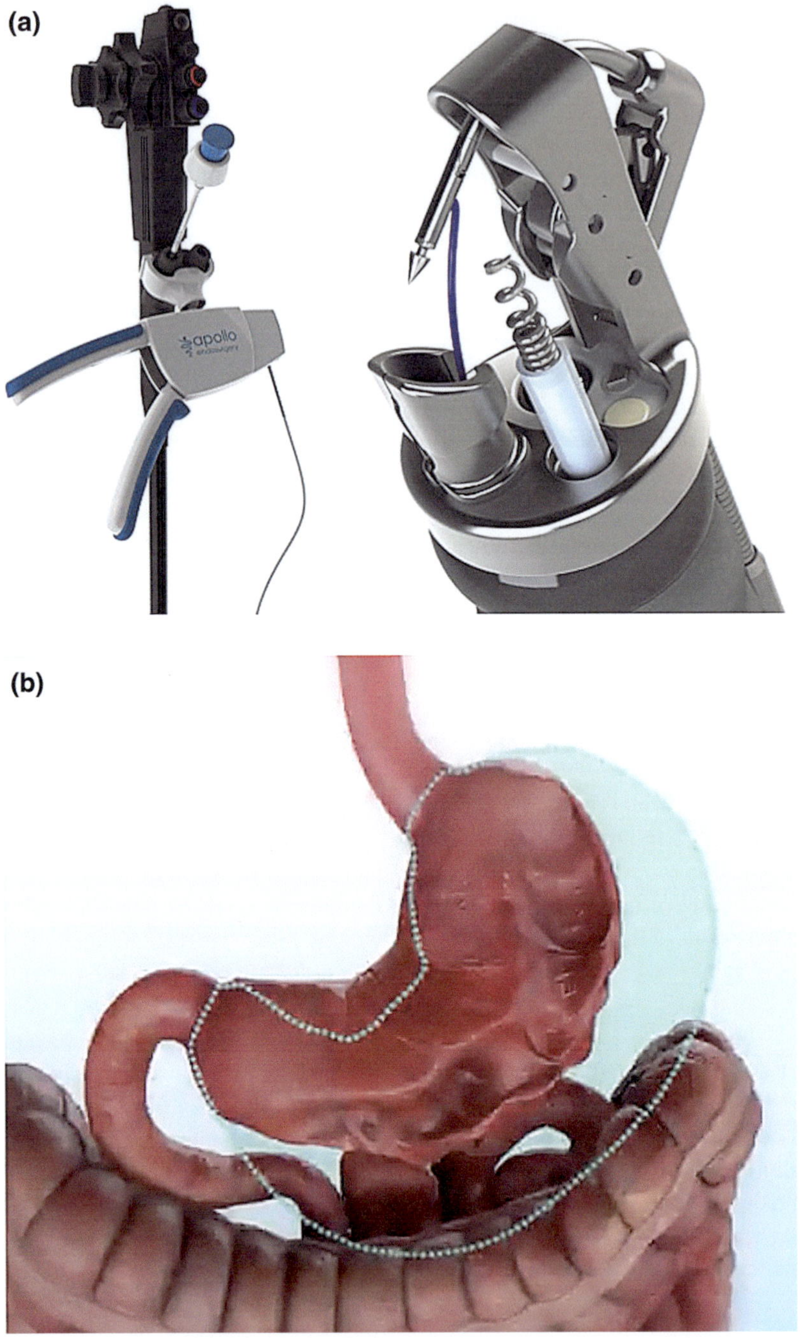

Fig. 10.4 **a** and **b** OverStitch™ for endoscopic sleeve gastroplasty (Courtesy of Apollo Endosurgery)

These studies suggest that ESG is a promising procedure for significant weight loss in patients seeking endoscopic alternatives to sleeve gastrectomy. However, more data are needed to evaluate long-term durability and safety of the endoscopic gastroplasty procedure. As with any stomach-excluding procedure, the risk of disease such as ulcers or gastric cancer in the remnant stomach remains. The Primary Obesity Multicenter Incisionless Suturing Evaluation (PROMISE) trial (NCT01662024) to study efficacy of ESG using OverStitch™ has been completed in the USA, but the results are not yet available. Finally, as with other EBTs, USA insurance companies do not yet cover this procedure, and thus, costs can be significant to the patient.

Incisionless Operating Platform for Primary Obesity Surgery Endoluminal (POSE)

The incisionless operating platform (IOP) used to perform the primary obesity surgery endoluminal (POSE) procedure uses a per-oral incisionless operating platform (USGI Medical, San Clemente, CA) to place 8–10, full-thickness, tissue anchor applications that reduce accommodation of the gastric fundus. Several applications are also placed in the distal gastric body to delay gastric emptying (Fig. 10.5a, b). The large overtube-style platform of the IOP is the TransPort®, which is steerable in 4 directions, with 4 working channels that accommodate a slim 4.9-mm endoscope and 3 specialized instruments. These include the g-Prox®, a flexible endoscopic grasper with a jawed gripper for creating serosa-to-serosa tissue folds and able to cut suture, the g-Lix™, a flexible tissue grasper with a distal helical tip designed to assist the g-Prox® in capturing target tissue for a full-thickness plication, and the g-Cath™, a suture–anchor delivery catheter system with a needle at its distal tip that, after advancement through the lumen of the g-Prox®, penetrates the target tissue deploying a pair of preloaded tissue anchors joined by suture material which holds the plication until serosal fusion occurs.

(a)

(b)

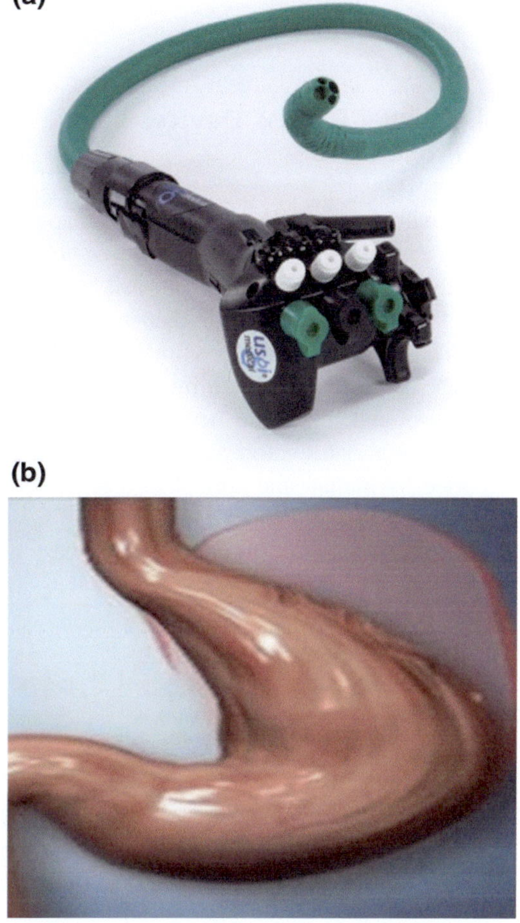

Fig. 10.5 **a** and **b** Incisionless operating platform for primary obesity surgery endoluminal (POSE) procedure (Courtesy of USGI Medical)

A single-center, open-label, prospective trial from Spain enrolling 45 obese patients with mean BMI of 36.7 kg/m^2 demonstrated the feasibility and safety of the POSE procedure [71]. At 6 months, BMI decreased by 5.8 kg/m^2, %EWL was 49.4%, and %TWL was 15.5% without any operative morbidity or mortality. Subjects reported less hunger and earlier satiety post-procedure. Liquid intake began 12 h post-procedure, with full solids by 6 weeks. The ESSENTIAL Trial (NCT01958385) is a US multicenter, randomized, sham-controlled, pivotal trial of the POSE procedure which has enrolled 332 subjects for goal follow-up of 12 months to evaluate safety and efficacy endpoints. Results of this trial are expected to be released shortly.

Small-Bowel Bypass Devices and Procedures

The proximal small bowel actively manages nutrient absorption and thus is believed to significantly mediate glucose homeostasis and play a role in the pathogenesis of diet-induced diabetes. Thus, bypass of the proximal small intestine is believed to contribute importantly to the weight loss and metabolic benefits experienced after certain bariatric surgeries. This rationale is supported by human and animal research evaluating duodenal exclusion [72–74]. EBTs have been developed and studied with hopes of reproducing this effect.

EndoBarrier® Duodenal-Jejunal Bypass Liner

The EndoBarrier® (GI Dynamics, Lexington, MA) is a duodenojejunal bypass sleeve (DJBS) consisting an impermeable sleeve of Teflon anchored in the bulb of the duodenum by a nitinol crown with barbs. The 65-cm sleeve and anchoring device are restrained within a delivery capsule that is advanced to the duodenal bulb over a stiff wire under endoscopic and fluoroscopic guidance and subsequently deployed. The sleeve extends into the jejunum and prevents food contents from contacting the mucosa of the proximal small intestine, allowing food to reach the mid-jejunum earlier. However, the sleeve allows pancreaticobiliary secretions to move along the outside of the device to the jejunum. The EndoBarrier® is removed endoscopically after 12 months via a custom device retrieval hood to help avoid trauma to the stomach or esophagus upon explantation. Out of seven studies involving EndoBarrier, the %EWL ranged between 12% and 22% at 12 weeks, 24 and 32% at 24 weeks, and 30 and 47% at 52 weeks [75–81]. A meta-analysis of four RCTs from these studies compared 12–24 weeks of treatment with the EndoBarrier® DJBS (90 patients) with a sham or control arm (84 patients). The mean %EWL difference compared with a control group was significant at 9.4% (95% CI, 8.26–10.65) [46]. Improvement in % hemoglobin A1c was significant compared with sham or control diabetic group, where the EndoBarrier® DJBS resulted in an additional 1% reduction compared to controls [46]. Regarding the safety profile of the EndoBarrier®, this same meta-analysis reviewed the 271 implantations in the literature and found a pooled early device removal rate of 18.4%. Serious adverse events included migration (4.9%), GI bleeding (3.86%), sleeve obstruction (3.4%), liver abscess (0.126%), cholangitis (0.126%), acute cholecystitis (0.126%), and esophageal perforation (0.126%) secondary to trauma from an uncovered barb at withdrawal. Notably, the multicenter US Pivotal ENDO Trial (NCT01728116) was placed on hold in March 2015 by the FDA after reports of 7 cases of hepatic abscess among the 325 patients already enrolled of the 500 initial sample size. Thus, the future clinical use of EndoBarrier in the USA is uncertain.

Other endoscopic bypass devices such as the gastroduodenojejunal bypass sleeve (ValenTx, Inc., Hopkins, MN) is a 120-cm long fluoropolymer sleeve that is secured at the gastroesophageal junction. It remains under investigational development.

Aspiration Therapy

Aspiration therapy is a novel therapeutic approach for weight loss that allows obese patients to dispose a significant portion of their ingested caloric intake via a specially designed percutaneous endoscopic gastrostomy (PEG) tube.

AspireAssist®

The AspireAssist® (Aspire Bariatrics, King of Prussia, PA) is a modified PEG tube with an external accessory for aspirating about one-third of the ingested meal ideally 20 min after

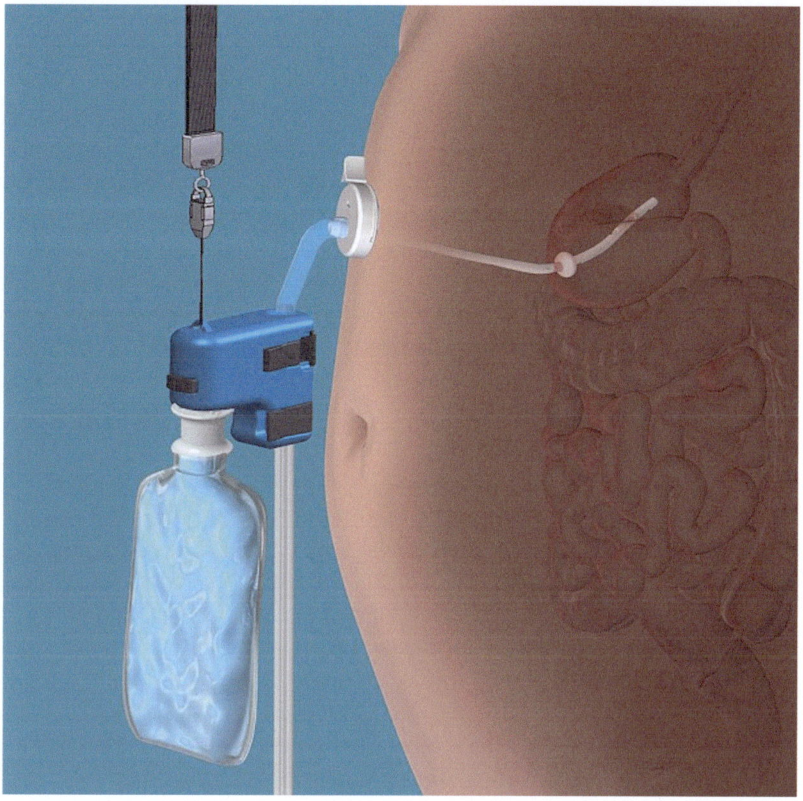

Fig. 10.6 AspireAssist®

consumption and takes about 5–10 min to complete (Fig. 10.6). The device includes a large-bore fenestrated silicone gastrostomy tube (A-Tube) which is attached to a skin port with a connector and valve placed at the skin. A 600-mL reservoir facilitates flushing and aspiration of gastric contents postprandially. A randomized, pilot, proof-of-concept study published by Sullivan et al. in 2013 studied 18 subjects with 11 assigned to AspireAssist® and 7 to the control group [82]. All patients underwent a 15-session diet and behavioral education program. Ten of the 11 subjects in the aspiration therapy group and 4 of the 7 subjects in the lifestyle therapy group completed the first year of the trial. After 12 months, the aspiration therapy group achieved TWL of 18.6% and EWL of 49.0% compared to 5.9% TWL and 14.9% EWL in the lifestyle therapy control arm. Seven of the 10 subjects in the AspireAssist® group decided to complete an additional 12 months of therapy and maintained a 20.1% TWL with 54.6% EWL. Notably, there was no evidence of binge eating behavior in the aspiration therapy group, nor evidence of increased food intake to compensate for aspirated food. Reported adverse events included abdominal pain at the PEG tube site, site infection in 3 patients, and persistent gastrocutaneous fistula, which eventually closed spontaneously, in 1 patient. A more recent study from Sweden evaluated 25 obese patients with mean BMI of 39.8 ± 0.9 kg/m^2 and found that after 6 months, mean weight lost was 16.5 kg and %EWL was 40.8 in the 22 subjects who completed 26 weeks of therapy. Two patients were hospitalized for adverse events including 1 subject for pain after PEG tube placement and another due to an aseptic intra-abdominal fluid collection 1 day after gastrostomy tube placement. Notably, there were no clinically significant changes in electrolytes. While aspiration therapy is an interesting and promising approach with preliminary results demonstrating high efficacy and safety, more long-term data will be needed given concern for possibly inducing eating disorders. The Pivotal

Aspiration Therapy With Adjusted Lifestyle Therapy Study (PATHWAY) prospective multicenter clinical trial in the USA is currently under way (NCT01766037).

Other Novel Endoscopic Bariatric Therapies

Revita™ Duodenal Mucosal Resurfacing (Fractyl Laboratories)

As previously mentioned, given that the proximal small intestine plays an extremely active role in glucose homeostasis, research has indicated that the duodenum may play a significant role in the pathogenesis of diet-induced diabetes [72, 73]. Enteroendocrine cells in the duodenum sense luminal nutrients and release gut peptides that are thought to mediate satiety and enhance insulin secretion [incretins, including gastric inhibitory polypeptide (GIP) and glucagon-like peptide-1 (GLP-1)] which may account for the fact that oral glucose administration promotes a much greater degree of insulin secretion compared to a parenteral glucose infusion (incretin effect) [83]. However, it is unclear whether a reduced incretin effect in type 2 diabetes is a cause or consequence of the diabetic state [84]. In the Revita™ Duodenal Mucosal Resurfacing (DMR) procedure (Fractyl Laboratories, Cambridge, MA), thermal ablation of the superficial duodenal mucosa is performed using radiofrequency energy after lifting it with a submucosal saline injection (Fig. 10.7a, b). It is believed that this procedure may result in mucosal remodeling and hypothetically reset duodenal enteroendocrine cells that have become diseased, thus restoring signaling that can improve diabetic control potentially through an incretin effect. Clinical investigations are underway.

Self-assembling Magnets for Endoscopy (GI Windows)

Self-assembling magnets for endoscopy (GI Windows, Boston, Mass) is a novel technology that generates incisionless magnetic compression anastomoses such as gastrojejunostomies, gastroileostomies, and duodenoileostomies [85]. This small-bowel malabsorptive procedure is intended to promote weight loss and improvement in diabetes via the ileal break phenomenon whereby infusion of nutrients and bile directly into the distal part of the small intestine alters gastrointestinal motility and inhibits food intake [86]. A recent 3-month porcine survival study evaluating 8 animals showed that large-caliber, leak-free, foreign-body-free, endoscopic intestinal bypass by using Incisionless Anastomosis System [IAS]. Magnets could be safely and rapidly performed using only intravenous sedation [87]. The mean 3-month weight gain was 45 kg in bypass pigs and 78 kg in controls ($P = 0.01$). Additional clinical trials are under way to evaluate the safety and efficacy of this device.

Future Frontiers in Endoluminal Bariatrics

With the armamentarium of endoluminal bariatric therapies growing each year and several devices awaiting FDA approval on the near horizon line, the bariatric endoscopist will have an increasing number of treatment options available to offer patients. Along these lines, there are several key elements which we feel may greatly shape the field of bariatric endoscopy in the future.

Novel Professional Collaborations and Personalized Endobariatrics

With the range of devices to treat obesity, as well as those targeting metabolic disease such as diabetes exclusively, new practice patterns will need to evolve as part of multidisciplinary expert teams for patients. One example of this is that endocrinologists at present do not refer patients directly to gastroenterologists for management of diabetes. But by generating increased awareness of EBTs as well as forming comprehensive

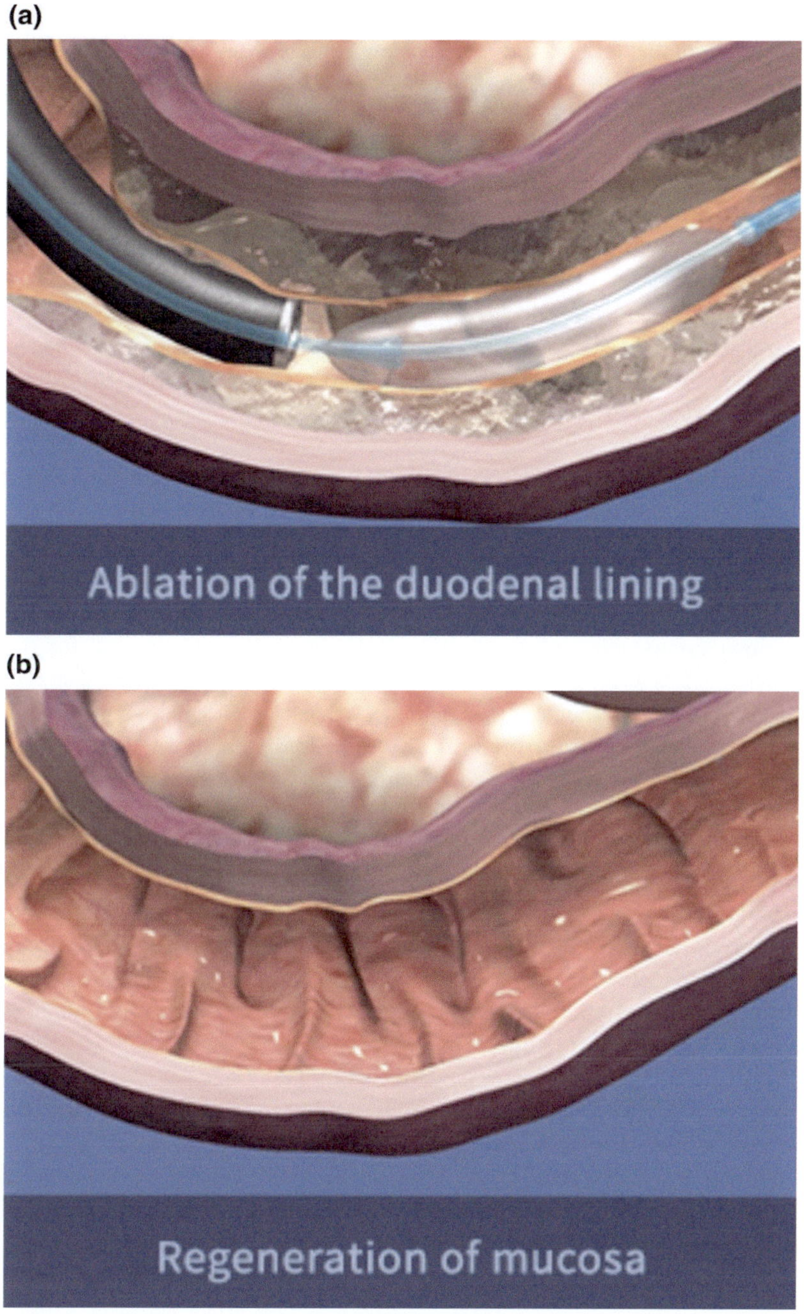

Fig. 10.7 **a** and **b** Revita™ duodenal mucosal resurfacing (Courtesy of Fractyl Laboratories)

weight centers designed to ensure expert patient selection and close follow-up for patients, such practice patterns may change. Full-service weight centers with collaborative input from gastroenterology, bariatric surgery, endocrinology, hepatology, psychology, exercise physiology, nutrition support, and internal medicine will be crucial to ensuring the best possible results for each individual patient. Along these lines, with the large number of EBTs which will likely be available, personalizing the right treatment for each patient will require significant expertise in a range of therapeutic options. Additionally, as better understanding behind the pathophysiology of each patient's obesity arises, we may be better equipped to target and individualize these therapies based on rational hypotheses. With the aid of team collaborations, bariatric endoscopists will need to create pathways of preprocedural, intraprocedural, and post-procedural care which may be unique to their previous work, including design of clinics and endoscopy suites for bariatric patients, as well as addressing best practices in venous thromboembolism prophylaxis.

Combination of Endoscopic and Adjunctive Medical Bariatric Therapies

With EBTs in development that deconstruct the various components of gold-standard bariatric surgical interventions such as the Roux-en-Y gastric bypass, combination therapies which target multimodal elements of surgical weight loss will likely be deployed. Rational combinations of EBTs such as joining IGB or ESG with endoscopic bypass technology or Revita™ dudoenal mucosal resurfacing have the potential to increase the levels of weight loss to those achieved with higher-morbidity bariatric surgeries. Such combination therapies will need to undergo rigorous safety and efficacy trials similar to the single-device studies previously done. Finally, more repeatability trials, which study the results of multiple sequential therapies such as repeat IGBs, will be important [88]. Just as combination of EBTs will likely arise, adjunctive therapies combining medications for weight-loss maintenance hold promise.

Comparative and Cost Effectiveness Research

As the bariatric surgery literature is replete with long-term data demonstrating favorable effects on reducing morbidity and mortality from obesity and metabolic disease, endoluminal bariatric therapies will need to be studied with similar rigor. Primary endpoints related to weight loss are necessary but not sufficient, as increased pressures to contain costs and promote comparative effectiveness research increase. To do this, it will be essential to establish national and international registries of patients which can track outcomes related to safety and efficacy. Given the apparent safety of the less invasive endoscopic methods, head-to-head trials between endoluminal and surgical bariatric procedures may not be necessary for complimentary technologies.

Reimbursement and Insurance Coverage

For EBTs to effectively bridge the gap between medical weight loss and bariatric surgery, insurance approval for these devices and procedures will be needed to expand the pool of candidate patients. At present, these devices in the USA are paid for out of pocket, limiting their use to patients with significant financial means. Governing bodies such as the American Society for Gastrointestinal Endoscopy (ASGE), the American Society for Metabolic and Bariatric Surgery (ASMBS), and Association for Bariatric Endoscopy (ABE) will likely play integral roles in dialogues between large insurers and patients requesting the devices.

Frameshift for a Healthier World

Finally, as we move from a reactive to proactive healthcare paradigm, a frameshift in our approach to obesity and obesity-related diseases must target prevention strategies. Thus, future trials with EBTs targeting BMI in the overweight category will be important toward this end given that by the time class I obesity begins, reversing pathophysiologic processes and behaviors likely becomes more challenging than early intervention. Endoluminal bariatric therapies hold great promise to improve worldwide health, and the bariatric endoscopist is poised to play a critical role in this positive change.

Disclosures Jonah Cohen has no disclosures to report related to this work.
Ram Chuttani is a senior medical advisor to Allurion Technologies.

References

1. Haslam DW, James WP. Obesity. Lancet. 2005;366 (9492):1197–209.
2. Flegal KM, Carroll MD, Ogden CL, Curtin LR. Prevalence and trends in obesity among US adults, 1999–2008. JAMA. 2010;303(3):235–41.
3. Flegal KM, Carroll MD, Kit BK, Ogden CL. Prevalence of obesity and trends in the distribution of body mass index among US adults, 1999–2010. JAMA. 2012;307(5):491–7.
4. Cawley J, Meyerhoefer C. The medical care costs of obesity: an instrumental variables approach. J Health Econ. 2012;31(1):219–30.
5. Flegal KM, Carroll MD, Ogden CL, Johnson CL. Prevalence and trends in obesity among US adults, 1999–2000. JAMA. 2002;288(14):1723–7.
6. Finkelstein EA, Trogdon JG, Cohen JW, Dietz W. Annual medical spending attributable to obesity: payer-and service-specific estimates. Health Aff (Millwood). 2009;28(5):w822–31.
7. Ogden CL, Carroll MD, Kit BK, Flegal KM. Prevalence of childhood and adult obesity in the United States, 2011–2012. JAMA. 2014;311(8):806–14
8. Obesity: preventing and managing the global epidemic. Report of a WHO consultation. World Health Organ Tech Rep Ser. 2000;894:i–xii, 1–253.
9. Ng M, Fleming T, Robinson M, Thomson B, Graetz N, Margono C, et al. Global, regional, and national prevalence of overweight and obesity in children and adults during 1980–2013: a systematic analysis for the Global Burden of Disease Study 2013. Lancet. 2014;384(9945):766–81.
10. Swinburn BA, Sacks G, Hall KD, McPherson K, Finegood DT, Moodie ML, et al. The global obesity pandemic: shaped by global drivers and local environments. Lancet. 2011;378(9793):804–14.
11. McTigue K, Larson JC, Valoski A, Burke G, Kotchen J, Lewis CE, et al. Mortality and cardiac and vascular outcomes in extremely obese women. JAMA. 2006;296(1):79–86.
12. Nguyen NT, Magno CP, Lane KT, Hinojosa MW, Lane JS. Association of hypertension, diabetes, dyslipidemia, and metabolic syndrome with obesity: findings from the National Health and Nutrition Examination Survey, 1999 to 2004. J Am Coll Surg. 2008;207(6):928–34.
13. Bhaskaran K, Douglas I, Forbes H, dos-Santos-Silva I, Leon DA, Smeeth L. Body-mass index and risk of 22 specific cancers: a population-based cohort study of 5.24 million UK adults. Lancet. 2014;384(9945):755–65.
14. Gortmaker SL, Must A, Perrin JM, Sobol AM, Dietz WH. Social and economic consequences of overweight in adolescence and young adulthood. N Engl J Med. 1993;329(14):1008–12.
15. Lau DC, Teoh H. Benefits of modest weight loss on the management of type 2 diabetes mellitus. Can J Diabetes. 2013;37(2):128–34.
16. Soleymani T, Daniel S, Garvey WT. Weight maintenance: challenges, tools and strategies for primary care physicians. Obes Rev. 2016;17(1):81–93.
17. Mathus-Vliegen EM. Endoscopic treatment: the past, the present and the future. Best Pract Res Clin Gastroenterol. 2014;28(4):685–702.
18. Clinical Guidelines on the Identification. Evaluation, and treatment of overweight and obesity in adults—the evidence report. National Institutes of Health. Obes Res. 1998;6(Suppl 2):51S–209S.
19. Swinburn BA, Caterson I, Seidell JC, James WP. Diet, nutrition and the prevention of excess weight gain and obesity. Public Health Nutr. 2004;7(1A):123–46.
20. Wadden TA, Webb VL, Moran CH, Bailer BA. Lifestyle modification for obesity: new developments in diet, physical activity, and behavior therapy. Circulation. 2012;125(9):1157–70.
21. Gregg EW, Chen H, Wagenknecht LE, Clark JM, Delahanty LM, Bantle J, et al. Association of an intensive lifestyle intervention with remission of type 2 diabetes. JAMA. 2012;308(23):2489–96.
22. Diabetes Prevention Program Research G, Knowler WC, Fowler SE, Hamman RF, Christophi CA, Hoffman HJ, et al. 10-year follow-up of diabetes incidence and weight loss in the Diabetes Prevention Program Outcomes Study. Lancet. 2009;374(9702):1677–86.
23. Look ARG. Eight-year weight losses with an intensive lifestyle intervention: the look AHEAD study. Obesity (Silver Spring). 2014;22(1):5–13.
24. Yanovski SZ, Yanovski JA. Long-term drug treatment for obesity: a systematic and clinical review. JAMA. 2014;311(1):74–86.
25. Sjostrom L, Lindroos AK, Peltonen M, Torgerson J, Bouchard C, Carlsson B, et al. Lifestyle, diabetes, and cardiovascular risk factors 10 years after bariatric surgery. N Engl J Med. 2004;351(26):2683–93.
26. Sjostrom L, Narbro K, Sjostrom CD, Karason K, Larsson B, Wedel H, et al. Effects of bariatric surgery on mortality in Swedish obese subjects. N Engl J Med. 2007;357(8):741–52.
27. Bariatric surgery lowers all-cause mortality in the morbidly obese. J Fam Pract. 2007;56(11):893.
28. Gloy VL, Briel M, Bhatt DL, Kashyap SR, Schauer PR, Mingrone G, et al. Bariatric surgery versus non-surgical treatment for obesity: a systematic review and meta-analysis of randomised controlled trials. BMJ. 2013;347:f5934.
29. Colquitt JL, Pickett K, Loveman E, Frampton GK. Surgery for weight loss in adults. Cochrane Database Syst Rev. 2014;8:CD003641.

30. Morino M, Toppino M, Forestieri P, Angrisani L, Allaix ME, Scopinaro N. Mortality after bariatric surgery: analysis of 13,871 morbidly obese patients from a national registry. Ann Surg. 2007;246 (6):1002–7 (discussion 7-9).
31. Flum DR, Dellinger EP. Impact of gastric bypass operation on survival: a population-based analysis. J Am Coll Surg. 2004;199(4):543–51.
32. Chang SH, Stoll CR, Song J, Varela JE, Eagon CJ, Colditz GA. The effectiveness and risks of bariatric surgery: an updated systematic review and meta-analysis, 2003–2012. JAMA Surg. 2014;149(3): 275–87.
33. Buchwald H, Oien DM. Metabolic/bariatric surgery worldwide 2011. Obes Surg. 2013;23(4):427–36.
34. Thompson CC. Bariatric endoscopy. Thompson CC, Ryan, M.B., editors. New York: Springer; 2013.
35. Kumar N. Endoscopic therapy for weight loss: gastroplasty, duodenal sleeves, intragastric balloons, and aspiration. World J Gastrointest Endosc. 2015;7 (9):847–59.
36. Cote GA, Edmundowicz SA. Emerging technology: endoluminal treatment of obesity. Gastrointest Endosc. 2009;70(5):991–9.
37. Stimac D, Majanovic SK. The position of endoscopic procedures in the treatment of obesity. Curr Clin Pharmacol. 2013;8(3):238–46.
38. Majumder S, Birk J. A review of the current status of endoluminal therapy as a primary approach to obesity management. Surg Endosc. 2013;27(7):2305–11.
39. van Hout G, van Heck G. Bariatric psychology, psychological aspects of weight loss surgery. Obes Facts. 2009;2(1):10–5.
40. Prospective Studies C, Whitlock G, Lewington S, Sherliker P, Clarke R, Emberson J, et al. Body-mass index and cause-specific mortality in 900 000 adults: collaborative analyses of 57 prospective studies. Lancet. 2009;373(9669):1083–96.
41. van de Laar A, de Caluwe L, Dillemans B. Relative outcome measures for bariatric surgery. Evidence against excess weight loss and excess body mass index loss from a series of laparoscopic Roux-en-Y gastric bypass patients. Obes Surg. 2011;21(6):763–7.
42. Dixon JB, McPhail T, O'Brien PE. Minimal reporting requirements for weight loss: current methods not ideal. Obes Surg. 2005;15(7):1034–9.
43. Dallal RM, Quebbemann BB, Hunt LH, Braitman LE. Analysis of weight loss after bariatric surgery using mixed-effects linear modeling. Obes Surg. 2009;19 (6):732–7.
44. Therapy AATFoEB, Ginsberg GG, Chand B, Cote GA, Dallal RM, Edmundowicz SA, et al. A pathway to endoscopic bariatric therapies. Gastrointest Endosc. 2011;74(5):943–53.
45. Genco A, Maselli R, Frangella F, Cipriano M, Paone E, Meuti V, et al. Effect of consecutive intragastric balloon (BIB(R)) plus diet versus single BIB(R) plus diet on eating disorders not otherwise specified (EDNOS) in obese patients. Obes Surg. 2013;23(12):2075–9.
46. Abu Dayyeh BK, Kumar N, Edmundowicz SA, Jonnalagadda S, Larsen M, Sullivan S, et al. ASGE Bariatric Endoscopy Task Force systematic review and meta-analysis assessing the ASGE PIVI thresholds for adopting endoscopic bariatric therapies. Gastrointest Endosc. 2015;82(3):425–38e5.
47. Genco A, Maselli R, Frangella F, Cipriano M, Forestieri P, Delle Piane D, et al. Intragastric balloon for obesity treatment: results of a multicentric evaluation for balloons left in place for more than 6 months. Surg Endosc. 2015;29(8):2339–43.
48. Lopez-Nava G, Galvao M, Bautista-Castano I, Fernandez-Corbelle JP, Trell M. Endoscopic sleeve gastroplasty with 1-year follow-up: factors predictive of success. Endosc Int Open. 2016;4(2):E222–7.
49. Genco A, Bruni T, Doldi SB, Forestieri P, Marino M, Busetto L, et al. BioEnterics intragastric balloon: the Italian experience with 2515 patients. Obes Surg. 2005;15(8):1161–4.
50. Gaur S, Levy S, Mathus-Vliegen L, Chuttani R. Balancing risk and reward: a critical review of the intragastric balloon for weight loss. Gastrointest Endosc. 2015;81(6):1330–6.
51. Nieben OG, Harboe H. Intragastric balloon as an artificial bezoar for treatment of obesity. Lancet. 1982;1(8265):198–9.
52. Dumonceau JM. Evidence-based review of the bioenterics intragastric balloon for weight loss. Obes Surg. 2008;18(12):1611–7.
53. Fernandes M, Atallah AN, Soares BG, Humberto S, Guimaraes S, Matos D, et al. Intragastric balloon for obesity. Cochrane Database Syst Rev. 2007(1): CD004931.
54. Gleysteen JJ. A history of intragastric balloons. Surg Obes Relat Dis. 2015.
55. Ponce J, Woodman G, Swain J, Wilson E, English W, Ikramuddin S, et al. The REDUCE pivotal trial: a prospective, randomized controlled pivotal trial of a dual intragastric balloon for the treatment of obesity. Surg Obes Relat Dis. 2015;11 (4):874–81.
56. Imaz I, Martinez-Cervell C, Garcia-Alvarez EE, Sendra-Gutierrez JM, Gonzalez-Enriquez J. Safety and effectiveness of the intragastric balloon for obesity. A meta-analysis. Obes Surg. 2008;18 (7):841–6.
57. Abu Dayyeh BK, Edmundowicz SA, Jonnalagadda S, Kumar N, Larsen M, Sullivan S, et al. Endoscopic bariatric therapies. Gastrointest Endosc. 2015;81 (5):1073–86.
58. Dastis NS, Francois E, Deviere J, Hittelet A, Ilah Mehdi A, Barea M, et al. Intragastric balloon for weight loss: results in 100 individuals followed for at least 2.5 years. Endoscopy. 2009;41(7):575–80.
59. Genco A, Lopez-Nava G, Wahlen C, Maselli R, Cipriano M, Sanchez MM, et al. Multi-centre European experience with intragastric balloon in overweight populations: 13 years of experience. Obes Surg. 2013;23(4):515–21.

60. Kotzampassi K, Grosomanidis V, Papakostas P, Penna S, Eleftheriadis E. 500 intragastric balloons: what happens 5 years thereafter? Obes Surg. 2012;22(6):896–903.
61. Lopez-Nava G, Rubio MA, Prados S, Pastor G, Cruz MR, Companioni E, et al. BioEnterics(R) intragastric balloon (BIB(R)). Single ambulatory center Spanish experience with 714 consecutive patients treated with one or two consecutive balloons. Obes Surg. 2011;21(1):5–9.
62. Genco A, Cipriano M, Bacci V, Maselli R, Paone E, Lorenzo M, et al. Intragastric balloon followed by diet vs intragastric balloon followed by another balloon: a prospective study on 100 patients. Obes Surg. 2010;20(11):1496–500.
63. Dumonceau JM, Francois E, Hittelet A, Mehdi AI, Barea M, Deviere J. Single vs repeated treatment with the intragastric balloon: a 5-year weight loss study. Obes Surg. 2010;20(6):692–7.
64. Mion F, Ibrahim M, Marjoux S, Ponchon T, Dugardeyn S, Roman S, et al. Swallowable Obalon (R) gastric balloons as an aid for weight loss: a pilot feasibility study. Obes Surg. 2013;23(5):730–3.
65. Machytka E, Chuttani R, Bojkova M, Kupka T, Buzga M, Stecco K, et al. Elipse, a procedureless gastric balloon for weight loss: a proof-of-concept pilot study. Obes Surg. 2016;26(3):512–6.
66. Machytka E, Klvana P, Kornbluth A, Peikin S, Mathus-Vliegen LE, Gostout C, et al. Adjustable intragastric balloons: a 12-month pilot trial in endoscopic weight loss management. Obes Surg. 2011;21(10):1499–507.
67. Brooks J, Srivastava ED, Mathus-Vliegen EM. One-year adjustable intragastric balloons: results in 73 consecutive patients in the U.K. Obes Surg. 2014;24(5):813–9.
68. Genco A, Dellepiane D, Baglio G, Cappelletti F, Frangella F, Maselli R, et al. Adjustable intragastric balloon vs non-adjustable intragastric balloon: case-control study on complications, tolerance, and efficacy. Obes Surg. 2013;23(7):953–8.
69. Sharaiha RZ, Kedia P, Kumta N, DeFilippis EM, Gaidhane M, Shukla A, et al. Initial experience with endoscopic sleeve gastroplasty: technical success and reproducibility in the bariatric population. Endoscopy. 2015;47(2):164–6.
70. Abu Dayyeh BK, Acosta A, Camilleri M, Mundi MS, Rajan E, Topazian MD, et al. Endoscopic sleeve gastroplasty alters gastric physiology and induces loss of body weight in obese individuals. Clin Gastroenterol Hepatol. 2015.
71. Espinos JC, Turro R, Mata A, Cruz M, da Costa M, Villa V, et al. Early experience with the Incisionless Operating Platform (IOP) for the treatment of obesity: the primary obesity surgery endolumenal (POSE) procedure. Obes Surg. 2013;23(9):1375–83.
72. Bradley D, Magkos F, Klein S. Effects of bariatric surgery on glucose homeostasis and type 2 diabetes. Gastroenterology. 2012;143(4):897–912.
73. Rubino F, Forgione A, Cummings DE, Vix M, Gnuli D, Mingrone G, et al. The mechanism of diabetes control after gastrointestinal bypass surgery reveals a role of the proximal small intestine in the pathophysiology of type 2 diabetes. Ann Surg. 2006;244(5):741–9.
74. Klein S, Fabbrini E, Patterson BW, Polonsky KS, Schiavon CA, Correa JL, et al. Moderate effect of duodenal-jejunal bypass surgery on glucose homeostasis in patients with type 2 diabetes. Obesity (Silver Spring). 2012;20(6):1266–72.
75. Tarnoff M, Rodriguez L, Escalona A, Ramos A, Neto M, Alamo M, et al. Open label, prospective, randomized controlled trial of an endoscopic duodenal-jejunal bypass sleeve versus low calorie diet for pre-operative weight loss in bariatric surgery. Surg Endosc. 2009;23(3):650–6.
76. Gersin KS, Rothstein RI, Rosenthal RJ, Stefanidis D, Deal SE, Kuwada TS, et al. Open-label, sham-controlled trial of an endoscopic duodenojejunal bypass liner for preoperative weight loss in bariatric surgery candidates. Gastrointest Endosc. 2010;71(6):976–82.
77. Schouten R, Rijs CS, Bouvy ND, Hameeteman W, Koek GH, Janssen IM, et al. A multicenter, randomized efficacy study of the endobarrier gastrointestinal liner for presurgical weight loss prior to bariatric surgery. Ann Surg. 2010;251(2):236–43.
78. de Moura EG, Martins BC, Lopes GS, Orso IR, de Oliveira SL, Galvao Neto MP, et al. Metabolic improvements in obese type 2 diabetes subjects implanted for 1 year with an endoscopically deployed duodenal-jejunal bypass liner. Diabetes Technol Ther. 2012;14(2):183–9.
79. Escalona A, Pimentel F, Sharp A, Becerra P, Slako M, Turiel D, et al. Weight loss and metabolic improvement in morbidly obese subjects implanted for 1 year with an endoscopic duodenal-jejunal bypass liner. Ann Surg. 2012;255(6):1080–5.
80. de Jonge C, Rensen SS, Verdam FJ, Vincent RP, Bloom SR, Buurman WA, et al. Endoscopic duodenal-jejunal bypass liner rapidly improves type 2 diabetes. Obes Surg. 2013;23(9):1354–60.
81. Koehestanie P, de Jonge C, Berends FJ, Janssen IM, Bouvy ND, Greve JW. The effect of the endoscopic duodenal-jejunal bypass liner on obesity and type 2 diabetes mellitus, a multicenter randomized controlled trial. Ann Surg. 2014;260(6):984–92.
82. Sullivan S, Stein R, Jonnalagadda S, Mullady D, Edmundowicz S. Aspiration therapy leads to weight loss in obese subjects: a pilot study. Gastroenterology. 2013;145(6):1245–52e1-5.
83. Nauck MA, Meier JJ. The incretin effect in healthy individuals and those with type 2 diabetes: physiology, pathophysiology, and response to therapeutic interventions. Lancet Diabetes Endocrinol. 2016.
84. Knop FK, Vilsboll T, Hojberg PV, Larsen S, Madsbad S, Volund A, et al. Reduced incretin effect in type 2 diabetes: cause or consequence of the diabetic state? Diabetes. 2007;56(8):1951–9.

85. Ryou M, Cantillon-Murphy P, Azagury D, Shaikh SN, Ha G, Greenwalt I, et al. Smart Self-Assembling MagnetS for ENdoscopy (SAM-SEN) for transoral endoscopic creation of immediate gastrojejunostomy (with video). Gastrointest Endosc. 2011;73(2):353–9.
86. van Avesaat M, Troost FJ, Ripken D, Hendriks HF, Masclee AA. Ileal brake activation: macronutrient-specific effects on eating behavior? Int J Obes (Lond). 2015;39(2):235–43.
87. Ryou M, Agoston AT, Thompson CC. Endoscopic intestinal bypass creation by using self-assembling magnets in a porcine model. Gastrointest Endosc. 2016;83(4):821–5.
88. Alfredo G, Roberta M, Massimiliano C, Michele L, Nicola B, Adriano R. Long-term multiple intragastric balloon treatment—a new strategy to treat morbid obese patients refusing surgery: prospective 6-year follow-up study. Surg Obes Relat Dis. 2014;10(2):307–11.

NOTES Transgastric Diaphragm Pacing

11

Raymond P. Onders

Abstract

Mechanical ventilation (MV) is a life-sustaining treatment in patients who are unable to maintain spontaneous ventilation. Failure to wean (FTW) from MV, or prolonged ventilation results in significant morbidity, mortality, and health care costs. Diaphragm pacing (DP) was initially developed to provide natural negative pressure ventilation in spinal cord injured (SCI) patients on MV. Its use has since expanded to ALS patients, as well as in critically ill patients to shorten MV time. A new technical development was that of a temporary and removable electrode. Since our group has experience with bedside NOTES with PEG rescue, we hypothesize that NOTES placement of DP electrodes is technically feasible and safe.

Keywords

Diaphragm pacing · Mechanical ventilation · Diaphragm pacing system · Failure to wean · Tracheostomy · Intensive care unit

Abbreviations

ALS	Amyotrophic lateral sclerosis
DP	Diaphragm pacing
DPS	Diaphragmatic pacing systems
EMG	Daily electromyogram
EPG	External pulse generator
FDA	Federal drug administration
FTW	Failure to wean
ICU	Intensive care unit

R.P. Onders (✉)
Margaret and Walter Remen Chair of Surgical Innovation, University Hospitals Case Medical Center, Case Western Reserve University School of Medicine, 11100 Euclid Avenue, Cleveland, OH 44106-5047, USA
e-mail: Raymond.onders@uhhospitals.org

J.R. Romanelli et al. (eds.), *NOTES and Endoluminal Surgery*, Clinical Gastroenterology, DOI 10.1007/978-3-319-50610-4_11

LTMV	Long-term mechanical ventilation
MV	Mechanical ventilation
NOTES	Natural orifice translumenal endoscopic surgery
PEG	Percutaneous endoscopic gastrostomy
SCI	Spinal cord injury/spinal cord injured
VIDD	Ventilator-induced diaphragm dysfunction

Background

Mechanical ventilation (MV) is a life-sustaining treatment in patients who are unable to maintain spontaneous ventilation. In the hospital setting, MV is utilized for treatment of acute respiratory failure, trauma, as well as intra-operatively and during post-operative recovery. Failure to wean (FTW) from MV or prolonged ventilation results in significant morbidity, mortality, and health care costs. The etiology of FTW is multifactorial, but inspiratory muscle atrophy has been shown to be a significant contributor to this condition. Research in animals and humans has shown that short exposure to MV leads to decreases in protein synthesis and increased proteolysis, which is histopathologically manifested as diaphragm muscle atrophy, with 50% diaphragm atrophy and conversion to the non-functional, fast-twitch, type-IIb muscle fibers in less than one day [1]. The severity of this muscle atrophy increases with increased time of MV exposure. This condition is called ventilator-induced diaphragm dysfunction (VIDD). There is an identified clinical need for treatments to prevent the muscle atrophy that leads to VIDD. Direct electrical stimulation of muscle has been shown to reduce muscle atrophy.

Diaphragm pacing (DP) was developed to provide natural negative pressure ventilation in spinal cord injured (SCI) patients on MV. DP involves laparoscopically placed electrodes at the motor point of each hemi-diaphragm where stimulation provides maximal contraction of the diaphragm. Essentially, DP electrically stimulates intact lower motor units in the spinal column replacing the upper motor neuron signal. DP has been approved by the Federal Drug Administration (FDA) in patients with high SCI and has been shown to facilitate weaning from MV and be the primary ventilatory support following successful removal from MV [2]. DP has also been approved for use in patients with amyotrophic lateral sclerosis (ALS). In this ALS patient cohort, DP has been shown to increase muscle thickness and, in comparison to historical controls, to prolong survival [3].

DP has also been used recently in helping to wean patients from MV without SCI using the standard laparoscopic approach, which required a separate trip to the operating room. Because many intensive care unit (ICU) patients already have bedside endoscopy performed for percutaneous endoscopic gastrostomies (PEG), natural orifice translumenal endoscopic surgery (NOTES) may be the logical next step for DP implantation. Although bedside laparoscopy has been performed in ICUs, it is not as well accepted as or as easy as bedside endoscopy. This chapter outlines current diaphragm pacing technology and the development of temporary diaphragm pacing electrodes implanted with NOTES at the time of a bedside PEG.

History of Standard Laparoscopic Diaphragm Pacing

Surgical implantation of standard DP begins with general anesthesia being administered without neuromuscular blocking agents so that muscle stimulation can occur. Short-acting agents such as propofol for amnesia, remifentanil for pain, along with inhalation agents are the preferred anesthetic management for patients undergoing DP [4]. Four laparoscopic ports are used: one supraumbilical, two lateral, and one 12-mm epigastric port for the implant instrument. The falciform ligament is divided allowing easier access of the implant instruments to the diaphragm and to provide an unimpeded exit for the pacing electrodes.

The next step of DP surgery is mapping of the diaphragm. This process identifies the motor point. The tip of a laparoscopic dissector is touched against the diaphragm muscle. A twitch stimulus is delivered from a clinical station to the instrument, and both qualitative and quantitative data are obtained. Quantitative changes in abdominal pressure are measured through tubing that is attached to one of the surgical ports and connected to the clinical station. A greater change in pressure indicates closer proximity to the motor point of the phrenic nerve, and a larger diaphragm muscle contraction. Qualitative visual observation of the diaphragm is made during stimulation. The area of electrode placement is chosen based on location of larger contraction, with strong preference for the posterior diaphragm to facilitate posterior lung lobe ventilation, which will decrease atelectasis. Two electrodes are then implanted into the right and left diaphragm muscle. Placement of two electrodes in each diaphragm provides redundancy and synergy for maximal muscle recruitment. The electrodes are implanted using an implant instrument (Fig. 11.1). The electrode is threaded through the instrument to the tip of needle. The needle at the end of the instrument is inserted into the muscle, and the polypropylene barb on the end of the electrode releases upon withdrawal of the needle. The four electrodes and an anode are then tunneled subcutaneously to an appropriate exit site.

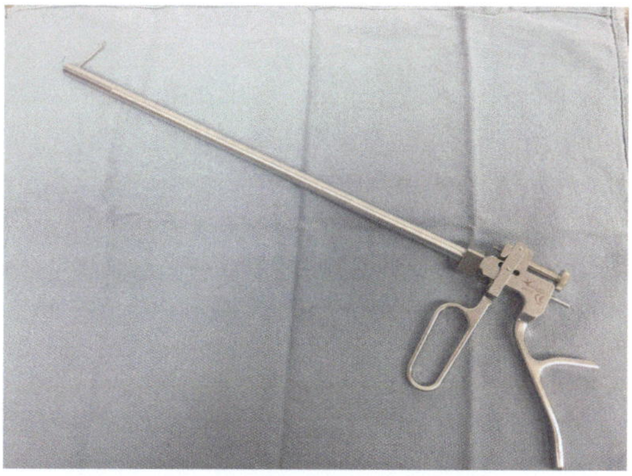

Fig. 11.1 Laparoscopic implant instrument houses the diaphragm pacing electrode, which is a double helix of 14 stainless steel wires that are Teflon coated. The needle of the implant instrument enters the diaphragm muscle and a polypropylene barb allows the electrode to be fixed in place

The implanted intramuscular electrodes are connected to a four-channel, external pulse generator (EPG). This stimulator provides capacitive coupled, charge-balanced, biphasic stimulation to each subcutaneous electrode. The EPG is programmed with patient-specific parameters of pulse amplitude, pulse duration, inspiratory time, pulse rate, and respiratory rate to maximize ventilation for SCI patients or for muscle training in other patient populations. DP users simply connect and turn the device on or off. The goal for patient settings is to use the highest settings that do not cause any patient discomfort. Once implanted, the device can be utilized immediately to begin diaphragm conditioning. DP conditioning will convert the atrophied muscle fibers from fast-fatigable type 2B muscle fibers to the better functioning, slow-twitch type 1.

The initial FDA, multicenter clinical trial of DP in SCI dependent on tracheostomy and MV showed that 100% of implanted patients with stimulatable diaphragms were able to breathe for 4 consecutive hours with DP alone. Over 50% of patients utilized DP for over 24 h of continuous use. While the objective of DP in SCI is to provide primary ventilatory support off MV for several hours, a course of short-duration diaphragm conditioning sessions is needed first in order to reverse disuse atrophy of the diaphragm as would be done in ICU patients. This trial reports no pneumonia deaths because of the improvement of posterior lobe ventilation with DP as opposed to MV. Therefore, DP may be beneficial for even short-term use in ICU patients.

Posluszny et al. [5] conducted a retrospective analysis of the interventional use of DPS in 29 traumatic cervical SCI patients at 10 centers who underwent early implantation in the ICU after their injury. Of the stimulable patients undergoing DP, 72% (16 of 22) were completely free of ventilator support in an average of 10.2 days. The study concluded that DP can shorten the duration of mechanical ventilation and, in many instances, allow for complete independence from mechanical ventilation in those patients with an intact phrenic system but without control of ventilation. Also, 30% of the patients recovered their own ability to breathe and no longer needed DP, therefore identifying the use of DP as a temporary device in the ICU.

In a pilot ALS study in which 16 patients were implanted with diaphragmatic pacers, there were a total of 452 implant months of follow-up, with a mean of 28.2 months per patient [6]. This study showed that the post-DP implant diaphragm muscle thickness, as evaluated by ultrasound, was consistently greater for all patients than at pre-implant. This showed the ability of DP to overcome disuse atrophy and improve diaphragm strength. Further, an evaluation of 86 ALS patients with chronic hypoventilation and preserved bilateral phrenic nerve function showed that DPS used with or without concurrent NIV improved survival when compared to historical controls (FDA: HDE H100006).

Recently, Onders et al. [7] reported on the extended use of diaphragm pacing in patients with diaphragm dysfunction leading to symptomatic hypoventilation. In this study, 21 patients with a mean of 36 months of respiratory symptoms were implanted with diaphragmatic pacers. Thirteen patients (62%) had clinically relevant respiratory improvements, and 4 had partial improvement. Four patients were able to be completely weaned from MV. In these patients, the DP system was removed, again highlighting the possibility of a temporary DP system for weaning patients from MV in the ICU.

Development of NOTES Diaphragm Pacing in the Intensive Care Unit

For NOTES DP to be successful for temporary use in the ICU, several key points needed to be addressed: adequate visualization of the diaphragm with NOTES, utilization of NOTES in the ICU, gastrotomy closure, concern of infection with a NOTES approach to diaphragm pacing, the development of temporary diaphragm electrodes for implantation and externalization, and ability to implant the diaphragm electrodes without laparoscopic mapping and still able to provide respiratory support.

Our group at University Hospitals and Case Western Reserve University has shown the feasibility both in animals and in humans for ICU NOTES. One of the first ICU NOTES cases was a PEG rescue showing the initial feasibility of ICU access to the peritoneal cavity with closure of the gastrostomy with a PEG [8]. In subsequent clinical experience in these cases, we could easily see both diaphragms in retroflexed view through the gastrotomy. In an initial pilot (and subsequently randomized) animal trial comparing NOTES with laparoscopy to assess for simulated ICU pathology, we showed that a positive identification via NOTES was highly specific, with a strong positive predictive value [9, 10]. The diaphragm was also easily visualized in these cases. We therefore believe that diaphragm visualization can be easily done with NOTES in the ICU setting.

Diagnostic and therapeutic flexible endoscopy at the bedside is a standard ICU procedure that requires minimal support from ancillary staff. Using the same equipment, NOTES can provide access to the peritoneal cavity and could decrease the number of patients with unrecognized intra-abdominal catastrophic events. The peritoneal cavity is accessed by a transgastric route through a modified percutaneous endoscopic gastrostomy (PEG) technique, which is a common ICU procedure. It is a technically familiar procedure and uses instruments and materials that are widely available. This appears to be the most dependable method, involving a Seldinger technique in which a guidewire is placed in the gastric lumen at a standard anterior site on the abdominal wall for a PEG. The endoscope and guidewire are then brought out through the mouth, and the endoscope is reinserted alongside the guidewire. A gastrotomy is performed at the site of the guide wire with needle-knife cautery to make the initial incision, followed by endoscopic balloon dilation to enlarge the gastrotomy. The endoscope is then advanced into the peritoneal cavity for visualization and can be retroflexed to visualize both diaphragms through the gastrotomy.

The optimal gastrotomy closure for NOTES is still to be determined. However, in the ICU, the gastrotomy does not have to be closed but can be managed with the use of a PEG. PEGs are commonly placed in patients on MV to optimize nutrition. Once the NOTES abdominal exploration is complete, the gastrotomy is managed by attaching a standard-pull PEG tube to the guidewire left in place during the NOTES procedure. The PEG is withdrawn back through the gastrotomy, leaving the internal mushroom bumper in the gastric lumen. When concern that the gastrotomy has become too large is an issue, additional sutures to affix the stomach to the anterior abdominal wall can be accomplished using a T-fastener technique. Therefore, the concern of closing the gastrotomy in NOTES DP is easily addressed.

In a group of ALS patients undergoing simultaneous DP and gastrostomy, a significant improvement was seen in both 30-day mortality and 1-year survival compared with PEG alone (76% survival at 1 year with DP and PEG vs. only 23% with PEG alone) [11]. Simultaneous diaphragm pacing and PEGs showed no increase in the infection rate of the implanted transperitoneal diaphragm wires when a gastrostomy was done, even though it became a contaminated case. This large experience of DP with PEGs, and no increase in infection with long-term DP use, confirms temporary DP wires placed via NOTES should not increase the infection risk, since NOTES is only used to visualize the percutaneous implantation of the electrodes.

One major change that was performed was to change the electrode to allow for easier removal. The distal end of the newly designed temporary diaphragm electrode (TransLoc, Synapse Biomedical, Oberlin, OH) is identical to the permanent diaphragm pacing electrode used in over 1500 humans (PermaLoc, Synapse Biomedical, Oberlin, OH) except that there is no polypropylene barb affixed to the stimulus end of the electrode (Fig. 11.2). The removal of the polypropylene barb from the electrode reduces the fixation of the electrode to the diaphragm that occurs during normal tissue encapsulation. This allows easy removal with no retained foreign bodies. It has also been reported in animal studies that a similar electrode can be placed successfully with the use of NOTES visualization [12]. This would also decrease the risk of contamination because the electrode does not traverse the gastric lumen.

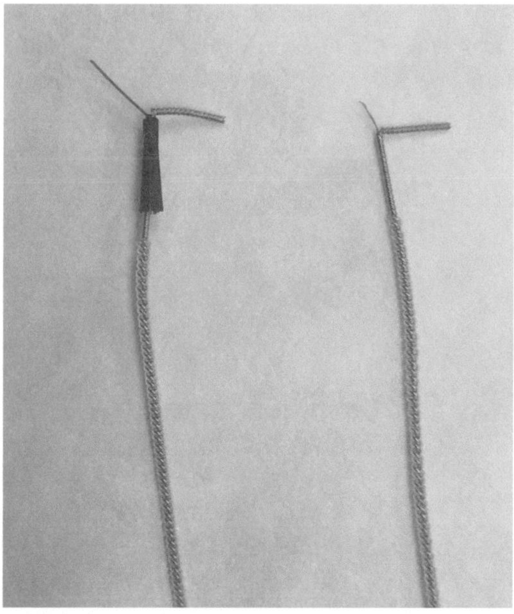

Fig. 11.2 Comparison of permanent diaphragm pacing electrode to temporary diaphragm pacing electrode

A human trial of this new electrode was recently completed. This was a prospective FDA study (IDE #G150040), was IRB-approved, and was listed on clinicaltrials.gov (NCT 02410798) that evaluated the feasibility of temporary diaphragm electrodes to provide ventilation with stimulation. At the end of the subject's primary surgical procedure, two temporary diaphragm pacing electrodes were placed intramuscularly in each hemi-diaphragm at the expected motor point where, with stimulation, diffuse diaphragm contraction would occur because of proximity to the phrenic nerve. This was done without mapping the diaphragm. The electrodes were removed from the abdominal or chest cavity with a Keith needle attached to the electrode or via the use of a percutaneous grasper for the laparoscopic cases. These removal methods would also be used after NOTES placement (Fig. 11.3). The electrodes exited the abdominal or chest cavity on each lateral side without tunneling to a central location, which is standard with the permanent system used in SCI and ALS patients. The electrodes that would be placed with the NOTES technique would be attached immediately at the bedside to an EPG with connecting cables to begin diaphragm conditioning (Figs. 11.4 and 11.5).

There were 8 males and 4 females who underwent 3 different approaches: 4 median sternotomy, 4 laparoscopy, and 4 laparotomy.

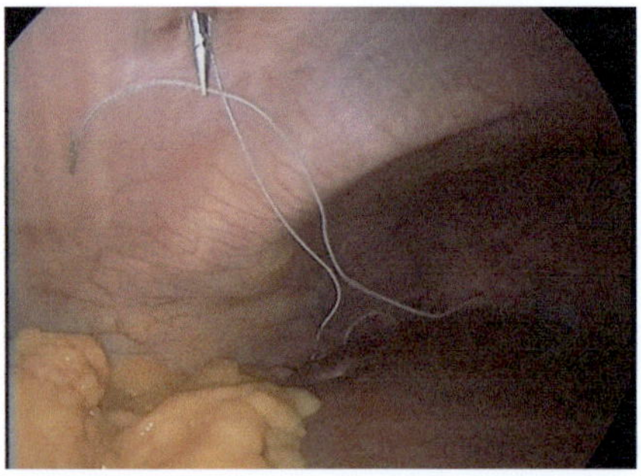

Fig. 11.3 Percutaneous retrieval of the temporary electrode using a suture grasper (Carter-Thompson) because direct external access can be visualized with NOTES

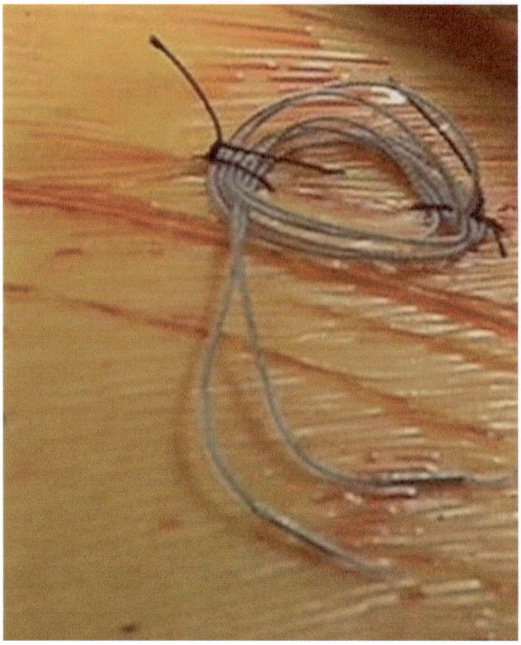

Fig. 11.4 The placed electrodes are sutured to the skin in a fashion similar to the ubiquitous temporary cardiac pacing wires

Subjects had multiple comorbidities, with ASA of 2–4 (2.9 average). In all patients, electrode stimulation exceeded ideal tidal volumes by an average of 37% (0–95%). This confirms that in this group of patients, mapping the diaphragm would not be necessary to adequately provide ventilation. A daily electromyogram was obtained to analyze respiratory function and confirming stability of placement until removal.

This study confirmed that these electrodes could be utilized throughout a patient's hospitalization to maintain diaphragm strength and prevent atrophy. There were no complications with the placement of the electrodes, and all 48 study electrodes remained in place until removal prior to discharge. There was complete intact removal of all 48 electrodes at the bedside. This trial demonstrates the ease of placement, removal, functionality, and safety of temporary DP electrodes [13].

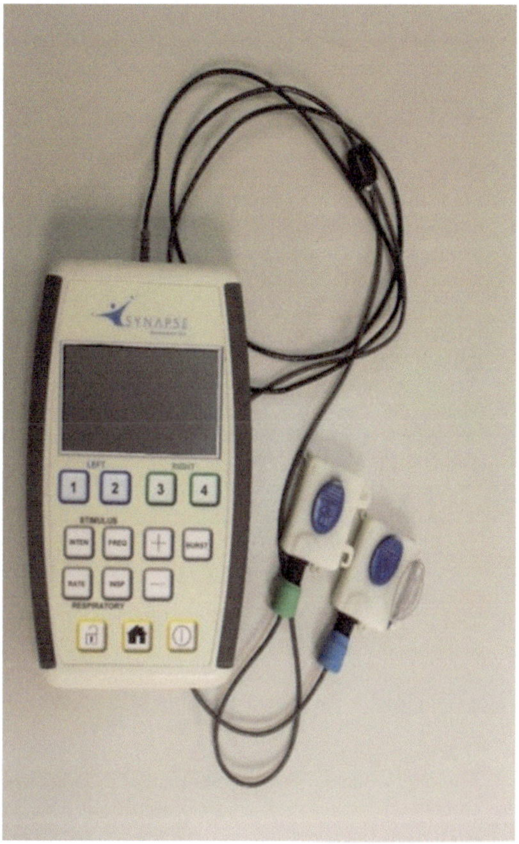

Fig. 11.5 To condition the diaphragm. the diaphragm electrodes would immediately be attached to an EPG via connecting cables to begin conditioning the diaphragm after the NOTES procedure (prototype from Synapse Biomedical, Oberlin, Ohio)

Conclusion

Up to 50% of ICU patients require mechanical ventilation, and 20% are on a ventilator for over 7 days. Over 40% of this time is spent weaning a patient from mechanical ventilation after the initial event that caused intubation. There are multiple etiologies contributing to FTW resulting in long-term mechanical ventilation (LTMV). LTMV has a 20–50% 1-year mortality rate, poor functional outcomes, and a median cost of $306,000.00. The number of LTMV patients is growing at 5.5% annually. It is estimated there will be 605,000 patients requiring LTMV by 2020 at a cost of $64 billion, making prevention and treatment of FTW a priority [14]. DP has been successfully used in SCI and in other causes of FTW to replace or decrease mechanical ventilation. Early implantation of DP has substantial benefits and as of yet no known drawbacks [5]. The concerns of NOTES DP have been addressed with engineering and clinical experience. NOTES DP can provide a novel adjunctive therapy, stimulating the diaphragm to maintain diaphragm muscle strength, translating to decreased ventilator wean times, and reducing long-term MV.

At the American Thoracic Society Meeting in May 2016, the group from University Hospitals in Cleveland reported the use of the DP system in a series of FTW patients. This was a retrospective review of compassionate, off-label use of an FDA-approved device under IRB approval [15]. Immediately after implantation, the DP system was used to drive ventilation, with subsequent weaning from mechanical ventilation. Ten patients were implanted laparoscopically with no complications. The primary diagnosis causing FTW was the result of: 7 patients who had a median sternotomy with acute phrenic nerve injury (2 heart transplant, 1 left ventricular device, 3 CABG, 1 atrial myxoma), 1 aspiration pneumonia, 1 liver transplant, and 1 idiopathic diaphragm paralysis. Mean duration of positive pressure mechanical ventilation prior to intervention was 44 days (range 4 to 148 days). All 10 were successfully weaned. Mean time to completely wean from invasive ventilation was 15 days (range 1–35). All tracheostomy patients were decannulated. In the 6 patients implanted 12 months or longer, there is an average survival of 34.84 months (14.4–58 months). All live at home, perform activities of daily living independently and are at or near pre-respiratory failure function.

The conclusion is that DP can be used as a therapy to treat FTW. The long-term survival and functionality of this group is significantly better than typical reports of prolonged MV patients. The last patient in this report was identified with significant diaphragm dysfunction post-median sternotomy with only 4 days of invasive ventilation. He was weaned with DP in one day, obviating the need for tracheostomy. This suggests that DP could alter the paradigm of PMV and should be studied more extensively in select groups of patients. The ability to implant DP with NOTES at the bedside would significantly decrease the morbidity and cost of going to the operating room. In the future, if NOTES DP can be shown to maintain diaphragm strength with diaphragm pacing as a powered muscle stimulator, and prevent the need for a tracheostomy as shown in our last patient, the common classification of a patient in an ICU may change from the need for a "tracheostomy and a PEG" to the need for a "PEG and NOTES DP." This could significantly decrease the over 100,000 temporary tracheostomies performed a year in the USA for FTW and might decrease the burden of long-term MV.

Conflict of Interest Disclosure Dr. Raymond Onders, University Hospitals of Cleveland and Case Western Reserve University School of Medicine have intellectual property rights involved with the diaphragm pacing system and equity in Synapse Biomedical who manufactures the device.

References

1. Levine S, Nguyen T, Taylor N, Friscia ME, Budak MT, Rothenberg P, et al. Rapid disuse atrophy of diaphragm fibers in mechanically ventilated humans. N Engl J Med. 2008;35:1327–35.
2. Onders RP, Khansarinia S, Weiser T, Chin C, Hungness E, et al. Multi-center analysis of diaphragm pacing in tetraplegic with cardiac pacemakers: positive implications for ventilator weaning in intensive care units. Surgery. 2010;148:893–7.
3. Onders RP, Elmo M, Khansarinia S, Bowman B, Yee J, et al. Complete worldwide experience in laparoscopic diaphragm pacing: results and differences in spinal cord injured patients and amyotrophic lateral sclerosis patients. Surg Endosc. 2009;23:1433–40.
4. Onders RP, Carlin AM, Elmo MJ, Sivashankaran S, Katirji B, Schilz R. Amyotrophic lateral sclerosis: the midwestern surgical experience with diaphragm pacing stimulation system shows that general anesthesia can be safely performed. Am J Surg. 2009;197:386–90.
5. Posluszny JA, Onders R, Kerwin AJ, Weinstein MS, Stein DM, et al. multicenter review of diaphragm pacing in spinal cord injury: successful not only in weaning from ventilators but also in bridging to independent respiration. J Trauma Acute Care Surg. 2014;76:303–10.
6. Onders R, Elmo M, Kaplan C, Katirji B, Schilz R. Final analysis of the pilot trial of diaphragm pacing in amyotrophic lateral sclerosis with long term follow-up: diaphragm pacing positively affects diaphragm respiration. Am J Surg. 2014;207:393–7.
7. Onders R, Elmo MJ, Kaplan C, Katirji B, Schilz R. Extended use of diaphragm pacing in patients with unilateral of bilateral diaphragm dysfunction: a new therapeutic option. Surgery. 2014;156:772–86.
8. Marks JM, Ponsky JL, Pearl JP, McGee MF. PEG "Rescue": a practical NOTES technique. Surg Endosc. 2007;21:816–9.
9. Onders RP, McGee MF, Marks J, Chak A, Rosen MJ, et al. Natural orifice transluminal endoscopic surgery (NOTES): as a diagnostic tool in the intensive care unit (ICU). Surg Endosc. 2007;21:681–3.
10. Trunzo JA, Poulose BK, McGee MF, Nikfarjam M, Schomisch SJ, et al. The diagnostic efficacy of natural orifice transluminal endoscopic surgery: is there a role in the intensive care unit? Surg Endosc. 2010;24:2485–91.
11. US Food and Drug Administration. NeuRx DPS™, diaphragm pacing system. Summary of safety and probable benefit (SSPB). 2011. Retrieved 15 Aug 2016 from FDA website: http://www.accessdata.fda.gov/cdrh_docs/pdf10/H100006b.pdf.
12. Onders R, McGee MF, Marks J, Chak A, Schilz R, et al. Diaphragm pacing with natural orifice transluminal endoscopic surgery (NOTES): potential for difficult to wean intensive care unit (ICU) patients. Surg Endosc. 2007;21:475–9.
13. Onders R, Markowitz A, Hardacre J, Prabhu A, Novitsky Y, Nearman H, Elmo M, Kaplan C. Completed FDA feasibility trial of surgically placed temporary diaphragm pacing electrodes: a promising option to prevent and treat respiratory failure. Am J Respir Crit Care Med. 2016;193:A7654. doi:10.1164/ajrccm-conference.2016.193.1_MeetingAbstracts.A7654 (First published online May 02, 2016).
14. Daniel Martin A, Smith B, Gabrielli A. Mechanical ventilation, diaphragm weakness and weaning: a rehabilitation perspective. Respir Physiol Neurobiol. 2013;189(2):377–83.
15. Onders R, Elmo M, Kaplan C, Nearman H, Schilz R. Diaphragm pacing as successful salvage therapy in failure to wean patients: should this novel technology be used earlier. Am J Respir Crit Care Med. 2016;193:A7653. doi:10.1164/ajrccmconference.2016.193.1_MeetingAbstracts.A7653 (First published online May 02, 2016).

NOTES Pancreatic Debridement

12

Ryan Law and Todd H. Baron

Abstract

Recent refinements in the nomenclature have attempted to simplify previous classification schemes regarding acute pancreatitis and its sequelae. Our understanding of the natural history of acute pancreatitis and its sequelae continues to evolve. A subset of patients with acute pancreatitis develops peripancreatic collections that, over time, may evolve into walled-off necrosis (WON). The currently available literature suggests that endoscopic management of WON is the preferred management strategy in the majority of cases. Treatment strategies range from simple drainage of liquefied contents to repeated direct endoscopic necrosectomy (DEN) of a complex necrotic collection, with each method requiring a variety of techniques and tools necessary to achieve success. In this chapter, we focus on the indications, techniques, and outcomes for endoscopic therapy of WON.

Keywords

Acute pancreatitis · Pancreatic necrosis/therapy · Endoscopic therapy · Minimally invasive · Pancreatitis/adverse events · Drainage/methods · Therapeutic irrigation

R. Law
Division of Gastroenterology and Hepatology,
University of Michigan, Ann Arbor, MI, USA
e-mail: rjlaw@umich.edu

T.H. Baron (✉)
Division of Gastroenterology and Hepatology,
University of North Carolina, 41041 Bioinformatics
Blvd, CB 7080, Chapel Hill, NC 27599-0001, USA
e-mail: todd_baron@med.unc.edu

J.R. Romanelli et al. (eds.), *NOTES and Endoluminal Surgery*,
Clinical Gastroenterology, DOI 10.1007/978-3-319-50610-4_12

Abbreviations

WON	Walled-off necrosis
CT	Computed tomography
DEN	Direct endoscopic necrosectomy
FNA	Fine needle aspiration
EUS	Endoscopic ultrasound
SEMS	Self-expandable metal stent
LAMS	Lumen-apposing metal stent
ERCP	Endoscopic retrograde cholangiopancreatography
VARD	Video-assisted retroperitoneal debridement
TTS	Through-the-scope

Introduction

Regardless of the mechanism, injury to the pancreas leads to parenchymal inflammation and often to disruption of the main pancreatic duct and/or its side branches. Ductal involvement following pancreas injury frequently leads to leakage of ductal contents and subsequent formation of pancreatic collections containing fluid with or without the presence of solid debris. Approximately 5–10% of patients with acute pancreatitis develop evidence of parenchymal necrosis, most commonly in conjunction with necrosis of surrounding structures [1]. Clinically severe acute pancreatitis is frequently secondary to necrosis of the pancreatic parenchyma and/or necrosis of surrounding peripancreatic tissues. Over the course of several weeks, this process evolves, culminating in walled-off necrosis (WON) (Fig. 12.1) [1, 2]. The basis of endoscopic therapy in this setting relies on drainage of liquefied contents and, when necessary, removal of necrotic debris. Endoscopic therapy is considered the current standard of care for management of WON after acute pancreatitis. Minimally invasive approaches have been adopted by most institutions, most commonly including flexible endoscopic and percutaneous intervention, either alone or in combination [3]. This chapter will focus on the indications, techniques, and outcomes of endoscopic therapy and management of WON.

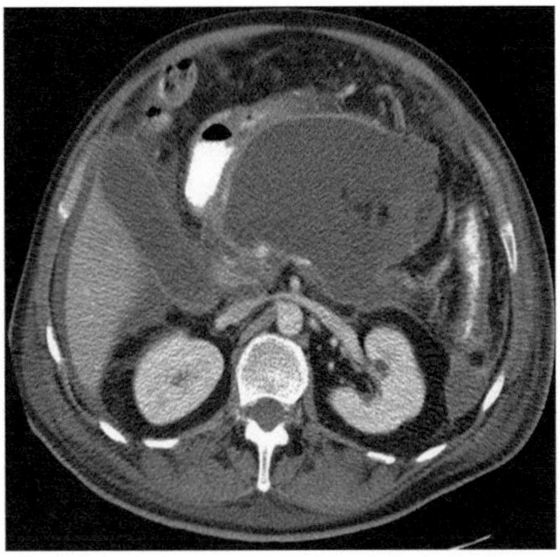

Fig. 12.1 CT scan of walled-off pancreatic necrosis 5 weeks after onset of acute necrotizing pancreatitis. A large collection replacing the pancreas is seen

Indications and Timing of Intervention

Cross-sectional imaging should be performed prior to initiation of endoscopic debridement to evaluate the characteristics of the collection (i.e., size, shape, wall thickness), discern any intervening vasculature, and determine the relationship to the lumen wall. The computed tomography (CT) appearance of WON can vary. Most commonly pancreatic necrosis is detected radiographically on contrast-enhanced CT by the presence of non-enhancement of the pancreatic parenchyma and surrounding structures. However, it may appear homogenous, similar to that of an acute pseudocyst, as underlying solid debris is frequently indistinct on CT. This may lead one to embark on standard pseudocyst drainage methods that inadequately remove the underlying solid material potentially resulting in serious infection.

In patients with evidence of classic WON on cross-sectional imaging, it is necessary to discern the infection status of the necrotic cavity, as clinical signs of infection (i.e., leukocytosis, fever) are frequently insufficient. Percutaneous fine needle aspiration (FNA) may be used to determine the infection status of the necrosis, though this is not often necessary or performed. Urgent endoscopic drainage and debridement mandated in patients with microbiologic evidence of infected necrosis.

The indications and timing of drainage of sterile pancreatic necrosis are more controversial. Generally, pancreatic necrosis is not amenable to endoscopic drainage until 4–6 weeks after onset of pancreatitis, allowing the process time to organize and encapsulate. As a general rule, endoscopic drainage and debridement should be delayed as long as possible in patients demonstrating clinical stability. The most common indications for drainage of sterile necrosis include the following: (1) persistent abdominal pain; (2) evidence of gastric outlet obstruction (clinical or radiologic) (Fig. 12.2); (3) biliary obstruction; or (4) failure to thrive (ongoing systemic illness, anorexia, and weight loss). The appearance (i.e., size, location) of the necrotic collection on cross-sectional imaging may not be indicative of the patient's clinical status and that finding alone is not an indication for intervention.

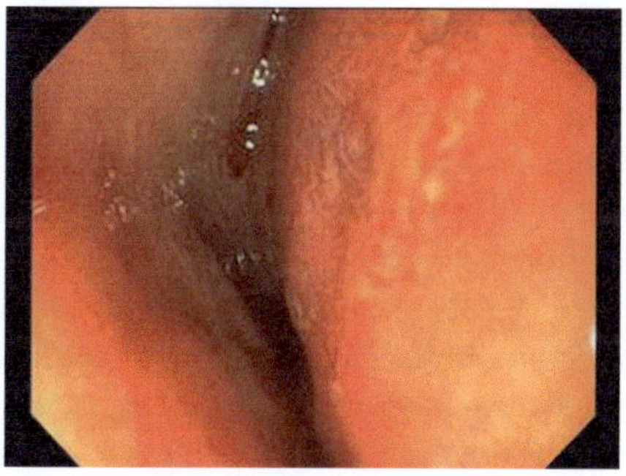

Fig. 12.2 Endoscopic view of extrinsic compression in the second duodenum from large walled-off pancreatic necrosis. The patient presented with gastric outlet obstruction

Procedural Technique

Basic pre-procedural tasks are also vitally important. The INR and platelet count should be obtained and corrected, as necessary. Pre-procedural, broad-spectrum antibiotics should be administered in patients not already receiving them. Intravenous penicillins (i.e., piperacillin/tazobactam), quinolones (i.e., levofloxacin), or carbapenems (i.e., meropenem) are considered recommended agents. Antibiotic therapy should be tailored based on microbiologic cultures obtained during the procedure. Of note, we perform all direct endoscopic necrosectomy (DEN) procedures with general anesthesia given the patient acuity, length of the procedure, and higher risk for intraprocedural adverse events. Given the risk of air embolism with conventional endoscopic insufflation, CO_2 insufflation is routinely used during endoscopic necrosectomy.

Careful review of cross-sectional imaging is vital. Coronal CT images can be very useful and often provide complementary information to standard axial images. Understanding the degree of necrosis, including extension into the paracolic gutters and communications between cavities, will direct the therapeutic plan and promote efficient therapy. Patients may appear to have multiple separate cavities, though these are generally extensions of the same area of necrosis. Non-dependent locules of air are also frequently seen within collections, though this finding in no way implies infection with a gas-forming organism but instead commonly represents a fistulous connection to the gastrointestinal lumen. In certain clinical scenarios, this fistulous tract can be used for transmural entry into the cavity to provide egress or to facilitate debridement as described below.

The endoscopic approach to the management of WON is predicated on evacuation of solid debris from the necrotic cavity. An initial transmural puncture through the gastric or duodenal wall is necessary to facilitate access to the collection, and to drain liquefied material. For WON located within or adjacent to the mid-body or tail of the pancreas, a transgastric route is preferable, while a transduodenal puncture may be necessary for collections confined to the pancreatic head. Non-endoscopic ultrasound (EUS)-guided punctures using fluoroscopic guidance can be successfully performed (>95%) with low adverse events (<5%) when an obvious luminal protrusion is observed endoscopically [4], though most experts agree that EUS guidance is preferred if available. EUS provides precise targeting of the lesion, potentially mitigates inadvertent damage to adjacent vasculature, and allows real-time assessment of the extent and volume of the necrotic cavity [5].

A variety of endoscopic accessories can be used to perform the transmural puncture, including electrocautery-based instruments such as needle knives and specialized fistulotomy devices (Cystotome, Cook Endoscopy, Winston-Salem, NC), and non-cautery accessories such as EUS-FNA needles. A newer stent with electrocautery-enhanced delivery system (described below) has recently become available. Entry into the cavity is confirmed by extravasation of cyst contents within the lumen during puncture, aspiration of cyst fluid through a needle, and/or the injection of radiopaque contrast in the cavity under fluoroscopy. One advantage of FNA or other aspiration needles is the ability for guidewire passage through the needle into the cavity using the Seldinger technique, following drainage of liquefied contents. We typically utilize a specialized 19-G FNA needle (EchoTip Ultra HD Ultrasound Access Needle, Cook Endoscopy) designed for such procedures.

After puncture and drainage, a guidewire is passed into the cavity and the transmural tract is dilated with a standard dilating balloon to a diameter of ≥15 mm. It is important to pass an ample length of guidewire into the collection in preparation for subsequent stent placement. If guidewire loss occurs inadvertently, it may be challenging to re-access the cavity and may increase the risk for adverse events while attempting to do so, even despite prior tract dilation.

Once a stable guidewire is placed, some endoscopists elect to place one (or more) double-pigtail plastic stents prior to performing necrosectomy. This technique is especially important with transgastric access, as it may be challenging to identify the puncture site among gastric folds. When using plastic stents, we recommend using two 10-Fr double-pigtail stents with a length of 3–5 cm to minimize the risk of stent migration into or out of the cavity, and stent impaction causing trauma to the lumen or cavity wall. Care must be taken not to deploy the entire plastic stent within the collection. We routinely place an endoscopically visible indelible mark at the midpoint of the stent prior to placement to guard against this situation. An alternative option is to place a large-bore (16–23 mm mid-body diameter) self-expandable metal stent (SEMS) across the dilated gastric or duodenal wall [6–10]. Transmural placement of large-diameter, covered esophageal SEMS facilitates subsequent DEN procedures and avoids the need for repeated balloon dilation prior to each debridement [7]. The use of esophageal SEMS is somewhat limited as the shortest SEMS lengths are 6–7 cm, resulting in excessive stent length within the gastrointestinal lumen or the necrotic cavity. The excess length can be trimmed using argon plasma coagulation to prevent impaction against the lumen or cavity wall, though care should be taken to minimize disruption of the SEMS interstices. An alternative option is to place a double-pigtail plastic stent within the deployed SEMS. The double-pigtail stent serves two purposes: (1) It acts as a bumper between the stent flange and the lumen/cavity wall, and (2) it

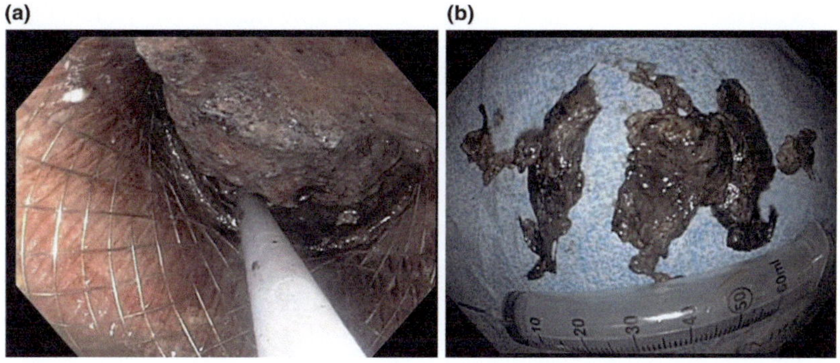

Fig. 12.3 **a** Endoscopic view of organized pancreatic necrosis with the endoscope positioned just within a fully covered self-expandable 15-mm luminal apposition stent. A snare is being used to evacuate solid debris. **b** Necrotic debris evacuated from same patient

prevents loose necrotic debris from obstructing the SEMS.

The recent development and FDA-approval of a lumen-apposing metal stent (LAMS) (AXIOS; Boston Scientific, Marlboro, MA) serves to overcome many of the limitations of our current drainage options (Fig. 12.3). These stents are available with mid-body luminal diameters of 10 and 15 mm and external flange diameters of 21 and 24 mm, with an overall stent length of ~1 cm. Two AXIOS stent delivery systems are available, one which requires placement via the standard technique (i.e., 1-puncture, 2-guidewire placement, 3-tract dilation, 4-stent deployment) and the other which is fitted with an electrocautery tip designed for simultaneous puncture and tract dilation followed by stent deployment without the need of guidewire placement. This short-length LAMS is ideal for DEN, as the 15 mm stent diameter accommodates repeated endoscope entry and exit necessary for adequate debridement, while providing apposition between the gastric wall and cavity wall [11, 12].

Spontaneous fistulous tracts can also be utilized to access, drain, and debride a necrotic collection [13]. Puncture and subsequent drainage is followed by balloon dilation of the tract to a diameter ≥15 mm. Dilation allows egress of the remaining liquid and solid material and facilitates DEN. Adjunctive transpapillary stenting can be considered; however, this technique only allows drainage of additional simple peripancreatic fluid and is inadequate as a conduit for removal of pancreatic debris.

A variety of techniques have been described for removal of solid debris from necrotic collections. Some endoscopists advocate for irrigation of the cavity through placement of a 7-Fr nasocystic irrigation tube within the collection, adjacent to the transmural stents, using one or more transmural exit sites [14, 15]. Up to 200 cc of normal saline (±3% hydrogen peroxide) is forcefully and rapidly infused via the tube every 2–4 h initially to lavage debris from the cavity. Many providers have abandoned the use of nasocystic irrigation tubes for current clinical practice, mainly due to patient intolerance [16]. A variation of this technique includes the combination of endoscopic and percutaneous therapy, termed "dual-modality therapy" [17]. This technique involves percutaneous drain placement, in lieu of a nasocystic tube, and endoscopic transmural drainage with irrigation via the percutaneous catheter and egress through the transmural tracts to promote ongoing debridement of the necrotic tissue [17].

In the majority of cases we advocate for DEN if clinically appropriate. DEN is a time-intensive procedure, which requires passage of an endoscope transmurally into the collection. Both diagnostic and therapeutic endoscopes can be used, each with inherent advantages and disadvantages. Diagnostic endoscopes can be advantageous when maximal flexibility is desired.

Therapeutic endoscopes offer a high-flow water jet which is particularly helpful in fragmentation and irrigation of necrotic tissue. The use of hydrogen peroxide lavage may be effective in liquefying necrotic tissue during DEN, though evidence from comparative trials is lacking [18]. Endoscopic debridement can be performed utilizing a variety of standard endoscopic accessories (i.e., stone retrieval baskets, polypectomy snares, polyp-retrieval nets, grasping forceps, etc.). Once the necrotic tissue is grasped, it is withdrawn from the cavity and deposited in the lumen. Alternatively, large pieces may be cut into smaller pieces using snare electrocautery and flushed from the cavity; this may avoid repeated entry into and withdrawal from the cavity. The consistency of necrotic debris varies from patient to patient, ranging from smooth, solid debris that is densely adherent, to tissue that is loose and easily removed. Some endoscopists routinely perform DEN following the initial transmural puncture, while others advocate for initial drainage with debridement commencing during a second procedure. No data exist to suggest a benefit of one strategy over the other. The goal of each DEN procedure should be to remove as much necrotic tissue as possible.

Following DEN, patients can resume (or initiate) oral intake the day of the procedure, assuming no intraprocedural adverse events have occurred. Per-oral antibiotics are generally continued for several weeks and in most cases until complete resolution of the cavity. Repeat procedures are almost always necessary and frequently include stent exchange and additional debridement. Subsequent procedures can be scheduled if the initial necrosectomy is known to be incomplete [19], or performed as necessary based on clinical status and/or cross-sectional imaging findings. Debilitated patients requiring hospitalization may need more frequent procedures (every 1–2 days), while outpatients who continually improve may tolerate 1–2 weeks between interventions. The interval between debridements is often predicated on the clinical scenario in conjunction with logistical issues (i.e., inpatient/outpatient status, distance from treatment center, and availability of an advanced therapeutic endoscopic team). In patients with continued collections despite multiple interventions, endoscopic retrograde cholangiopancreatography (ERCP) should be considered for evaluation of an ongoing pancreatic duct disruption. As resolution ensues, external drains should be removed before internal drains to prevent formation of gastro-/enterocutaneous fistulae. Internal drains are then endoscopically removed after complete resolution of the collection.

Outcomes

Many case series have demonstrated the efficacy of DEN [16, 20–23]. Patients with WON are a heterogeneous group with notable variation in the following: (1) size of the necrotic collection, (2) total burden of necrosis, (3) the presence of paracolic gutter extension(s), (4) comorbid medical illnesses, and (5) time from onset of necrosis to intervention. Thus, comparison of outcomes between reported series remains challenging as definitions for outcomes vary substantially. Successful resolution can be defined as complete non-surgical resolution (including percutaneous drainage) or resolution due to flexible endoscopy alone [16].

Two recent systematic reviews, including 233 and 455 patients, respectively, have demonstrated complete resolution of pancreatic necrosis in 81% of patients using endoscopy alone [24, 25]. The mean number of procedures necessary for resolution was 4 in both studies, while the adverse event rates were 21 and 36%, respectively. Two large retrospective studies of DEN showed successful resolution in approximately 90% of patients with an adverse event rate of approximately 14% [16, 21].

Outcomes' data regarding the use of esophageal SEMS and LAMS to facilitate DEN have begun to emerge but remain limited to small cohort studies. A recently published, retrospective study performed at two US academic medical centers, including 17 patients, demonstrated resolution in 88% of patients when utilizing an esophageal SEMS to maintain transmural access [26]. In this cohort, a mean of 5 DEN procedures were needed to obtain complete endoscopic resolution with an adverse event rate of 6%. A similar study including 10 patients published by Attam et al. [27] yielded similar results (90% resolution, median 3 procedures). Outcomes following LAMS placement have reported even more recently have shown high rates of technical (>95%) and clinical success (>80%), with low risk of serious adverse events (<7%) [28, 29].

Currently, no guidelines exist regarding the use of double-pigtail plastic stents versus NC 27599-0001 SEMS/LAMS to establish and maintain tract patency in patients undergoing DEN. Both techniques permit high clinical resolution rates (>80%). Clinical judgment should be utilized to determine the optimal strategy on a case-by-case basis. In general, we advocate for the use of esophageal SEMS or LAMS in patient with larger necrotic collections (>6 cm) as multiple DEN sessions will likely be necessary to achieve resolution. Procedural efficiency and safety can be improved using SEMS/LAMS, as tract dilation is not required during prior to each session. For smaller collections, the use of pre-DEN tract dilation and maintenance of the tract with double-pigtail stents is likely sufficient. The main advantage of LAMS or SEMS is the shorter length ($\sim$1 cm) and lack of exposed edges (involuted at full expansion). As mentioned, the length of SEMS (6–7 cm) can be problematic in certain cases, as impaction on the opposing gastric or cavity wall is not uncommon.

Alternative Treatment Strategies

Management of WON is usually based upon local expertise and severity of comorbid medical illnesses. Ideally, these patients are best managed by a multidisciplinary approach in tertiary centers. Alternatives to endoscopic drainage include nutritional support using parenteral or enteral formulations, percutaneous drainage, and/or surgical drainage. An ongoing multicenter, randomized, controlled trial (TENSION trial) has been designed to compare outcomes between endoscopic step-up approach (transmural drainage ± DEN) and a surgical step-up approach (percutaneous drainage ± surgical necrosectomy) [30].

Percutaneous DEN has been described through external placement of a large-bore, fully covered SEMS (20–25 mm diameter) or a modified flexible overtube to facilitate debridement of WON [31, 32]. The exact timing between percutaneous drain placement and SEMS placement is not known. After placement, the SEMS remains in situ, with an ostomy appliance placed over the stent between interventions and can be removed when the cavity collapses. This approach is similar to video-assisted retroperitoneal debridement (VARD) performed by gastrointestinal surgeons, who pass rigid endoscopes through percutaneous tracts to access necrotic collections [33]. This method is an ideal adjunct to DEN and may be most useful in treating paracolic gutter extensions, areas that have already been accessed with percutaneous drains but demonstrate inadequate drainage, and those collections that cannot be accessed transluminally. Paracolic gutter extensions can be difficult to treat, particularly when extending into the pelvis and often remain unresolved with endoscopic therapy alone.

Adverse Events Associated with Endoscopic Intervention of Pancreatic Collections

Life-threatening adverse events can occur both intraprocedurally or post-procedurally when attempting endoscopic therapy for WON. A recent systematic review identified a mortality rate of 6% in patients undergoing DEN following necrotizing pancreatitis [34]. It is generally recommended that these endoscopic procedures be performed with the availability of surgical and interventional radiology support. The most dreaded adverse events of transmural therapy include bleeding and perforation.

Bleeding most frequently occurs at the puncture site, though can occur after any step in the process (i.e., transmural puncture, dilation, or during drainage). Supportive measures are often sufficient as bleeding is typically self-limited with cessation by the end of the procedure. Endoscopic hemostasis, surgical intervention, or angiographic embolization may be necessary in rare circumstances. Refractory bleeding during the procedure can be managed by dilute epinephrine injection, balloon tamponade, through-the-scope (TTS) endoclips, or electrocautery. Torrential bleeding at the entry site can be treated by placement of a large-diameter, fully covered esophageal SEMS [35, 36]. Intracavitary bleeding during DEN also occurs and is usually self-limited, though severe intracavitary bleeding can be life-threatening.

Perforations can occur at the entry site or within the cavity wall. Entry site perforations generally occur due to dehiscence of the lumen wall from the apposed cavity wall. This can generally be managed with TTS endoclips or placement of a large-caliber SEMS [36], similar to management of entry-related bleeding. If egress of gastric contents is avoided, the gastric wall closes rapidly, and many patients will improve with conservative measures (i.e., nasogastric suction, antibiotics) alone. Some endoscopists believe that transduodenal perforation may also be managed conservatively, since the perforation is retroperitoneal. Large intracavity perforations are more concerning and often require surgical or percutaneous drainage. Intraprocedural perforations can rarely result in tension pneumoperitoneum, a life-threatening emergency requiring needle decompression [37].

Infectious adverse events occur from inadequate drainage of fluid and/or solid debris. Therefore, the need for sufficient removal of fluid and solid debris is essential. Following endoscopic intervention, patients should be maintained on antibiotics. Patients who demonstrate evidence of infection (i.e., leukocytosis, fever/chills, culture positivity) may require broadening of their antimicrobial regimen. Occasionally, patients may require adjuvant placement of percutaneous drainage and/or irrigation catheters to manage infectious adverse events. This occurs most commonly in patients with WON extending to the paracolic gutters [14].

Uncommon adverse events include stent migration and air embolism. Migration of both double-pigtail plastic stents and SEMS into the collection (distal migration) may occur during or after endoscopic placement. Endoscopic retrieval is feasible assuming migration is identified promptly. Delayed recognition allows collapse of the collection and closure of the transmural puncture site. Premature proximal migration (out of the cavity and back into the lumen) may also occur, increasing the risk of infection.

Fatal air embolism has been described following DEN [38]. This has prompted the use of CO_2 rather than air for insufflation during endoscopic intervention of pancreatic collections as many believe this alternative prevents air embolism. Indeed, use of CO_2 is now considered mandatory by most endoscopists who perform these procedures.

Author Contributions Ryan Law, DO, prepared the draft of the manuscript and approved the final manuscript. Todd H. Baron, MD, provided the conception of article, conducted a critical review, and approved the final manuscript.

Conflict of Interest Ryan Law, DO, has no conflict of interest.Todd H. Baron, MD: W.L. Gore, Boston Scientific, Olympus, Cook Endoscopy.

References

1. Banks PA, Bollen TL, Dervenis C, Gooszen HG, Johnson CD, et al. Classification of acute pancreatitis—2012: revision of the Atlanta classification and definitions by international consensus. Gut. 2013;62(1):102–11.
2. Bakker OJ, van Santvoort H, Besselink MG, Boermeester MA, van Eijck C, et al. Extrapancreatic necrosis without pancreatic parenchymal necrosis: a separate entity in necrotising pancreatitis? Gut. 2013;62(10):1475–80.
3. van Santvoort HC, Besselink MG, Bakker OJ, Hofker HS, Boermeester MA, et al. A step-up approach or open necrosectomy for necrotizing pancreatitis. N Engl J Med. 2010;362(16):1491–502.

4. Chahal P, Papachristou GI, Baron TH. Endoscopic transmural entry into pancreatic fluid collections using a dedicated aspiration needle without endoscopic ultrasound guidance: success and complication rates. Surg Endosc. 2007;21(10):1726–32.
5. Jurgensen C, Arlt A, Neser F, Fritscher-Ravens A, Stolzel U, et al. Endoscopic ultrasound criteria to predict the need for intervention in pancreatic necrosis. BMC Gastroenterol. 2012;12:48.
6. Antillon MR, Bechtold ML, Bartalos CR, Marshall JB. Transgastric endoscopic necrosectomy with temporary metallic esophageal stent placement for the treatment of infected pancreatic necrosis (with video). Gastrointest Endosc. 2009;69(1):178–80.
7. Belle S, Collet P, Post S, Kaehler G. Temporary cystogastrostomy with self-expanding metallic stents for pancreatic necrosis. Endoscopy. 2010;42(6): 493–5.
8. Itoi T, Nageshwar Reddy D, Yasuda I. New fully-covered self-expandable metal stent for endoscopic ultrasonography-guided intervention in infectious walled-off pancreatic necrosis (with video). J Hepatobiliary Pancreat Sci. 2013;20(3):403–6.
9. Krishnan A, Ramakrishnan R. EUS-guided endoscopic necrosectomy and temporary cystogastrostomy for infected pancreatic necrosis with self-expanding metallic stents. Surg Laparosc Endosc Percutan Tech. 2012;22(5):e319–21.
10. Sarkaria S, Sethi A, Rondon C, Lieberman M, Srinivasan I, et al. Pancreatic necrosectomy using covered esophageal stents: a novel approach. J Clin Gastroenterol. 2014;48(2):145–52.
11. Siddiqui AA, Adler DG, Nieto J, Shah JN, Binmoeller KF, et al. EUS-guided drainage of peripancreatic fluid collections and necrosis by using a novel lumen-apposing stent: a large retrospective, multicenter U.S. experience (with videos). Gastrointest Endosc. 2016;83(4):699–707.
12. Shah RJ, Shah JN, Waxman I, Kowalski TE, Sanchez-Yaque A, et al. Safety and efficacy of endoscopic ultrasound-guided drainage of pancreatic fluid collections with lumen-apposing covered self-expanding metal stents. Clin Gastroenterol Hepatol. 2015;13(4):747–52.
13. Kang SG, Parkdo H, Kwon TH, Park JY, Park SH, et al. Transduodenal endoscopic necrosectomy via pancreaticoduodenal fistula for infected peripancreatic necrosis with left pararenal space extension (with videos). Gastrointest Endosc. 2008;67(2):380–3.
14. Papachristou GI, Takahashi N, Chahal P, Sarr MG, Baron TH. Peroral endoscopic drainage/debridement of walled-off pancreatic necrosis. Ann Surg. 2007;245(6):943–51.
15. Varadarajulu S, Phadnis MA, Christein JD, Wilcox CM. Multiple transluminal gateway technique for EUS-guided drainage of symptomatic walled-off pancreatic necrosis. Gastrointest Endosc. 2011;74 (1):74–80.
16. Gardner TB, Chahal P, Papachristou GI, Bege SS, Petersen BT, et al. A comparison of direct endoscopic necrosectomy with transmural endoscopic drainage for the treatment of walled-off pancreatic necrosis. Gastrointest Endosc. 2009;69 (6):1085–94.
17. Ross A, Gluck M, Irani S, Hauptmann E, Fotoohi M, et al. Combined endoscopic and percutaneous drainage of organized pancreatic necrosis. Gastrointest Endosc. 2010;71(1):79–84.
18. Abdelhafez M, Elnegouly M, Hasab Allah MS, Elshazli M, Mikhail HM, et al. Transluminal retroperitoneal endoscopic necrosectomy with the use of hydrogen peroxide and without external irrigation: a novel approach for the treatment of walled-off pancreatic necrosis. Surg Endosc. 2013;27 (10):3911–20.
19. Coelho D, Ardengh JC, Eulalio JM, Manso JE, Monkemuller K, et al. Management of infected and sterile pancreatic necrosis by programmed endoscopic necrosectomy. Dig Dis. 2008;26(4):364–9.
20. Charnley RM, Lochan R, Gray H, O'Sullivan CB, Scott J, et al. Endoscopic necrosectomy as primary therapy in the management of infected pancreatic necrosis. Endoscopy. 2006;38(9):925–8.
21. Gardner TB, Coelho-Prabhu N, Gordon SR, Gelrud A, Maple JT, et al. Direct endoscopic necrosectomy for the treatment of walled-off pancreatic necrosis: results from a multicenter U.S. series. Gastrointest Endosc. 2006;73(4):718–26.
22. Seewald S, Groth S, Omar S, Imazu H, Seitz U, et al. Aggressive endoscopic therapy for pancreatic necrosis and pancreatic abscess: a new safe and effective treatment algorithm (videos). Gastrointest Endosc. 2005;62(1):92–100.
23. Voermans RP, Veldkamp MC, Rauws EA, Bruno MJ, Fockens P. Endoscopic transmural debridement of symptomatic organized pancreatic necrosis (with videos). Gastrointest Endosc. 2007;66 (5):909–16.
24. Puli SR, Graumlich JF, Pamulaparthy SR, Kalva N. Endoscopic transmural necrosectomy for walled-off pancreatic necrosis: a systematic review and meta-analysis. Can J Gastroenterol Hepatol. 2014;28(1):50–3.
25. van Brunschot S, Fockens P, Bakker OJ, Besselink MG, Voermans RP, et al. Endoscopic transluminal necrosectomy in necrotising pancreatitis: a systematic review. Surg Endosc. 2014;28(5):1425–38.
26. Sarkaria S, Sethi A, Rondon C, Lieberman M, Srinivasan I, et al. Pancreatic necrosectomy using covered esophageal stents: a novel approach. J Clin Gastroenterol. 2014;48(2):145–52.
27. Attam R, Trikudanathan G, Arain M, Nemoto Y, Glessing B, et al. Endoscopic transluminal drainage and necrosectomy by using a novel, through-the-scope, fully covered, large-bore esophageal metal stent: preliminary experience in 10 patients. Gastrointest Endosc. 2014;80(2):312–8.
28. Walter D, Will U, Sanchez-Yague A, Brenke D, Hampe J, et al. A novel lumen-apposing metal stent

for endoscopic ultrasound-guided drainage of pancreatic fluid collections: a prospective cohort study. Endoscopy. 2015;47(1):63–7.
29. Rinninella E, Kunda R, Dollhopf M, Sanchez-Yague A, Will U, et al. EUS-guided drainage of pancreatic fluid collections using a novel lumen-apposing metal stent on an electrocautery-enhanced delivery system: a large retrospective study (with video). Gastrointest Endosc. 2015;82(6):1039–46.
30. van Brunschot S, van Grinsven J, Voermans RP, Bakker OJ, Besselink MG, et al. Transluminal endoscopic step-up approach versus minimally invasive surgical step-up approach in patients with infected necrotising pancreatitis (TENSION trial): design and rationale of a randomised controlled multicenter trial [ISRCTN09186711]. BMC Gastroenterol. 2013;13:161.
31. Navarrete C, Castillo C, Caracci M, Vargas P, Gobelet J. Wide percutaneous access to pancreatic necrosis with self-expandable stent: new application (with video). Gastrointest Endosc. 2011;73(3): 609–10.
32. Yamamoto N, Isayama H, Takahara N, Sasahira N, Miyabayashi K, et al. Percutaneous direct-endoscopic necrosectomy for walled-off pancreatic necrosis. Endoscopy. 2013;45(Suppl 2 UCTN):E44-5.
33. Horvath K, Freeny P, Escallon J, Heagarty P, Comstock B, et al. Safety and efficacy of video-assisted retroperitoneal debridement for infected pancreatic collections: a multicenter, prospective, single-arm phase 2 study. Arch Surg. 2010;145(9):817–25.
34. van Brunschot S, Fockens P, Bakker OJ, Besselink MG, Voermans RP, et al. Endoscopic transluminal necrosectomy in necrotising pancreatitis: a systematic review. Surg Endosc. 2014;28(5):1425–38.
35. Akbar A, Reddy DN, Baron TH. Placement of fully covered self-expandable metal stents to control entry-related bleeding during transmural drainage of pancreatic fluid collections (with video). Gastrointest Endosc. 2012;76(5):1060–3.
36. Iwashita T, Lee JG, Nakai Y, Samarasena JB, Chang KJ. Successful management of arterial bleeding complicating endoscopic ultrasound-guided cystogastrostomy using a covered metallic stent. Endoscopy. 2012;44(Suppl 2 UCTN):E370-1.
37. Baron TH, Wong Kee Song LM, Zielinski MD, Emura F, Fotoohi M, et al. A comprehensive approach to the management of acute endoscopic perforations (with videos). Gastrointest Endosc. 2012;76(4):838–59.
38. Seifert H, Biermer M, Schmitt W, Jürgensen C, Will U, et al. Transluminal endoscopic necrosectomy after acute pancreatitis: a multicentre study with long-term follow-up (the GEPARD Study). Gut. 2009;58(9):1260–6.

NOTES Pancreatic Pseudocystgastrostomy

13

Mersadies Martin, David J. Desilets and John R. Romanelli

Abstract

A pancreatic pseudocyst is a collection of fluid encapsulated within or around the pancreas. This often needs to be drained due to symptoms. Surgical drainage typically results in an anastomosis to the stomach or jejunum. Endoscopic treatment of pancreatic pseudocysts has been well described and consists of drainage and/or debridement of necrotic tissue. Endoscopic puncture of pseudocyst across the gastric wall are also well described. Inspired by the less-invasive concept of NOTES, and using a flexible endoscopic stapler, a stapled pancreatic pseudocystgastrostomy can be created utilizing a per-oral approach. This often follows endoscopic drainage, although it has been described doing both concurrently. Further development of flexible stapling tools, as well as endoscopic suturing tools, may make the procedure easier to perform and afford the widespread adoption of this procedure.

Keywords

NOTES · Pancreatic pseudocyst · Endoscopic drainage · Pancreatic pseudocystgastrostomy · Transmural drainage · Anastomosis

M. Martin
Department of Surgery, Kaiser Permanente, 4405 Vandever Ave, 4th floor, San Diego, CA 92120, USA
e-mail: Mersadies.MartinMD@baystatehealth.org

D.J. Desilets
Department of Medicine, Gastroenterology, Baystate Medical Center, Springfield, MA 01199, USA
e-mail: David.Desilets@baystatehealth.org

J.R. Romanelli (✉)
Department of Surgery, University of Massachusetts Medical School, Baystate Medical Center, Springfield, MA 01199, USA
e-mail: john.romanelli@baystatehealth.org

J.R. Romanelli et al. (eds.), *NOTES and Endoluminal Surgery*, Clinical Gastroenterology, DOI 10.1007/978-3-319-50610-4_13

A pancreatic pseudocyst is a collection of fluid encapsulated within or around the pancreas. The walls of the pseudocyst do not have an epithelial lining but instead consist of reactive granulation tissue that turns into fibrous tissue. The fluid within the cyst may be rich in pancreatic enzymes, inflammatory debris, blood, or necrotic tissue that leaked from damaged parenchyma or the pancreatic duct. The wall of the pseudocyst usually takes up to 6 weeks to form completely. Pancreatic pseudocysts are complications of pancreatitis or progressive ductal obstruction that may develop weeks or months after an attack of acute pancreatitis, chronic pancreatitis, or pancreatic trauma.

The treatment of pancreatic pseudocyst is dependent upon surgeon experience, pseudocyst location, size, and associated complications. Treatment options include laparoscopic or open pseudocystenterostomy, endoscopic transpapillary or transmural drainage, and percutaneous catheter drainage. Although surgery has been the standard technique for drainage of pancreatic pseudocysts, the use of endoscopic methods is increasing.

The historic landmark in the surgery of pancreatic pseudocysts occurred in 1882, when Gussenbauer [1] introduced marsupialization as a method of treatment. Shortly thereafter, external drainage with or without marsupialization proved satisfactory for decompression of pancreatic pseudocysts. In 1915, excision of part of the pancreatic cyst and anastomosis to the posterior stomach was accomplished [2]. In 1927, a reported cystojejunal anastomosis was successfully performed [3]. By 1946, the Roux-en-Y principle was introduced to decompress a pancreatic pseudocyst [4]. Open stapled pseudocystgastrostomy was first described in 1979 [5]. The first report of laparoscopic stapled cystgastrostomy was published in 1995 [6].

Human cases of NOTES procedures emerged in 2005 via transgastric appendectomy cases [7]. An emerging minimally invasive endoscopic drainage procedure for the treatment of pancreatic pseudocystgastrostomy is NOTES stapled cystgastrostomy. This is an entirely endoscopic, per-oral procedure that is less invasive than laparoscopic and open cystgastrostomy and has shown excellent outcomes. In 2008, a stapled pseudocystgastrostomy via the NOTES approach was successfully performed by our group [8]. The decision to perform this type of procedure was based on the fact that this patient, who had a large, infected pseudocyst which had already failed endoscopic transgastric catheter drainage, was too sick and unstable to tolerate even laparoscopic cystgastrostomy. A less invasive, more physiologically friendly approach was needed. The most recent and emerging procedure is the natural orifice translumenal endoscopic surgery (NOTES) stapled cystgastrostomy. This operation is completed entirely through an existing cystgastrostomy site with no incisions, thus avoiding the peritoneal cavity altogether.

Definitive treatment of pancreatic pseudocysts has evolved considerably over time. Optimal management may vary for an individual patient, but several options have evolved through a series of experiments that have utilized both external and internal drainage. In this chapter, the focus will be on the evolution, diagnosis, workup, indications, rationale, and methodology for intervention in regards to pancreatic pseudocysts, and specifically, the transoral, stapled pseudocystgastrostomy procedure.

Diagnosis and Workup

The majority of pancreatic pseudocysts are asymptomatic and do not require treatment. When symptomatic, patients often complain of abdominal pain, distention, vomiting, or poor digestion of food. Often the patient can present many weeks or months after recovery from acute or chronic pancreatitis. Complications of pancreatic pseudocysts include infection, abscess formation, hemorrhage, obstruction, and rupture. For obstruction, the pseudocyst can cause compression of the gastrointestinal tract from the stomach to colon, compression in the urinary tract, biliary system, or the circulatory system.

Diagnosis of a pancreatic pseudocysts is based on fluid analysis and imaging. The most useful imaging tools are computerized tomography (CT), ultrasonography, and magnetic resonance cholangiopancreatography (MRCP). The gold standard for initial assessment and follow-up is typically a CT scan. A common picture seen on CT is a fluid-filled mass around the pancreas. With fine-cut (3-mm) CT or MRCP, the pancreatic ducts can be identified in relationship to the pseudocyst, which may affect the type of treatment. It is important to note that in some patients, pancreatic cystic tumors such as mucinous cystadenoma may masquerade as a benign pseudocyst. It is therefore important to elicit a prior history of acute or chronic pancreatitis prior to embarking on endoscopic or surgical drainage. Endoscopic ultrasound (EUS) with transenteric puncture and stent placement is emerging as the endoscopic treatment of choice for pseudocysts and other peripancreatic fluid collections that abut the gastrointestinal (GI) tract. In addition, endoscopic retrograde cholangiopancreatography (ERCP) with pancreatic stent placement (so-called transpapillary drainage) may also be of benefit for pseudocysts that communicate with the pancreatic ducts.

Fluid analysis after EUS-guided aspiration of benign pancreatic pseudocysts should yield low carcinoembryonic antigen (CEA), low viscosity, and high amylase. On the other hand, a malignant cyst may show high CEA (greater than 192 ng/mL), high viscosity, and low amylase.

Indications for Intervention

All pancreatic cysts do not require treatment. In many cases, pseudocysts may improve and resolve on their own. In a patient with a small (less than 6 cm) pseudocyst that is not causing any symptoms, careful observation with periodic ultrasound or other cross-sectional imaging is indicated. On the other hand, an asymptomatic but large (greater than 6 cm) or enlarging pseudocysts may warrant internal, external, or endoscopic drainage due to the risk of rupture or hemorrhage.

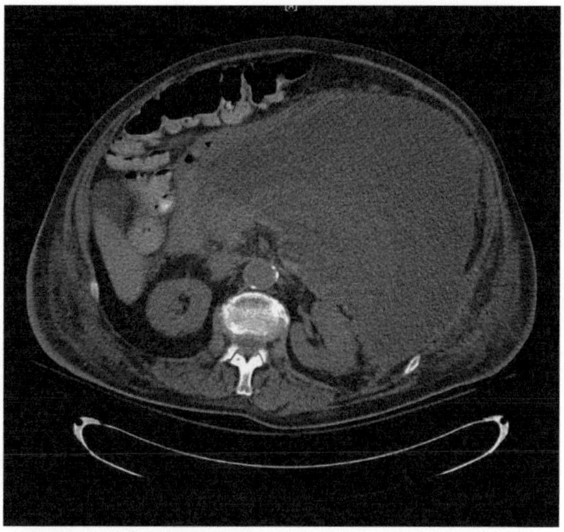

Fig. 13.1 CT scan of a large pancreatic pseudocyst. The heterogeneity indicates the likelihood of necrotic debris

In a significant number of patients, the pseudocyst will decrease and resolve without intervention. However, pseudocysts that are older than 6 weeks are unlikely to resolve spontaneously. These can become quite large and create a mass effect on other organs (Figs. 13.1 and 13.2). If a pseudocyst is persistent over many months, or if it is causing symptoms, treatment is required. Other factors that make spontaneous regression unlikely include the presence of multiple cysts, location of the pseudocyst in the tail of the pancreas, wall thickness is greater than 1 cm, lack of communication with Wirsung's duct, proximal ductal stenosis, or traumatic etiology, or an increase in size upon follow-up [9].

Ideally, pseudocysts should be observed initially, as it takes approximately 6 weeks for the wall to mature. The most suitable pseudocysts for endoscopic treatment are those with a wall thickness of more than 5 mm and less than 1 cm [5]. Drainage at less than 6 weeks may be indicated when clinical pancreatitis fails to improve despite aggressive medical management.

Pancreatic pseudocysts complicating chronic pancreatitis usually result from pancreatic duct side-branch disruption, or pancreatic duct outflow obstruction. This can be due to a pancreatic duct stone, stricture, or protein plug. Such

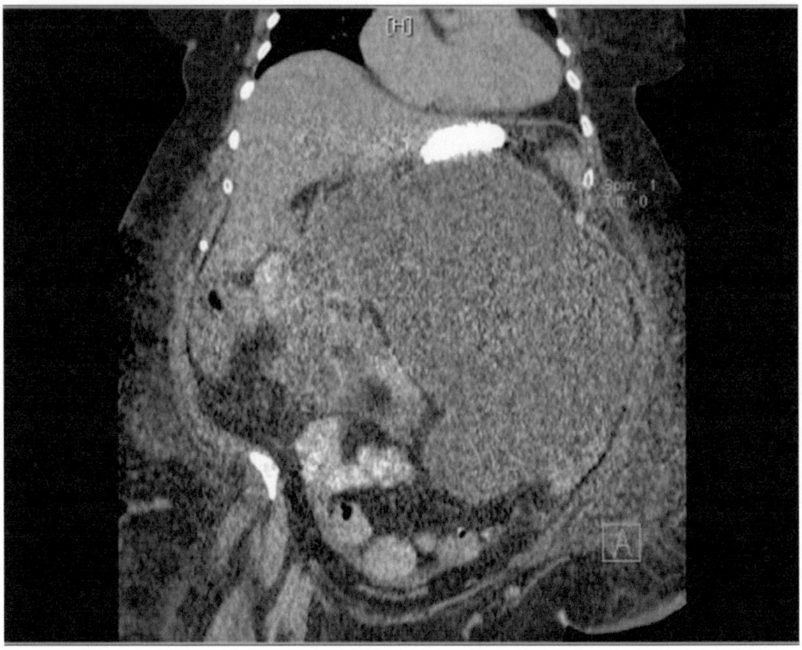

Fig. 13.2 A large pancreatic pseudocyst seen on coronal CT imaging

pseudocysts rarely resolve without intervention. In such cases, drainage is indicated to relieve acute symptoms associated with a mass effect and neighboring organ compression such as pain, gastric outlet obstruction, and even jaundice. Drainage is also indicated when pseudocysts become infected or there is bleeding within the pseudocyst.

Differentiation between a pancreatic pseudocyst and a cystic malignancy can be difficult. Unlike benign pancreatic pseudocysts, cystic malignant or premalignant tumors require complete resection. Cystic malignant tumors may present with weight loss, a palpable mass, lack of prior pancreatitis, or unilocular cysts. These tumors are also less commonly calcified, more often over 1 cm thick, and may have nodular components.

A number of different types of treatment are available for pseudocysts. Therefore, the treatment of pancreatic pseudocyst is complex and ideally should be performed in an institution where a multidisciplinary team of experienced pancreatic surgeons, gastroenterologists, and radiologists work together. The optimal procedure is dependent on the team's experience, type of cyst, and anatomy of the pseudocyst in relation to other organs.

Anatomic Considerations

The surgical approach may vary depending on surgeon/gastroenterologist experience. The treatment of pseudocysts can be performed open, laparoscopic, endoscopic, or via interventional radiologic procedure. The three most common open or laparoscopic procedures are pancreatic pseudocystgastrostomy, pseudocystjejunostomy (either loop or Roux-en-Y), and the pseudocyst-duodenostomy. The strategy for drainage of a benign pancreatic pseudocyst is to create a connection between the cyst and a path of least resistance, which is usually an adjacent part of the gastrointestinal tract (i.e., stomach, duodenum, or jejunum), or via percutaneous drainage when the GI tract is not accessible. In general, percutaneous drainage should be avoided, as a persistent pancreaticocutaneous fistula is possible. Internal drainage is much preferred. Complete excision of a benign pseudocyst has been associated with numerous morbidities compared to drainage alone and thus is not the standard of care.

The type of surgical procedure also depends on the location of the pseudocyst. For pseudocysts that occur in the body and tail of the pancreas, either a pseudocystjejunostomy or pseudocystgastrostomy can be performed. For pseudocysts that occur in the head of the pancreas a cystduodenostomy is usually preferred. For a pseudocyst abutting the stomach, the cystgastrostomy procedure is typically the approach of choice.

Endoscopic transpapillary approaches to the pseudocyst are the least invasive of procedures. Therefore, when a pancreatic pseudocyst is found to have a connection to Wirsung's duct, the preferred treatment is often transpapillary insertion of a stent for internal drainage. Endoscopic transmural (transgastric or transduodenal) approaches to the pseudocyst are alternatives to transpapillary drainage of the pseudocyst if such drainage is not possible. Transmural drainage can be done for pseudocyst that are both communicating and non-communicating with the pancreatic duct.

Another factor that must be considered when deciding whether to perform surgical or endoscopic drainage of a pseudocyst is the presence of necrotic material within the pseudocyst. Often necrotic debris is best treated with surgical debridement. We have found that discontinuation of acid suppression and exposure of complex cyst contents to gastric acid can aid in the resolution of peripancreatic fluid collections with solid debris or clot. Endoscopic debridement is an option but is less definitive, and often results in multiple procedures [10]. Therefore, we prefer drainage into the stomach as a primary endoscopic or surgical route of drainage whenever possible. Such an approach may be more effective if the patient ceases proton pump inhibitors or H_2 blockers, which many patients with foregut symptoms are commonly prescribed.

NOTES pseudocystgastrostomy, which provides definitive treatment of the pseudocyst, is comparable to previously described surgical approaches but is less invasive than laparoscopic or open pseudocystgastrostomy. Critical to the decision about this approach is the proximity of the pseudocyst to the gastrointestinal junction (Fig. 13.3). In our index case [8], the bulge of the pseudocyst seen posteriorly was about 2 cm from gastroesophageal junction, which made accessing the pseudocyst transorally an ideal approach.

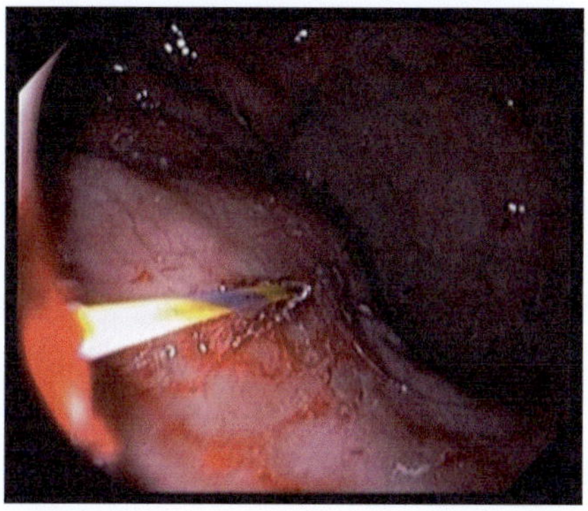

Fig. 13.3 Bulging pseudocyst, just distal to gastroesophageal junction, with guidewire placed into pseudocyst

Rationale for Surgical Intervention

The most common indications for surgical treatment of a pancreatic pseudocyst are unresolving pain, chronic infection, or obstruction of the gastric outlet or biliary tract. Decompression of the pseudocyst by internal or percutaneous drainage is advocated for symptomatic patients, and internal drainage can be performed by endoscopic or surgical pseudocystgastrostomy. The majority of patients who require treatment for their pseudocyst are treated by a definitive open, laparoscopic, or endoscopic surgery. Surgical drainage by pseudocystgastrostomy or pseudocystjejunostomy (either by a loop or Roux-en-Y) has been the standard treatment. The success rate is high, but surgical management requires an adequately mature pseudocyst wall that will hold sutures.

Percutaneous drainage has several drawbacks including skin discomfort and infection, and may leave a cutaneous fistula after drainage tube removal. In fact, percutaneous drainage is usually indicated only as an emergency procedure for acute fluid retention or infected cysts, as the recurrence rate after this form of treatment ranges as high as 70%, and percutaneous fistula are common complications (more than 20% of cases) [11].

Rationale for Endoscopic Intervention

Although surgery has been the standard technique for permanent drainage of pancreatic pseudocysts, endoscopic methods are increasingly becoming the standard of care. Endoscopic drainage is appealing, because it creates a similar result to internal surgical drainage, is less invasive, and can sometimes be used to treat immature pseudocysts.

In regards to the endoscopic procedure, an endoscopist drains the pseudocyst through the stomach by creating a small opening between the cyst and the stomach. The disadvantage of this technique is that if there is debris in the pseudocyst cavity, or if the cyst is very large, then infection or failure of pseudocyst resolution with this technique may occur. Given that, the cystgastrostomy is typically stented open with double-pigtail stents, which can be removed transorally at a subsequent endoscopic procedure. The application of endoscopic ultrasound to guide pseudocyst puncture through the stomach or duodenal wall has improved the success and safety of endoscopic pseudocyst drainage, and avoids inadvertent puncture of a major vascular structure.

Tools/Equipment Needed

A double-channel endoscope and a linear-array echoendoscope (Olympus America, Center Valley, PA) are used for viewing and locating an avascular area on the pseudocyst wall.

We use a 19-gauge needle (Cook Endoscopy, Winston-Salem, NC) to puncture the gastric/pseudocyst wall, and a 0.035 flexible, Teflon-coated guidewire (Tracer Metro wire, Cook Endoscopy) is passed into the pseudocyst cavity via the needle. Often, a Soehendra stent extractor (Cook Endoscopy) is needed to drill through the fibrotic wall of the pseudocyst. Alternatively, a 4F to 6F step-up biliary dilating catheter can be used to dilate the tract enough to allow passage of an endoscopic balloon dilation catheter across the gastric and cyst walls. The tract is dilated (up to 18 mm) using an esophageal dilation balloon (Microvasive, Boston Scientific, Natick, MA) over the guidewire. Finally, 2 or 3 double-pigtail, 10-French stents are placed to allow the pseudocysts contents to drain into the stomach.

Pseudocyst debridement can be undertaken using devices such as a biliary stone extraction basket (4 wire/2 × 4 cm, or 8 wire/3 × 6 cm web basket, Cook Endoscopy). A Roth net (US Endoscopy, Mentor, OH) can also be deployed to help remove debris.

In our NOTES pseudocyst drainage, the salient feature of the technique is to insert a linear, cutting stapler into the pseudocyst cavity through an existing endoscopically created cystgastrostomy, and performing a stapled cystgastrostomy analogous to that which is created during laparoscopic cystgastrostomy. An overtube is necessary to pass the stapling device transorally. We employed a 20-mm-diameter, gastric-length overtube (U.S. Endoscopy, Mentor, OH) for this purpose. The overtube back loaded onto the gastroscope prior to endoscopy at the time of the NOTES pseudocystgastrostomy.

The SurgAssist SLC™ (Power Medical Interventions, Langhorne, PA) is a flexible linear surgical stapling device that was mounted on a colonoscope-type shaft. The greatest width is 15 mm, which is at the junction of the stapling cartridge and the shaft. The rigid segment of the stapler shaft is 14 cm long. The device itself has no optics but can be inserted transorally through an overtube which is later backed up onto the shaft of the device. A standard gastroscope (GIF 160, Olympus America) can then be placed side-by-side with the stapler for vision. The stapler fires two triple rows of surgical staples and cuts between the two rows. Two 55-mm cartridges may be needed depending on the size of the pseudocyst, to form a pseudocystgastrostomy anastomosis with 4.8 mm staples for optimum hemostasis.

Given that the SurgAssist™ is no longer available, a possible alternative technique to consider includes utilizing a needle knife cautery, and the OverStitch™ Endoscopic Suturing System (Apollo EndoSurgery, Austin, TX) to endoscopically suture the edges of the pseudocystgastrostomy. This is similar to the classic description of open pseudocystgastrostomy with running locking sutures employed for hemostasis.

Additionally, standard endoscopic hemostatic clips (Olympus America, Cook Endoscopy, or Microvasive) should be available if there are small bleeding vessels that are disrupted either by firing the stapler, or opening the anastomosis with a needle knife.

Lastly, the use of fluoroscopy in the operating room can be helpful to ensure that the guidewire has entered the pseudocyst cavity. Contrast administration through the 19-gauge needle can also help to determine the actual size at the time of surgery which can be helpful with operative planning.

Description of NOTES Technique

The NOTES procedure should be performed in the operating room with the patient under general anesthesia and endotracheal intubation, with the plan to proceed with laparoscopic or open cystgastrostomy in the event of an adverse event or procedure failure. A therapeutic echoendoscope (Olympus America, Center Valley, PA) is inserted transorally into the stomach and is used to assess the pseudocyst sonographically. In addition, sonography can be used to measure wall thickness. In general, the distance from the gastric lumen to the cyst lumen should be not greater than 1 cm; otherwise, it can be difficult to dilate the cystgastrostomy tract after puncture (the so-called 1-cm rule). Next, color Doppler interrogation can be used to scan the proposed puncture site for vessels that may be in the needle path (Fig. 13.4).

Having determined the site for puncture, the pseudocyst is punctured with a 19-gauge needle (EchoTip® Ultra, Cook Endoscopy, Winston-Salem, NC) through the gastric and cyst walls, and a sample of the pseudocyst contents is aspirated. If the cyst appears infected, an aspirate should be sent for a Gram stain and culture. Contrast injection under fluoroscopy is

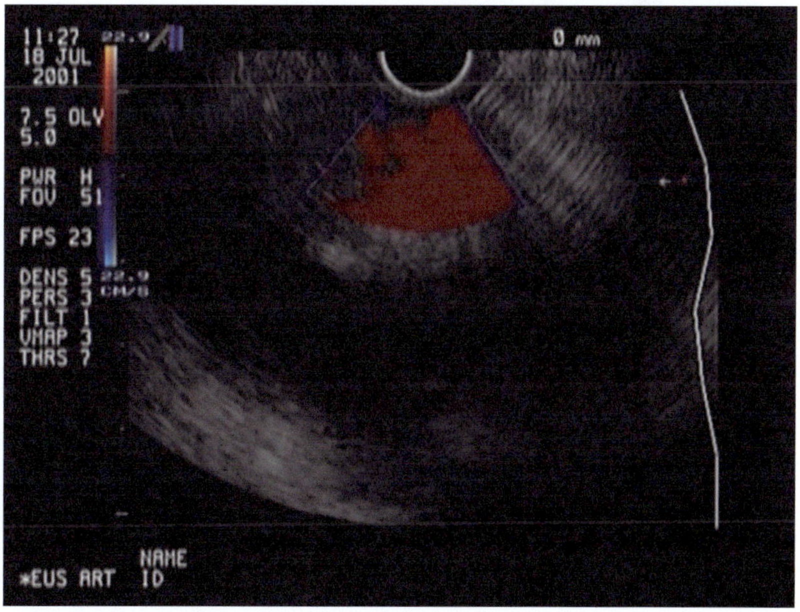

Fig. 13.4 *Colored area* indicates vascularity; the *dark area* near the bottom of the image represents the pseudocyst cavity

performed to document the size and anatomical boundaries of the cyst, and to identify a possible communication with the pancreatic duct. A 0.035-in. guidewire (Tracer Metro, Cook Endoscopy) is then inserted, and a Soehendra stent extractor is placed over the wire to dilate the opening into the pseudocyst (Fig. 13.5). Alternatively, and lately more effectively, we use a 4F to 6F step-up Soehendra biliary dilating catheter over the guidewire, which provides an excellent tract for subsequent balloon catheter passage. The drainage tract is then dilated with an 18- or 20-mm balloon catheter (CRE™ Balloon Dilatation Catheter, Boston Scientific, Marlborough, MA) (Fig. 13.6). At this point, the echoendoscope is usually swapped out over the guidewire for a standard gastroscope (GIF 160, Olympus). The endoscope should then be able to be passed directly into the pseudocyst lumen through the dilated tract (Fig. 13.7). Endoscopic necrosectomy and debridement are performed when possible, followed by transoral surgical anastomosis under endoscopic visualization with the SurgAssist™ SLC 55 4.8-mm stapler (Power Medical Interventions, Langhorne, PA) as described below. The stapler fires two triple rows of surgical staples and cuts between the two rows. Two 55-mm green load cartridges may be needed depending on the size of the pseudocyst to form a pseudocystgastrostomy anastomosis with 4.8 mm staples for optimum hemostasis.

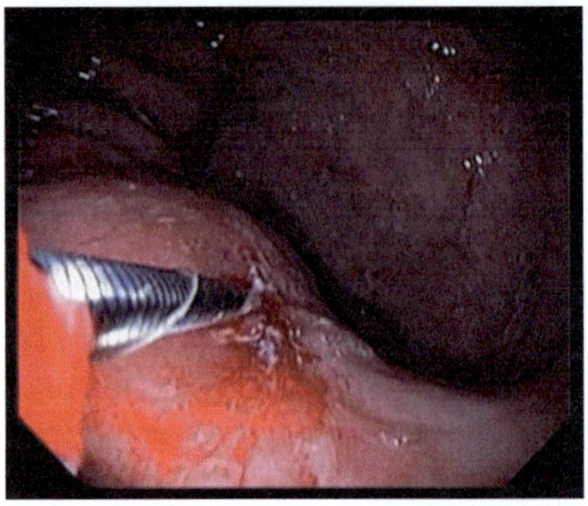

Fig. 13.5 A Soehendra stent extractor (Cook Endoscopy, Winston-Salem, NC) is used to enlarge the opening into the pseudocyst

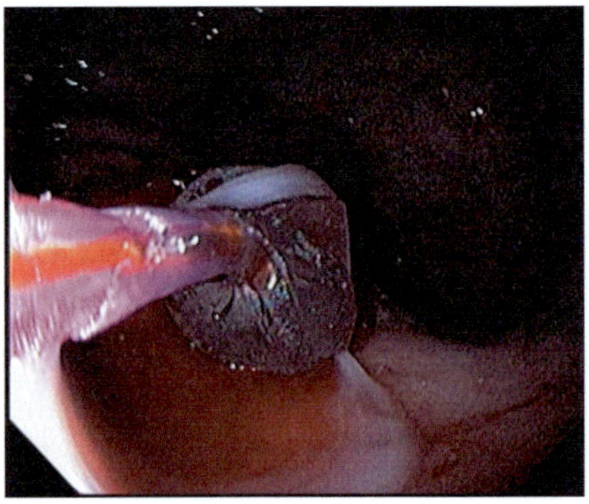

Fig. 13.6 An esophageal dilation balloon is placed across the newly created pseudocystgastrostomy. Note the purulent drainage below and around the balloon

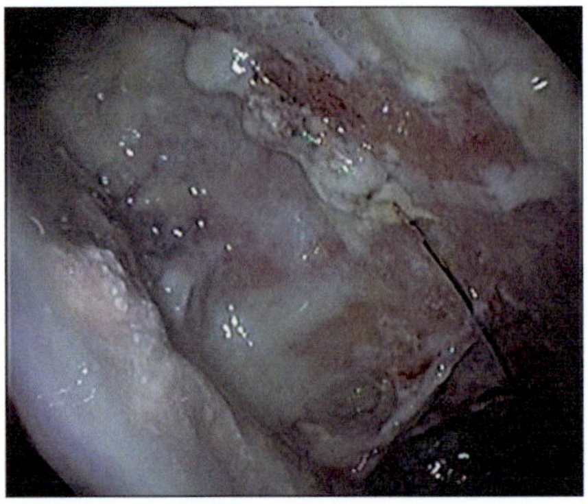

Fig. 13.7 Endoscopic view of a pseudocyst cavity. Note the guidewire present in the cavity

Once the cyst cavity has been inspected and lavaged or debrided as necessary, the standard gastroscope is removed, leaving the guidewire in place. A gastric length, 20-mm-diameter, endoscopic overtube (U.S. Endoscopy, Mentor, OH) is back loaded onto the gastroscope shaft, and the gastroscope is reinserted into the stomach over the guidewire. The guidewire is maintained in the pseudocyst throughout until the stapler is to be fired, so as to maintain access to the pseudocyst lumen. The lubricated overtube is then advanced over the endoscope shaft until its distal end is in the lumen of the stomach. The gastroscope is once again removed leaving the wire in the overtube.

The SurgAssist™ SLC 55 4.8-mm stapler is lubricated and then inserted through the overtube alongside the wire. It is often necessary to extend the patient's neck so as to keep the overtube as straight as possible and allow for passage of the device, which will not pass if the overtube is bent or curved. The overtube is necessary to allow the distal aspect of the stapler and cartridge to pass through the gastroesophageal junction, which tends to have too sharp an angle if not straightened by the overtube. The overtube is then backed out onto the shaft of the SurgAssist™. The diagnostic gastroscope is reinserted alongside the stapler until it enters the stomach. The endoscope is reinserted because the stapler has no optics, and because, although the distal end of the Power Medical stapler can be deflected somewhat with its motorized controls, additional endoscopic manipulation of the cartridge is needed to get one arm through the cystgastrostomy to facilitate stapling. The endoscope reinsertion and the use of the endoscope to manipulate the tip of the stapler are the two most difficult aspects of the procedure. Any means necessary can be employed to use the scope to manipulate the stapler to include scope pushing it with the scope tip, using snares or forceps, retroflexing, and looking backwards.

Once one of the jaws of the stapler is across the cyst wall and the other remains in the stomach, the device is advanced further until as much of the cyst/gastric wall as possible is between the walls of the stapler. The stapler is fired, forming a stapled pseudocystgastrostomy that measures about 5.5 cm. Depending on the size of the pseudocyst, the entire process can be repeated for a second firing. In this way, we have formed stapled cystgastrostomies up to 8 cm in length. Once the anastomosis is created, the necrotic debris in the pseudocyst should be visible from the stomach (Fig. 13.8). Fluoroscopic guidance can also be helpful in visualizing that the stapler is passing into the pseudocyst cavity (Fig. 13.9). If bleeding occurs during or after the anastomosis creation, hemostasis may be achieved using hemostatic clips (Fig. 13.10).

Aside from transoral anastomosis, other options are to place double-pigtail stents to drain the cyst into the stomach or duodenum. If the cyst appears infected or contains necrotic debris, a nasocystic catheter can be inserted for cyst

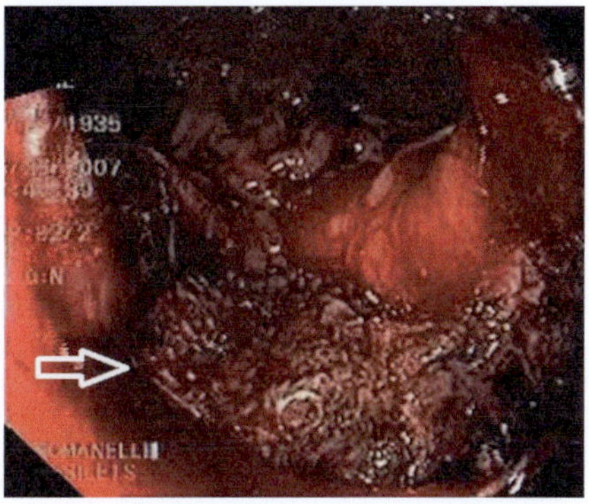

Fig. 13.8 Necrotic pancreatic debris (*arrow*), as seen from the endoscope after completion of the stapled anastomosis

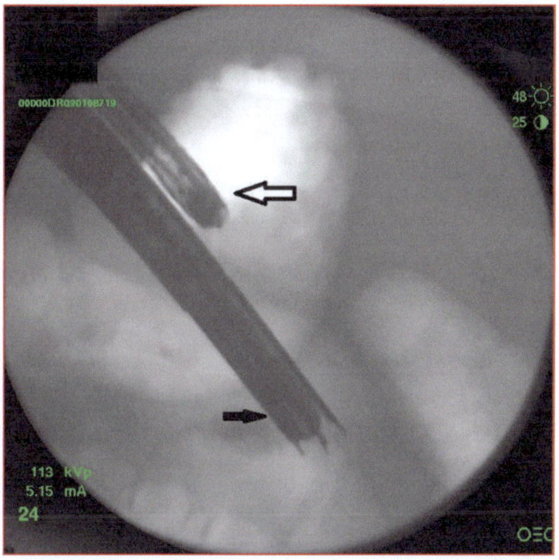

Fig. 13.9 Radiograph of the stapler (*black arrow*) and endoscope (*white arrow*), side-by-side, with the stapler cartridge in the pseudocyst

irrigation. Once the cyst contents are clear, the nasocystic catheter is exchanged for a stent to maintain drainage.

For endoscopic procedures, patients are kept on antibiotics and taken off acid-suppression medications until complete cyst resolution is documented by CT. Most pseudocysts will resolve 10–14 days after drainage. If a stent is placed, the stent is usually removed 6–8 weeks after cyst resolution to allow the cyst wall to scar

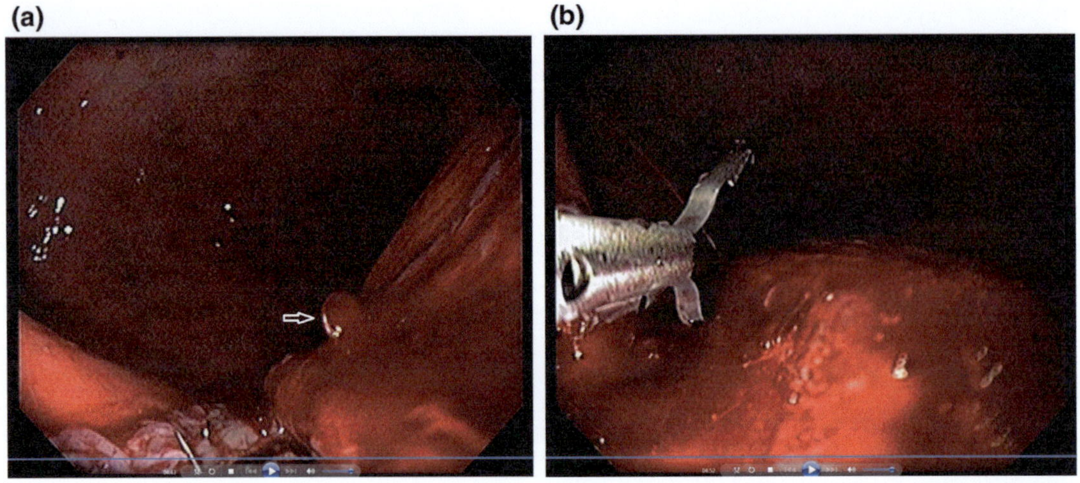

Fig. 13.10 a, b Note the bleeding vessel on the right edge of the anastomosis (*white arrow*) (**a**). This can easily be clipped with a hemoclip (**b**)

down. Routine esophagogastroduodenoscopy is recommended at 1 and 6 weeks postoperatively to evaluate patency, and a CT scan is recommended at 2–3 months to demonstrate resolution of the pseudocyst.

Results

Although surgery is the standard technique for drainage of pancreatic pseudocysts, the use of endoscopic methods is increasing. Endoscopic pseudocystgastrostomy has treatment success rates of 82–100%, and a mortality rate of less than 1% [8, 12–14]. Surgical pseudocystgastrostomy has technical and treatment success rates of greater than 90% and a mortality rate of 5–10% [14, 15]. In a randomized trial comparing endoscopic and surgical pseudocystgastrostomy for pancreatic pseudocyst drainage, none of the 20 patients in the endoscopy group had pseudocyst recurrence during the follow-up period; therefore, there is no evidence that surgical pseudocystgastrostomy is superior. However, endoscopic treatment was associated with shorter hospital stays, better physical and mental health of patients, and lower cost [12].

NOTES pseudocystgastrostomy is comparable to previously described surgical approaches, yet is as minimally invasive as endoscopic drainage procedures previously described for management of pseudocysts. The NOTES pseudocystgastrostomy procedure is also less invasive than laparoscopic or open pseudocystgastrostomy and provides definitive treatment. A study by our group performed on 6 patients concluded that all patients had significant decrease in pseudocyst size with a patent anastomosis postoperatively [13]. In that study, however, one patient required endoscopic anastomotic dilatation due to continued symptoms 6 weeks after the operation, but the patients pseudocyst completely resolved by 4 months [13].

Conclusion

An interdisciplinary approach is best suited for the safe and effective stage-specific treatment of pancreatic pseudocysts. The decision whether to treat a patient with a pancreatic pseudocyst, as well as when and with what technique, can be difficult. The endoscopic and minimally invasive therapeutic procedures for the drainage of pancreatic pseudocysts are superior to open surgical techniques with respect to their success rates, morbidity, and mortality, but they cannot always be performed. The choice of technique depends very heavily on the experience of the treatment center. Consideration for a NOTES approach to permanent drainage of a pancreatic pseudocyst relies on favorable anatomy, familiarity with the instrumentation, and a team with both advanced laparoscopic and advanced therapeutic endoscopic skills.

References

1. Gussenbauer C. Zur Operativen Behandlung der Pankreaszysten. Arch furklin Chir. 1883;29:355.
2. Jedlicka R. Eine Neue Operationsmethode der Pankreascysten. Zentralblatt fur Chir. 1923;501:132.
3. Beitragzur Hahn O, de Pankreasfistein Behandlung. Arch fur kiln Chir. 1928;143:73.
4. Konig E. Der inneren Anastomose in der Behandlung der Pankreascyste. Der Chir. 1946;17/18:24.
5. Taghizadeh F, Bower RJ, Kiesewetter WB. Stapled cystogastrostomy. A method of treatment for pediatric pancreatic pseudocyst. Ann Surg. 1979;190:166–9.
6. Trias M, Targarona EM, Balague C, et al. Intraluminal stapled laparoscopic cystogastrostomy for treatment of pancreatic pseudocyst. Br J Surg. 1995;82:403.
7. Rao GV, Reddy DN. "Transgastric appendectomy," video presentation. Society of gastrointestinal endoscopic surgeons annual meeting. April 2005, Ft. Lauderdale, FL.
8. Romanelli JR, Desilets DJ, Earle DB. Pancreatic pseudocystgastrostomy with a peroral, flexible stapler: human natural orifice transluminal endoscopic surgery anastomoses in 2 patients (with videos). Gastrointestinal Endosc. 2008;981–6.
9. Beckingham IJ, Krige JE, Bornman PC, Terblanche J. Long term out-come of endoscopic drainage of pancreatic pseudocysts. Am J Gastroenterol. 1999;94:71–4.
10. Varadarajulu S, Phadnis MA, Christein JD, Wilcox CM. Multiple transluminal gateway technique for EUS-guided drainage of symptomatic walled-off pancreatic necrosis. Gastrointest Endosc. 2011;74 (1):74–80.
11. Lerch MM, Stier A, Wahnschaffe U. Pancreatic pseudocysts. Dtsch Arztebl Int. 2009;106(38):614–21.
12. Varadarajulu S, Bang JY, Sutton BS, et al. Equal efficacy of endoscopic and surgical cystogastrostomy for pancreatic pseudocyst drainage in a randomized trial. Gastroenterology. 2013;145(3):583–90.
13. Pallapothu R, Earle DB, Desilets DJ, Romanelli JR. NOTES stapled cystgastrostomy: a novel approach for surgical management of pancreatic pseudocysts. Surg Endosc. 2011;23(3):883–9.
14. Bergman S, Melvin WS. Operative and nonoperative management of pancreatic pseudocysts. Surg Clin North Am. 2007;87:1447–60.
15. Johnson MD, Walsh RM, Henderson JM, et al. Surgical versus nonsurgical management of pancreatic pseudocysts. J Clin Gastroenterol. 2009;43:586–90.

Transgastric Peritoneoscopy

14

Peter Nau and Jeffrey Hazey

Abstract

The initial description of a deliberate passage of an endoscope across the wall of a hollow viscus came in 2004 with Kalloo's seminal report describing endoscopic transgastric peritoneoscopy. A year later, a video of a human transgastric appendectomy was revealed to the world and thus was born the concept of natural orifice translumenal endoscopic surgery (NOTES). Attempts at transgastric peritoneoscopy were replicated in the animal model in both survival and long-term studies. Human case series have been reported in patients undergoing other abdominal procedures. Infectious concerns, which developed from some of the animal work, have not proven to be a problem in human surgery. Visualization of the peritoneal cavity via an endoscope has been shown to be almost equivalent to laparoscopic examination.

Keywords

Natural orifice surgery · Natural orifice translumenal endoscopic surgery · NOTES · Transgastric peritoneoscopy · Endoscopic surgery

P. Nau (✉)
University of Iowa Hospitals and Clinics, 200 Hawkins Drive, Iowa City, IA 52242, USA
e-mail: peter-nau@uiowa.edu

J. Hazey
Wexner Medical Center, The Ohio State University, 410 West 10th Avenue, Columbus, OH 43210-1228, USA
e-mail: jeffrey.hazey@osumc.edu

J.R. Romanelli et al. (eds.), *NOTES and Endoluminal Surgery*, Clinical Gastroenterology, DOI 10.1007/978-3-319-50610-4_14

Introduction/Background

The concept of a diagnostic endoscopy was first described by Philip Bozzini in 1806 with his introduction of the "Lichtleiter." Utilizing an aluminum tube lit by candlelight, he was able to investigate the urogenital tract applying minimally invasive principles [1]. Alternatively, Konrad Langenbeck established the concept of transvaginal access to the abdomen in 1813 with his description of the transvaginal hysterectomy [2]. The colpotomy is reliably closed and provides for a safe approach to the peritoneal cavity. Its acceptance has been limited by its gender specificity and cultural perceptions of a transvaginal procedure [3, 4].

It was with this concept of an alternative approach to abdominal pathology that Kalloo pioneered the idea of a transgastric diagnostic peritoneoscopy in 2004 [5]. Following the publication of Kalloo's manuscript, the field of natural orifice translumenal endoscopic surgery (NOTES) experienced a revolution of innovation including potential operations and various techniques to access the abdominal cavity [6–10]. An unpublished but infamous video of a transgastric appendectomy from India helped ignite the interest and academic pursuits in natural orifice surgery. While it is unlikely that nephrectomy or incisional hernia repair will ever be completed utilizing solely NOTES techniques, other procedures have been tremendously successful including the transanal approach to colorectal cancer and per-oral endoscopic myotomy (POEM) for achalasia.

Notwithstanding the relative youth of the field of natural orifice surgery, there have been several approaches employed to access the abdominal cavity. As previously mentioned, the transanal technique in the setting of a resection for colorectal malignancies has been well described by Sylla and Lacy [11, 12]. To date, however, the morbidity of an elective colotomy has limited the advancement of the technique.

Perhaps nowhere has the future of natural orifice surgery been better realized that with the per-oral methodology. With case series reported in excess of 500 patients, POEM is now the first-line approach to the treatment of achalasia at many institutions [13]. Given the propensity to withstand the shearing forces of endoscopic manipulation as well as its central location in the abdomen, the transgastric approach to the abdominal cavity has also been extensively evaluated. We describe the validation of transgastric peritoneoscopy as a viable technique to explore the peritoneal cavity.

Establishing Transgastric Access

When laparoscopic cholecystectomy was initially embraced as an alternative to maximally invasive laparotomy, there was a sharp rise in the complication rate of what was otherwise a very well-tolerated procedure [14, 15]. Rather than replicate history through the adoption of NOTES without appropriate training milestones, leaders in the field of minimally invasive surgery and therapeutic endoscopy convened to discuss the challenges of safely implementing NOTES. The result of this meeting was the creation of the Natural Orifice Surgery Consortium for Assessment and Research (NOSCAR) working group and, perhaps more importantly, its work product, the White Paper [16]. In this document, the authors identified many of the perceived barriers to the widespread acceptance of natural orifice techniques. Chief among these issues was the achievement of a safe technique for accessing the abdominal cavity.

Blind access to the abdominal viscera via a transgastric approach was first introduced by Gauderer and Ponsky in 1981 with their description of the percutaneous endoscopic gastrostomy (PEG) tube [17]. For NOTES to succeed, however, the surgical endoscopist must be able to access safely and accurately the contents of the peritoneal cavity rather than simply placing a feeding tube. Initial transgastric peritoneoscopies were performed in animal models [5, 7, 18]. Utilizing both nonsurvival models as well as long-term subjects followed for complications, researchers validated the transgastric approach for endoscopic peritoneoscopy. Gastrotomy creation was noted to be both reproducible and safe.

Notwithstanding the technique used, all animal experiments involved novel and unproven methods for gastrotomy closure. Given this paucity of options for safe and consistent repair of a gastric defect, the initial work in a human model was completed in the setting of primary procedures which otherwise required a gastrotomy [19]. Others were completed in hybrid procedures during which the gastric defect was closed with standard laparoscopic techniques [20].

Perhaps the most thorough approach to the question of gastrotomy creation and transgastric passage of an endoscope was completed by the group from The Ohio State University [19]. In this collection of experiments, the ability to establish transgastric access safely and reliably was systematically assessed with gradually decreasing safeguards against iatrogenic injury. The initial 20 cases were completed in a population undergoing surgical treatment of pancreatic cancer. After having safely entered the peritoneal cavity laparoscopically, the process of endoscopic gastrotomy creation was directly observed. In this study, the authors demonstrated that endoscopic gastrotomy placement was safe and accurate in its positioning [21]. Next, in a population of forty patients undergoing laparoscopic Roux-en-Y gastric bypass, they accessed the abdominal cavity endoscopically and performed a transgastric endoscopic peritoneoscopy (TEP) [22]. There were two arms to this study. The initial 20 patients had pre-insufflation established via a Veress needle placed in the left upper quadrant. The second group had no pre-insufflation of the abdomen. Ten patients in each arm had no past surgeries in their abdomen. The other ten had previous abdominal operations. In these experiments, the authors were able to show that a gastrotomy can be safely created blindly, without pre-insufflation of the abdomen, and in those with a prior history of abdominal surgery. Only minor complications, such as superficial burns to the anterior abdominal wall or undersurface of the left lateral lobe of the liver, were encountered.

There have been many different techniques described for the establishment of transgastric access. The preponderance of transgastric procedures have been completed employing a modified version of that which was described by Kalloo and Nau (Table 14.1) [5, 22]. A single-channel therapeutic endoscope is introduced through the patient's oropharynx and into the stomach. Next a needle knife papillotome (Boston Scientific, Natick, MA) is passed through the therapeutic channel and, using external abdominal wall palpation, a site is chosen for gastrotomy creation. With short bursts of energy from a standard electrosurgical generator, a small gastrotomy is created. A 450-cm Jagwire (Boston Scientific) is next passed into the peritoneal cavity through this gastrotomy (Fig. 14.1). Over

Table 14.1 Instrumentation necessary for successful establishment of transgastric access for transgastric peritoneoscopy

Instruments for the NOTES toolbox
• Single-channel therapeutic endoscope
• Needle knife papillotome
• 450-cm Jagwire
• 18–20 mm wire-guided balloon dilation catheter
• Standard electrosurgical generator

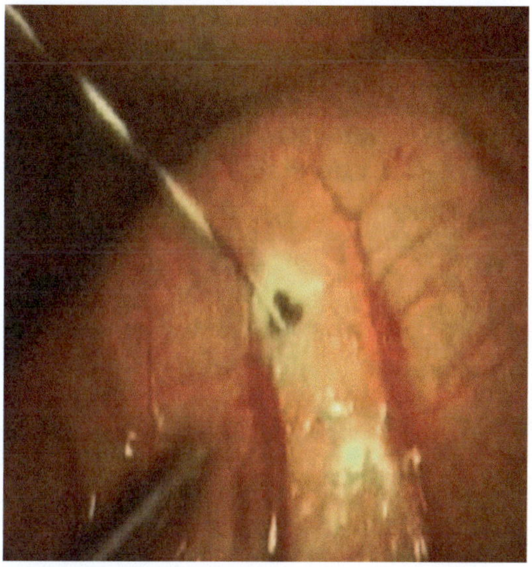

Fig. 14.1 Picture of Jagwire passing through the pinpoint gastrotomy made with needle knife. This flexible wire is used to facilitate balloon placement for dilation of the gastrotomy

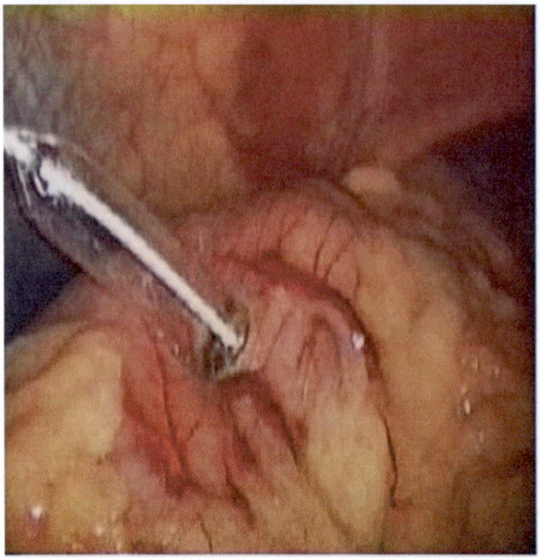

Fig. 14.2 Radially dilating balloon enlarging gastrotomy to accommodate transgastric passage of endoscope

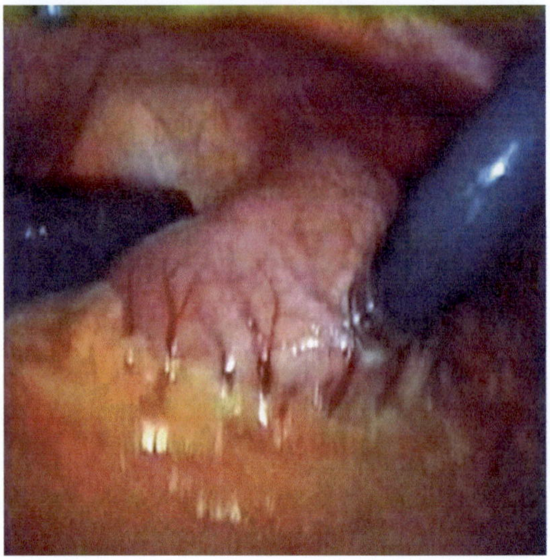

Fig. 14.3 Transgastric passage endoscope through the endoscopically created gastrotomy

this wire, an 18–20-mm wire-guided balloon dilator (Boston Scientific) is passed (Fig. 14.2). It is critical to place the gastric wall at the "waist" of the balloon so as to keep the balloon seated on the gastric wall during dilation. Visualization of the dilation process can be facilitated by marrying the end of the scope to the balloon so as to see through the balloon into the peritoneal cavity. After gastrotomy creation is completed, the balloon and scope are both advanced into the peritoneal cavity (Fig. 14.3). Alternatively, a sphincterotome can be used to enlarge the defect so as to accommodate the endoscope.

It should be noted that the aforementioned technique was described in a population that was undergoing a procedure that would otherwise necessitate a gastrotomy secondary to the lack of safe options for reliable endoscopic closure during an elective gastrotomy. While not completed in a human population, Pauli et al. described the creation of a submucosal tunnel for transgastric access similar to what is performed during a POEM [23]. Their self-approximating transluminal access technique, or STAT, employs principles of endoscopic submucosal resection. The procedure begins with the injection of 10 mL of saline into the gastric submucosa. Using a needle knife, a 1–1.5-cm incision is made in the mucosa. Submucosal dissection is then completed with the assistance of a grasping forceps for a total of 10–12 cm. Having achieved an appropriately long tunnel, the needle knife is again used to breach the muscular wall of the stomach. Similar to the technique used by Nau et al. [21], a radial dilating balloon is then used to create a gastrotomy large enough to accommodate the endoscope. The mucosal defect is closed with endoscopic clips and the seromuscular incision is left alone. While of uncertain clinical significance, it is notable that there were infections found in 40% of the animals on necropsy following a two-week survival period (one microabscess and one submucosal abscess). Given that Khashab et al. have recently described a per-oral endoscopic pyloromyotomy in a human patient and the submucosal tunnel is routinely used for the POEM, this description may likely be a reasonable approach to accessing the peritoneal cavity [24].

The transgastric approach to the peritoneal cavity is ideal in that it affords the surgeon unhindered access to many of the structures within the abdomen. The muscular wall of the stomach is also well suited to resist the shearing forces associated with a transgastric procedure. Gastrotomy positioning is reliable and safe. To date, however, there is no safe and reliable method for gastrotomy closure. Certainly the technique described by Pauli et al. [23] and the successes of the POEM procedure suggest that a tunneling technique may be a reasonable alternative to accessing the abdominal wall directly. Given the morbidity and mortality of a gastric leak, however, this aspect of the transgastric procedure must be consistent and safe prior to offering the approach to a population that does not otherwise need a gastrotomy.

Insufflation of the Abdominal Cavity

With the introduction and widespread adoption of laparoscopy as a viable approach to treating abdominal pathology, a new collection of issues arose. Principle among those was the technique for insufflating the abdomen and the physiologic consequences associated with this act. The cardiopulmonary implications of pneumoperitoneum established using laparoscopic techniques are well established [25–28]. Peritoneal insufflation to a pressure of more than 15 mm Hg may affect increases in aortic pressure, decreased urine blood flow and a respiratory acidosis secondary to systemic carbon dioxide absorption. With that said, laparoscopic surgery can be safely completed utilizing modern anesthetic techniques even in critically ill patients [29]. Establishing the safety and efficacy of the endoscopic creation of pneumoperitoneum is necessary if the NOTES approach is to be validated.

Initial studies completed in animal models replicated the techniques utilized for standard laparoscopy. Using a Veress needle, Ko et al. were able to access and insufflate the abdominal cavity allowing for effective gastrotomy creation for a diagnostic peritoneoscopy in a swine model [10]. This practice was replicated in the initial human series at the Ohio State University, safely and effectively establishing pneumoperitoneum with classic laparoscopic techniques, allowing for a natural orifice procedure [19].

In an effort to assess for a stand-alone NOTES procedure, von Delius et al. evaluated the effect of pneumoperitoneum established using the on-demand endoscopic air pump [30]. Using a swine model, they noted a wide variation in the intra-abdominal pressures with maximal pressures of 22 mm Hg and pressures greater than 15 mm Hg in 21% of the measurements. Meireles et al. witnessed similar results when comparing laparoscopic insufflation to on-demand endoscopic insufflation, again noting elevated intra-abdominal pressures in the endoscopic cohort with values exceeding 30 mm Hg [31]. It is with this deficiency in mind that the group from the Ohio State University assessed for the accuracy and safety of insufflating the abdomen using a hybrid technique [32]. To complete this investigation, the authors obtained blind peritoneal access as described above. Next, the laparoscopic insufflator was connected to the therapeutic channel of the endoscope and the abdomen insufflated to a pressure of 10 mm Hg. The pressure reading was then verified by connecting the insufflator to a Veress needle passed through the left upper quadrant. In a population of twenty patients, the authors noted that the mean pressure reading was 9.8 mm Hg (range 5–17 mm Hg) through the endoscope and 9.8 mm Hg through the Veress needle (range 4–17 mm Hg). This difference was not statistically significant ($P = 0.9$) and the absolute mean pressure difference between the 2 methods on a case-by-case basis was only 1.0 mm Hg.

Given the well-established deleterious effects of pneumoperitoneum on the cardiopulmonary and renal systems, the establishment of responsible methods for insufflating the abdominal cavity is critical to the success of NOTES. There is excellent literature supporting laparoscopy in critically ill cardiac patients. It stands to reason that the same technology utilized from a NOTES platform would have a similar safety profile. It is with that premise that the use of the laparoscopic insufflator through the working channel of the endoscope was validated as safe technique for establishing pneumoperitoneum in a NOTES procedure.

Infectious Implications

Critical to the validation of natural orifice approach is the establishment of the safety and efficacy of the technique. Flexible endoscopy as a diagnostic and therapeutic modality is well established from an intra-luminal approach. Traversing the gastric wall presents a new set of risks, including the risk of cross-contamination of the abdominal cavity with gastric flora. The gastric milieu is necessarily contaminated, and the risk that this poses to the patient must be negligible in order for a transgastric NOTES to be a viable option.

The question of the infectious implications of a transgastric procedure has been addressed from numerous different viewpoints using animal models. McGee et al. investigated the systemic inflammatory response of a transgastric procedure using pigs [33]. This group evaluated for changes in markers for inflammation including TNF-α and IL-6 following different interventions. They noted that systemic inflammation was similar when comparing a NOTES population to one undergoing both an exploratory laparotomy as well as exploratory laparoscopy.

Others have attempted to address the question of whether some degree of gastric decontamination is necessary to prevent cross-contamination of the peritoneal cavity with gastric flora. Again employing pigs, Eickhoff investigated a complex gastric decontamination protocol versus only gastric irrigation [34]. The authors found a statistically significant increase in the intra-abdominal bacterial burden in the control population. Perhaps more significant, however, was the finding that there was no difference in the rate of microscopic or macroscopic peritonitis between the two groups. McGee et al. also found no difference in the number of positive peritoneal cultures or intra-abdominal infections when comparing gastric lavage to an antibiotic-enriched lavage [35]. Contrasting this, Giday et al. noted a significant increase in both the number of abscesses as well as positive peritoneal cultures following a transgastric procedure without pre-procedural decontamination [36]. While it is clear that the gastric effluent is contaminated, there is no definitive information on the infectious implications in the animal studies to date.

It is with this ambiguity in mind that the Ohio State group investigated that infectious burden of a transgastric procedure in a human population. In each case, a single intravenous dose of preoperative prophylactic antibiotics was administered. No irrigation or decontamination of the stomach was completed. The endoscope was cleaned with glutaraldehyde per a standardized protocol, but was not considered sterile. The initial study completed assessed the infectious risks associated with the creation of a gastrotomy or jejunotomy during a laparoscopic Roux-en-Y gastric bypass (RYGB) [37]. Aspirates were collected from the stomach, from the peritoneum prior to violation of the intestines, and from the same location after completion of the operation. In this experiment, they found five of twenty possible cases of cross-contamination defined by similar bacterial isolates from the stomach found in the peritoneal samples. Most importantly, they identified no iatrogenic infections in any patient enrolled.

In the second experiment, the degree of contamination of the scope and the role of transgastric passage of this device was evaluated [21]. To do this, cultures were taken from sterile washes of the scope prior to the procedure, and then, cultures were drawn from the peritoneal cavity prior to, and following, transgastric passage of the endoscope. In this cohort, they found no difference in the bacterial burden following the gastrotomy, nor did they identify any instances of cross-contamination of the peritoneal cavity with gastric flora. In their final experiment, they evaluated the infectious risks of a stand-alone NOTES procedure via cultures taken from the stomach and then again from the peritoneal cavity after transgastric passage of the endoscope [38]. In each case, the cultures were collected by completing sterile washes through the therapeutic channel of the endoscope. In this study, the median level of bacteria present was significantly higher in the gastric samples (980 vs. 320 CFU/ml, $p = 0.001$). Cross-contamination from the stomach to the peritoneal cavity was documented in 21% of the cases. Interestingly, there was a higher bacterial burden in the stomach in those patients on proton pump inhibitors (PPI's) ($n = 25$) (7,800,000 vs. 340 CFU/ml; $p = 0.01$). However, in no instance was there an infectious complication noted in either the group using PPI's or the group as a whole.

This question is the crux of the issue of infectious implications of a transgastric operation. Inherent in any procedure that violates the gastrointestinal tract is the potential for translocation of intra-luminal bacteria to the peritoneal cavity. It is the clinical significance of this translocation that must be considered rather than the absolute bacterial load or cross-contamination of species. The work by Hazey et al. [19] has shown that this risk is minimal and should not deter the development of this approach.

Visualization

An important step in the validation of a transgastric approach to the peritoneal cavity is the ability to adequately visualize the structures of the abdomen. This fact was not lost on Kalloo et al. in their initial description of a diagnostic peritoneoscopy, during which they were able to explore the abdomen endoscopically [5]. Wang et al. also addressed the adequacy of an endoscopic exploration [39]. In their experiment, the ability to visualize the structures of the abdominal cavity was compared using a standard laparoscope, a 5.5-mm endoscope and a 12.8-mm endoscope. Using a grading scale of one to five, two independent investigators surveilled the abdominal organs including liver, gallbladder, spleen, stomach, small intestine, colon, bladder, fallopian tube, ovary, omentum, and peritoneum. They noted no difference in their ability adequately to visualize the structures in any of the three techniques. Nau et al. published their work on the diagnostic accuracy of an endoscopic exploration in a total of eighty humans [40]. Their initial study was completed in a population undergoing an exploration for pancreatic cancer metastases. In that cohort, findings from the endoscopic procedure correlated with the laparoscopic findings in 95% of the cases. The only discordance was a peritoneal implant that was not visualized endoscopically as it had been removed during the initial laparoscopic exploration. In their next experiment, the investigators compared the ability to surveil the abdomen in a population of 60 obese patients undergoing laparoscopic RYGB. Using a scale of one to five with five being unhindered visualization, the mean score was 4.8. Additionally, there was no difference in the ability to explore the different quadrants of the abdomen based on the presence or absence of prior surgical procedures (4.82 vs. 4.77; $p = 0.6$). While there have been many options proposed for an endoscopic exploration of the stomach, most have been limited in either their applicability to the population as a whole, or in the ability to visualize all quadrants of the abdomen. This cannot be said about the transgastric approach. Employing both animal and human models, the transgastric peritoneoscopy has consistently provided accurate and complete visualization of the intra-abdominal structures.

Conclusion

The introduction of NOTES was greeted with a great deal of enthusiasm and clinical investigation. While there has been a degree of disenchantment due to the lack of progression of the technique, it cannot be overstated the importance that NOTES has played in treating surgical disease. The indications for interventional endoscopy have expanded greatly. For example, POEM has supplanted the Heller myotomy in many institutions as the first-line treatment for achalasia. These developments can be traced back to Kalloo's discussion of a transgastric peritoneoscopy [5]. Since that manuscript, investigators have shown that this is a safe and reliable method for accessing and surveilling the abdominal cavity. In the event that a reproducible endoscopic method for closing the gastrotomy is developed, this technique will certainly allow for another option to explore the abdomen.

References

1. Morgenstern L. The 200th anniversary of the first endoscope: Philipp Bozzini (1773-1809). Surg Innov. 2005;12(2):105–6.
2. de Sousa LH, de Sousa JA, de Sousa Filho LH, de Sousa MM, de Sousa VM, et al. Totally NOTES (T-NOTES) transvaginal cholecystectomy using two endoscopes: preliminary report. Surg Endosc. 2009;23(11):2550–5.
3. Teoh AY, Ng EK, Chock A, Swanstrom L, Varadarajulu S, et al. Asian-Chinese patient perceptions of natural orifice transluminal endoscopic surgery cholecystectomy. Dig Endosc. 2014;26(3):458–66.
4. Bucher P, Ostermann S, Pugin F, Morel P. Female population perception of conventional laparoscopy, transumbilical LESS, and transvaginal NOTES for cholecystectomy. Surg Endosc. 2011;25(7):2308–15.
5. Kalloo AN, Singh VK, Jagannath SB, et al. Flexible transgastric peritoneoscopy: a novel approach to diagnostic and therapeutic interventions in the peritoneal cavity. Gastrointest Endosc. 2004;60(1):114–7.
6. Allemann P, Perretta S, Asakuma M, Dallemagne B, Mutter D, et al. NOTES retroperitoneal transvaginal distal pancreatectomy. Multimedia manuscript. Surg Endosc. 2009;23:882–3.
7. Isariyawongse JP, McGee MF, Rosen MJ, Cherullo EE, Ponsky LE. Pure natural orifice transluminal endoscopic surgery (NOTES) nephrectomy using standard laparoscopic instruments in the porcine model. J Endourol. 2008;22:1087–91.
8. Leroy J, Cahill RA, Perretta S, Forgione A, Dallemagne B, et al. Natural orifice translumenal endoscopic surgery (NOTES) applied totally to sigmoidectomy: an original technique with survival in a porcine model. Surg Endosc. 2009;23:24–30.
9. Simopoulos C, Kouklakis G, Zezos P, Ypsilantis P, Botaitis S, et al. Peroraltransgastric endoscopic procedures in pigs: feasibility, survival, questionings, and pitfalls. Surg Endosc. 2009;23:394–402.
10. Ko CW, Shin EJ, Buscaglia JM, Clarke JO, Magno P, et al. Preliminary pneumoperitoneum facilitates transgastric access into the peritoneal cavity for natural orifice transluminal endoscopic surgery: a pilot study in a live porcine model. Endoscopy. 2007;39:849–53.
11. Sylla P, Bordeianou LG, Berger D, Han KS, Lauwers GY, et al. A pilot study of natural orifice transanal endoscopic total mesorectal excision with laparoscopic assistance for rectal cancer. Surg Endosc. 2013;27(9):3396–405.
12. de Lacy AM, Rattner DW, Adelsdorfer C, Tasende MM, et al. Transanal natural orifice transluminal endoscopic surgery (NOTES) rectal resection: "down-to-up" total mesorectal excision (TME)–short-term outcomes in the first 20 cases. Surg Endosc. 2013;27(9):3165–72.
13. Inoue H, Sato H, Ikeda H, Onimaru M, Sato C, et al. Per-oral endoscopic myotomy: a series of 500 patients. J Am Coll Surg. 2015;221(2):256–64.
14. Moore MJ, Bennett CL. The learning curve for laparoscopic cholecystectomy. The Southern surgeons club. Am J Surg. 1995;170(1):55–9.
15. Deziel DJ, Millikan KW, Economou SG, Doolas A, Ko ST. Complications of laparoscopic cholecystectomy. A national survey of 4292 hospitals and an analysis of 77 604 cases. Am J Surg. 1993;165(1):9–14.
16. ASGE/SAGES Working group on natural orifice translumenal endoscopic surgery white paper. Gastrointest Endosc. 2006;63:199–203.
17. Gauderer MW, Ponsky JL. A simplified technique for constructing a tube feeding gastrostomy. Surg Gynecol Obstet. 1981;152(1):83–5.
18. Kantsevoy SV, Jagannath SB, Niiyama H, Isakovich NV, Chung SS, et al. A novel safe approach to the peritoneal cavity for per-oral transgastric endoscopic procedures. Gastrointest Endosc. 2007;65:497–500.
19. Hazey JW, Narula VK, Renton DB, Reavis KM, Paul CM, et al. Natural-orifice transgastric endoscopic peritoneoscopy in humans: initial clinical trial. Surg Endosc. 2008;22:16–20.
20. Auyang ED, Hungness ES, Vaziri K, Martin JA, Soper NJ. Human NOTES cholecystectomy: transgastric hybrid technique. J Gastrointest Surg. 2009;13(6):1149–50.
21. Nau P, Anderson J, Yuh B, Muscarella P Jr, Ellison EC. Diagnostic transgastric endoscopic peritoneoscopy: extension of the initial human trial for staging of pancreatic head masses. Surg Endosc. 2010;24(6):1440–6.
22. Nau P, Anderson J, Happel L, Yuh B, Narula VK. Safe alternative transgastric peritoneal access in humans: NOTES. Surgery. 2011;149(1):147–52.
23. Pauli EM, Moyer MT, Haluck RS, Mathew A. Self-approximating transluminal access technique for natural orifice transluminal endoscopic surgery: a porcine survival study (with video). Gastrointest Endosc. 2008;67:690–7.
24. Khashab MA, Stein E, Clarke JO, Saxena P, Kumbhari V. Gastric peroral endoscopic myotomy for refractory gastroparesis: first human endoscopic pyloromyotomy (with video). Gastrointest Endosc. 2013;78(5):764–8.
25. Chiu AW, Chang LS, Birkett DH, et al. The impact of pneumoperitoneum, pneumoretroperitoneum, and gasless laparoscopy on the systemic and renal hemodynamics. J Am Coll Surg. 1995;181:397–406.
26. Nguyen NT, Wolfe BM. The physiologic effects of pneumoperitoneum in the morbidly obese. Ann Surg. 2005;241:219–26.

27. O'Malley C, Cunningham AJ. Physiologic changes during laparoscopy. Anesthesiol Clin North Am. 2001;19:1–19.
28. Safran DB, Orlando R 3rd. Physiologic effects of pneumoperitoneum. Am J Surg. 1994;167:281–6.
29. Carroll BJ, Chandra M, Phillips EH, Margulies DR. Laparoscopic cholecystectomy in critically ill cardiac patients. Am Surg. 1993;59(12):783–5.
30. von Delius S, Huber W, Feussner H, Wilhelm D, Karagianni A. Effect of pneumoperitoneum on hemodynamics and inspiratory pressures during natural orifice transluminal endoscopic surgery (NOTES): an experimental, controlled study in an acute porcine model. Endoscopy. 2007;39(10):854–61.
31. Meireles O, Kantsevoy SV, Kalloo AN, Jagannath SB, Giday SA. Comparison of intraabdominal pressures using the gastroscope and laparoscope for transgastric surgery. Surg Endosc. 2007;21(6):998–1001.
32. Nau P, Anderson J, Needleman B, Ellison EC, Melvin WS, et al. Endoscopic peritoneal access and insufflation: natural orifice transluminal endoscopic surgery. Gastrointest Endosc. 2010;71(3):485–9.
33. McGee MF, Schomisch SJ, Marks JM, et al. Late phase TNF-α depression in natural orifice translumenal endoscopic surgery (NOTES) peritoneoscopy. Surgery. 2008;143(3):318–28.
34. Eickhoff A, Vetter S, von Renteln D, et al. Effectivity of current sterility methods for transgastric NOTES procedures: results of a randomized porcine study. Endoscopy. 2010;42(9):748–52.
35. McGee MF, Marks JM, Onders RP, et al. Infectious implications in the porcine model of natural orifice transluminal endoscopic surgery (NOTES) with PEG-tube closure: a quantitative bacteriologic study. Gastrointest Endosc. 2008;68(2):310–8.
36. Giday SA, Dray X, Magno P, et al. Infection during natural orifice transluminal endoscopic surgery: a randomized, controlled study in a live porcine model. Gastrointest Endosc. 2010;71(4):812–6.
37. Narula VK, Hazey JW, Renton DB, Reavis KM, Paul CM. Transgastric instrumentation and bacterial contamination of the peritoneal cavity. Surg Endosc. 2008;22(3):605–11.
38. Memark VC, Anderson JB, Nau PN, Shah N, Needleman BJ. Transgastric endoscopic peritoneoscopy does not lead to increased risk of infectious complications. Surg Endosc. 2011;25(7):2186–91.
39. Wang ZK, Yang YS, Zhang XL, Sun G, Hyder Q, et al. Comparison in efficacy between pure NOTES peritoneoscopy with small or large endoscope and laparoscopy. J Dig Dis. 2014;15(11):628–35.
40. Nau P, Ellison EC, Muscarella P Jr, Mikami D, Narula VK, et al. A review of 130 humans enrolled in transgastric NOTES protocols at a single institution. Surg Endosc. 2011;25(4):1004–11.

NOTES Hernia Repair

15

David B. Earle, John R. Romanelli and Erica D. Kane

Abstract

Hernias are one of the most commonly treated general surgical problems, with over 20 million procedures per year. Despite the frequency of occurrence, modern techniques remain troubled by long-term recurrence and chronic pain syndromes postoperatively. Innovative techniques such as employing a natural orifice approach to the abdomen have the potential to reduce some of the concerns about current hernia operations. While there are scattered case reports about human NOTES hernia repairs, there has been an abundance of animal work demonstrating safety and feasibility. Work remains before widespread adoption of such a technique could take place.

Keywords

Natural orifice translumenal endoscopic surgery · Hernia · Hernia repair

Abbreviations

IPOM	Intraperitoneal onlay mesh
NOTES	Natural orifice translumenal endoscopic surgery
PEG	Percutaneous endoscopic gastrostomy
SILS	Single-incision laparoscopic surgery

D.B. Earle
Lowell Surgical Associates, Lowell General Hospital, 20 Research Place, Suite 130, North Chelmsford, MA 01863, USA
e-mail: davidearle59@gmail.com

E.D. Kane
Department of Surgery, Baystate Medical Center, 759 Chestnut Street, S3656, Springfield, MA 01199, USA
e-mail: erica.kanemd@baystatehealth.org

J.R. Romanelli (✉)
University of Massachusetts Medical School - Baystate, Worcester, MA, USA
e-mail: john.romanelli@baystatehealth.org

J.R. Romanelli et al. (eds.), *NOTES and Endoluminal Surgery*, Clinical Gastroenterology, DOI 10.1007/978-3-319-50610-4_15

Introduction

Hernia disease represents a heterogeneous group of defects at any location throughout the abdominal wall. This common malady is responsible for the largest number of operations—over 20 million per year—for a single disease performed by general surgeons worldwide [1]. According to the Centers for Disease Control, the prevalence of incisional, umbilical, and other hernias is approximately five million for Americans alone [2]. While operations for hernia repair are safe overall, there is still substantial room for improvement in preventing recurrence and avoiding chronic pain [3–5]. Taking inguinal hernia alone, laparoscopic repair is only used for approximately 27% use of all inguinal hernia repairs in the USA [5, 6] despite multiple studies [7–13] showing superiority of the laparoscopic approach in terms of length of hospital stay, chronic pain, and equivalence or even decrease in recurrence. This is likely due to operators' limited laparoscopic skill and unfamiliarity with the laparoscopic groin anatomy. Robotic-assisted surgical devices are now becoming more popular for hernia repair but currently do not have the capability of overcoming the obstacle of the unfamiliar anatomic perspective inherent in the laparoscopic approach.

We believe that a transgastric approach to hernia repair may have the potential to offer a solution that reduces morbidity and recurrence, particularly for inguinal hernia repair. As inguinal hernias occur primarily in men, this approach is applicable to a larger group of patients as compared to a transvaginal approach. In addition, entering the abdomen through the stomach will allow for forward access to the groin and/or abdominal wall. In the future, this may simplify the repair in most patients, along with the development of new prosthetic materials and delivery methods.

Current Status

Multiple animal studies have been published documenting the feasibility of hernia repair via a natural orifice approach. The first report was published by Hu et al. [14] from the Apollo group in 2007. They performed a ventral hernia repair on two 50-kg pigs through a transgastric approach. A needle knife was used to make an incision in the abdominal wall. A prototype endoscopic suturing device, which was then dubbed the "Eagle Claw" but went on to be marketed as the OverStitch™ (Apollo EndoSurgery, Austin, TX), was used to fix the mesh to the abdominal wall.

A second report, which emerged later in 2007, utilized a transcolonic approach in a pig model [15]. In this novel publication, small pieces of mesh with pre-placed endoscopic clips were translocated endoscopically to the anterior abdominal wall, and magnets were employed to help position the mesh. Percutaneous transfascial T-tags were then used to fix the mesh to the abdominal wall.

Miedema et al. described a study with five pigs in which biologic mesh was delivered to the abdomen by a transgastric approach [16]. The mesh was fixed to the anterior abdominal wall with pre-placed sutures being externalized using a suture grasper with endoscopic guidance. This technique closely follows a standard method utilized in laparoscopic ventral hernia repair. Important to note was that abscesses were present at the mesh site in 3 of 5 animals at necropsy. A subsequent survival study by the same group with six pigs resulted in one perioperative death and one premature sacrifice due to extensive infection [17]. Nevertheless, the 4 pigs that survived 4 weeks showed complete coverage of the hernia defect. All pigs had abscesses or a positive mesh culture.

Sherwinter et al. also positioned mesh transgastrically for an inguinal hernia in a canine model [18]. In this experiment, the mesh was placed using a procedure which mimicked the intraperitoneal onlay mesh (IPOM) technique advocated by some surgeons in laparoscopic inguinal hernia repair. The mesh was fixed to the groin space using biologic glue. This intriguing proof-of-concept study demonstrated that mesh could be deployed to the groin region via the stomach and that a NOTES approach to inguinal hernia might be feasible. A follow-up survival study with 5 mongrel dogs revealed successful coverage of the myopectineal orifice in all animals, and no evidence of gross or microscopic infection [19].

Lomanto et al. [20] published a series of 5 pigs that underwent transvaginal placement of mesh, which was fixed in a manner similar to that described by Miedema [16]. In this two-week survival study, all animals were found to have successful mesh placement, but one did have a subcutaneous abscess. Kantsevoy et al. also performed transgastric ventral hernia repair in 5 pigs using polytetrafluoroethylene mesh [21]. The first pig had a mesh infection found at necropsy, but following experiments utilized a sterile mesh cover, and no further infections were found in the remaining 4 animals.

Our group published a series of five non-survival pigs using a similar technique, with a modified esophageal stent introducer to deliver the mesh in a sterile fashion [22]. We fixed polypropylene to the abdominal wall using pre-placed sutures and a proprietary endoscopic tack (Cook Medical, Winston-Salem, NC). Further details on this technique appear later in this chapter. A subsequent survival study in ten pigs revealed an abscess in the first pig, a microscopic infection in the second with no gross infections, and no other gross or microscopic infections in the remaining six animals that survived the experiment [23]. One pig died from peritonitis due to failed gastric closure, and one other died from an unknown cause, presumed to be a stress reaction or adverse reaction to anesthesia, with no obvious findings at necropsy.

To date, human cases of hernia repair have been limited to a transvaginal approach for small ventral hernias [24–29]. The first report emerged from Jacobsen et al. in 2010 and detailed a transvaginal repair of a recurrent umbilical hernia with the aid of one laparoscopic trocar [24]. The first known incisional hernia repair via a transvaginal approach was published by Wood et al. in 2013 for a trocar site hernia following a laparoscopic cholecystectomy [25]. They described an innovative technique using a single-incision laparoscopic surgery (SILS™) port (Medtronic, Minneapolis, MN) to pass 5- and 12-mm laparoscopic instruments. The mesh was placed in a specimen retrieval bag prior to entry into the vagina and thus was not contaminated. A second report from the same group described their first 6 cases. Notably, the first case involved a rectal injury which was recognized and repaired [26]. Two patients also reported transient urinary retention.

A publication from Spain reported a case of a recurrent epigastric hernia repaired with mesh via a transvaginal approach, with 2 laparoscopic trocars for assistance [27]. A report from Turkey [28] described two cases of hybrid transvaginal incisional hernias, where synthetic mesh was passed through the vagina without protection, and no infections were reported. A group from Switzerland recently published their experience with 6 cases of hybrid transvaginal epigastric and/or umbilical hernia repairs [29]. These were performed with two side-by-side transvaginal trocars (5 and 12 mm) and one laparoscopic trocar. Although no infections were reported, one early recurrence was detected in an obese patient.

Early studies using a NOTES approach to ventral or inguinal hernia repair have had mixed results regarding infection. Certainly, infections seem to be an almost omnipresent problem in the porcine model [16, 17, 20, 21, 23], although that may speak to the model and not necessarily to the technique. In human data infections do not seem as ubiquitous a problem, although one would note that all of the cases described were transvaginal and not transgastric. One recent study not only demonstrated that a prepped vaginal conduit was sterile and safe for mesh passage into the abdomen, but that the prepped vaginal mucosa was more sterile than prepped skin [30].

History

Our group has successfully developed a technique for mesh introduction and placement via the transgastric approach in a survival swine model [23]. While this model placed the mesh on the ventral abdominal wall, we believe this approach could be used for inguinal hernia repair as well. We developed a mesh delivery device by modifying an esophageal stent introducer (Dua Esophageal Antireflux Stent introducer, Cook Endoscopy, Winston-Salem, NC). Once a working prototype had been successfully used in a non-survival swine model [22], we performed an experiment with swine stomach explants in order to determine whether the device would reduce contamination [31]. We coated the lumen of the stomach with 60 cc of an ultraviolet light-sensitive cream commonly used for teaching hand-washing technique (GlitterBug, Brevis Corporation, Salt Lake City, UT). The control group had the mesh placed through the stomach without the device and had an average of 57% of the surface contaminated with the cream. The group using the delivery device had an average surface area of 0.01% contaminated with the cream. With the knowledge that the device could dramatically reduce contamination, we designed and experiment to determine whether this reduction in contamination would result in a decreased incidence of clinical infection. We performed ten consecutive transgastric hernia mesh placements in swine that were survived for two weeks [23]. In each case, a 10 cm × 15 cm plain polypropylene mesh was placed as an intraperitoneal onlay utilizing four transfascial fixation sutures and four endoscopically delivered nitinol tacks. The first animal developed subclinical abscesses at the suture anchor sites. We modified the technique to flush povidone-iodine solution into the working channels of the double-channel therapeutic gastroscope after which no gross abscesses developed in the remaining animals. The second pig had a positive culture swab at necropsy, but the remaining mesh implants were sterile.

Technique

In our swine model, we prepared the animals by fasting them overnight and administering prophylactic, preoperative, and intravenous antibiotics. The mouth and oropharynx were sprayed with povidone-iodine solution, and a double-channel therapeutic gastroscope (GIF-2T100, Olympus America, Center Valley, PA) was used to inspect the stomach. Each time the scope traversed the oropharynx, we irrigated the working channels with povidone-iodine by flushing this solution through the channels into the lumen of the stomach.

Gastrotomy was performed by a modification of percutaneous endoscopic gastrostomy (PEG) placement [32]. A double-channel gastroscope (Olympus America) was inserted transorally into the stomach, and both channels were flushed with Betadine solution. After sterile prep of the abdomen, also with Betadine, an 18-Ga spinal needle was inserted percutaneously into the stomach under endoscopic vision. A 0.035-in, Teflon-coated guidewire (Tracer Metro; Cook Medical, Winston-Salem, NC) was inserted into the stomach through the needle and brought out through the right scope channel with a snare (Fig. 15.1). An additional area on the abdominal wall was sterilely prepped, and a Veress needle was then inserted into the abdomen. Capnoperitoneum was then initiated with carbon dioxide (CO_2) to a pressure of 10 mm Hg. Once capnoperitoneum was achieved and space was created in the abdominal cavity, and with the tip of the endoscope against the gastric mucosa, extra wire was fed into the peritoneal cavity by pushing firmly at the skin entry site while fixing the wire in place at the biopsy channel cap. This serves to "knuckle" the guidewire into the space created by

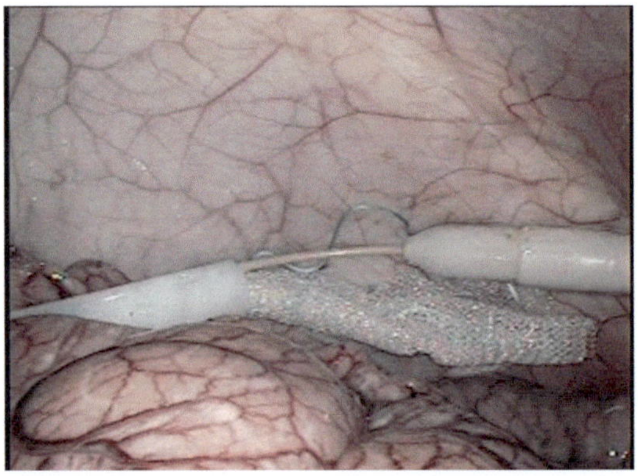

Fig. 15.1 Mesh deployed into the abdominal cavity (the photograph shows an earlier prototype of the mesh delivery system)

capnoperitoneum. An 18-mm, wire-guided, balloon dilation catheter was then pushed through the gastric wall along the guidewire and then inflated (Fig. 15.2). Once inflated, the balloon was pulled firmly against the tip of the scope, which was then advanced into the peritoneal cavity. The balloon was removed, and the peritoneal cavity was inspected for injury from the Veress needle placement and for the location of the mesh placement.

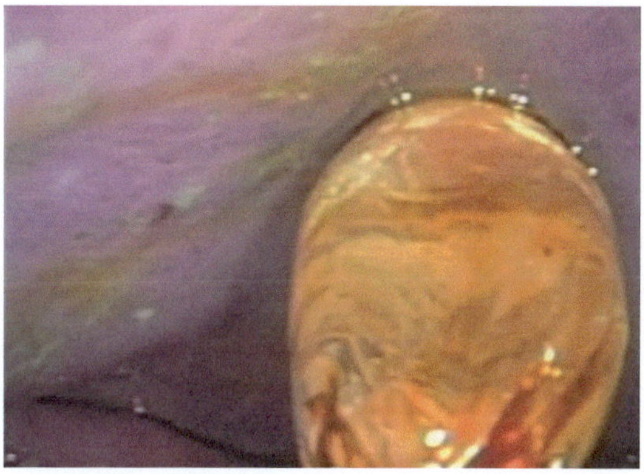

Fig. 15.2 A 20-mm balloon was placed across the gastrotomy to dilate the opening large enough to pass an endoscope

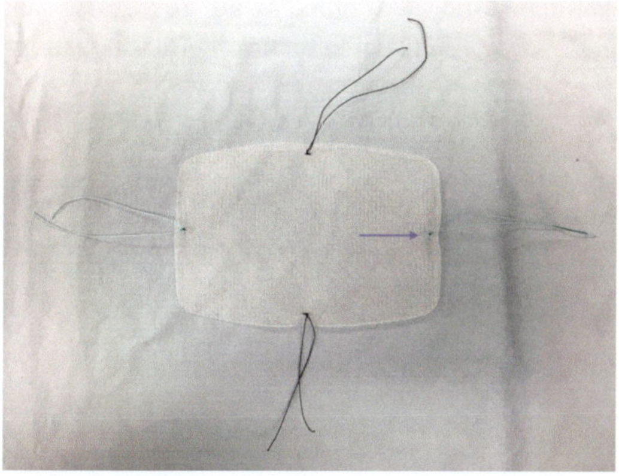

Fig. 15.3 The mesh with four pre-placed sutures

At this point, a new wire was inserted into the abdomen with the 18-Ga needle, low down in the pelvis, under direct endoscopic vision. The wire was grasped with a snare and pulled out through the mouth, scope, and all. This allowed for a "monorail" guidewire, which served the dual purpose of guiding the mesh delivery device into the abdomen when inserted transorally, and also to act as a guide to help locate the gastrotomy in the collapsed stomach (the stomach collapses because of the gastrotomy and the capnoperitoneum).

The mesh was fashioned with 4 full-thickness anchoring sutures (Fig. 15.3) and was placed into the delivery system, which was essentially a modified esophageal stent deployment device (Fig. 15.4). The device was then placed over the guidewire and inserted into the peritoneal cavity by pulling traction on both the oral and percutaneous/pelvic ends of the wire, which serves to make it taught (the "monorail" effect) and which easily allows the device to pass through the gastrotomy into the abdomen. The mesh is then deployed by extruding it from the introducer in a fashion analogous to the deployment of an esophageal stent (Fig. 15.1). The double-channel scope was then reinserted into the peritoneal cavity (after flushing the channels with povidone-iodine solution) to ensure proper mesh deployment. The presence of the

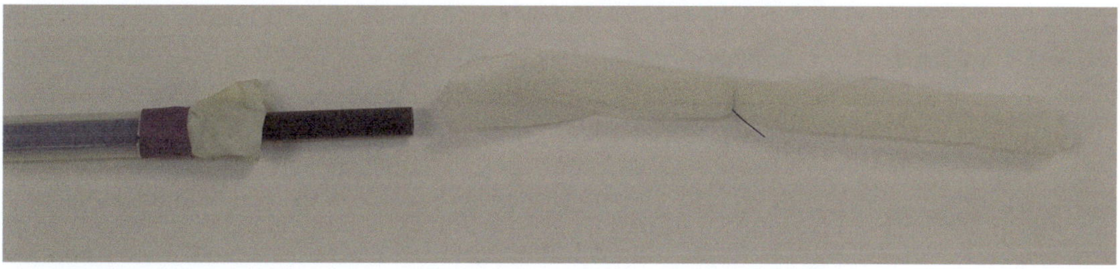

Fig. 15.4 The modified esophageal stent introducer (photograph courtesy of Cook Medical), used to pass mesh into the abdominal cavity in a sterile fashion

indwelling wire allowed for rapid identification of the gastrotomy.

The sutures were identified by color and removed through corresponding stab incisions on the abdominal wall using a looped spinal needle technique [33]. Any needle-sized suture grasper could be used for this part of the procedure. We pre-placed the sutures at the twelve, three, six, and nine o'clock positions around the "defect." (Of note, we did not create a defect as the aim of the experiment was to place mesh successfully on the abdominal wall without infection). Once the sutures were tied down to the fascia, nitinol tacks (Cook Medical; Fig. 15.5) were endoscopically placed at the four corners of the mesh (Fig. 15.6). These tacks have a double-sided, treble-hook configuration and are placed across the abdominal wall using a 19-gauge delivery needle.

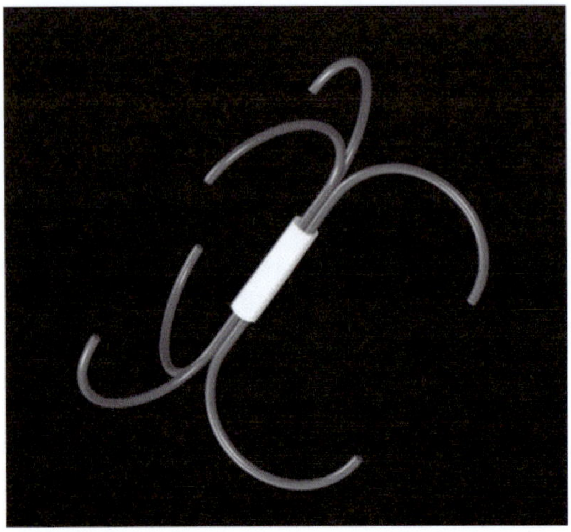

Fig. 15.5 Endoscopic tacks (photograph courtesy of Cook Medical)

Once the mesh placement was complete, the endoscope was removed, and the gastrotomy was closed. We typically used an endoscopically deployed clip, such as the Padlock-G™ (Aponos Medical, Kingston, NH), but any method of gastrotomy closure can be employed. It is beyond the scope of this chapter to discuss details of gastric closure.

We performed a necropsy at 2 weeks and examined the abdominal wall for gross and microscopic signs of infection; Fig. 15.7 shows an example of abscesses at the tack sites.

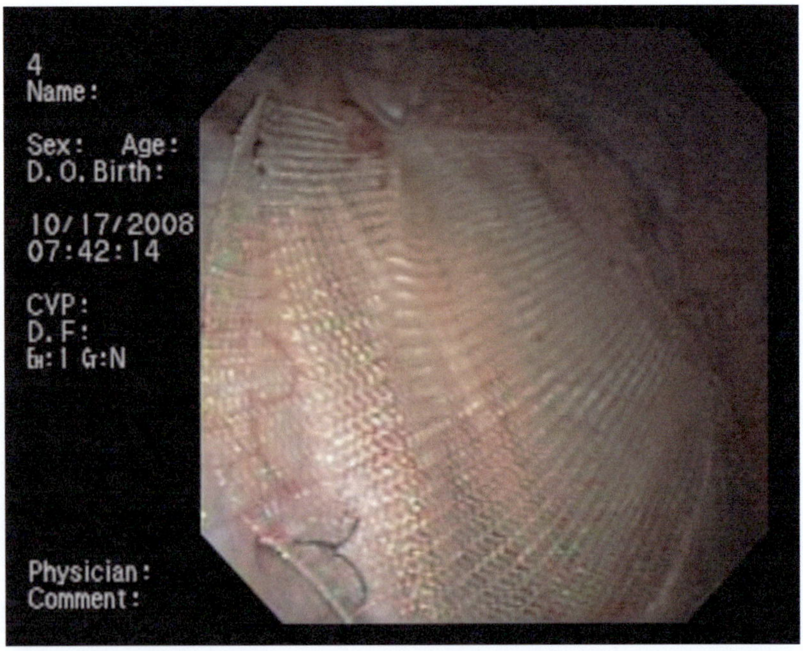

Fig. 15.6 The mesh located on the abdominal wall after sutures are tied and tacks are deployed

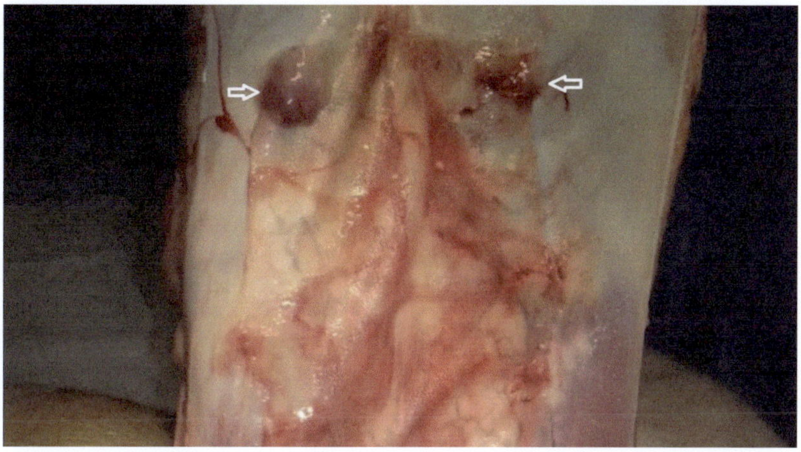

Fig. 15.7 The mesh at necropsy. White arrows indicate abscesses

The Future

In the future, we hope to develop a technique for transgastric endoscopic groin dissection in the cadaver model for inguinal hernia repair and also help to develop new prosthetics and fixation techniques. We believe this will culminate in an inguinal hernia repair that will be less invasive and potentially with fewer recurrences than our contemporary open and laparoscopic approaches. Further, we are optimistic that smaller ventral and incisional hernias will be able to be repaired in a sterile fashion via transgastric or transvaginal approaches, which will likely lead to faster recovery and less postoperative pain for our patients.

References

1. Kingsnorth AN, LeBlanc KA. Hernias: inguinal and incisional. The Lancet. 2003;362:1561–71.
2. Park AE, Roth JS, Kavic SM. Abdominal wall hernia. Curr Probl Surg. 2006;43:326–75.
3. Eklund AS, Montgomery AK, Rasmussen IC, Sandbue RP, Bergkvist LA, Rudberg CR. Low recurrence rate after laparoscopic (TEP) and open (Lichtenstein) inguinal hernia repair: a randomized, multicenter trial with 5-year follow-up. Ann Surg. 2009;249:33–8.
4. Flum DR, Horvath K, Koepsell T. Have outcomes of incisional hernia repair improved with time? A population-based analysis. Ann Surg. 2003;237(1):129–35.
5. Alexander MA, Scott DJ. Laparoscopic ventral hernia repair. Surg Clin N Am. 2013;93:1091–110.
6. Colavita PD, Tsirline VB, Belyansky I, Walters AL, Lincourt AE, Sing RF, Heniford BT. Prospective, long-term comparison of quality of life in laparoscopic versus open ventral hernia repair. Ann Surg. 2012;256:714–23.
7. McCormack K, Scott NW, Go PM, Ross S, Grant AM; EU Hernia trialists collaboration. Laparoscopic techniques versus open techniques for inguinal hernia repair. Cochrane Database Syst Rev. 2003;(1): CD001785.
8. O'Reilly EA, Burke JP, O'Connell PR. A Meta-analysis of surgical morbidity and recurrence after laparoscopic and open repair of primary unilateral inguinal hernia. Ann Surg. 2012;255:846–53.
9. Tadaki C, Lomelin D, Simorov A, Jones R, Humphreys M, daSilva M, Choudhury S, Shostrom V, Boilesen E, Kothari V, Oleynikov D, Goede M. Perioperative outcomes and costs of laparoscopic versus open inguinal hernia repair. Hernia. 2016.
10. Pierce RA, Spitler JA, Frisella MM, Matthews BD, Brunt LM. Pooled data analysis of laparoscopic vs. open ventral hernia repair: 14 years of patient data accrual. Surg Endosc. 2007;21(3):378–86.
11. Sajid MS, Bokhari SA, Mallick AS, Cheek E, Baig MK. Laparoscopic versus open repair of incisional/ventral hernia: a meta-analysis. Am J Surg. 2009;197(1):64–72.
12. Sauerland S, Walgenbach M, Habermalz B, Seiler CM, Miserez M. Laparoscopic versus open surgical techniques for ventral or incisional hernia repair. Cochrane Database Syst Rev. 2011;(3): CD007781.
13. Awaiz A, Rahman F, Hossain MB, Yunus RM, Khan S, Memon B, Memon MA. Meta-analysis and systematic review of laparoscopic versus open mesh repair for elective incisional hernia. Hernia. 2015;19(3):449–63.

14. Hu B, Kalloo AN, Chung SS, Cotton PB, Gostout CJ, et al. Peroral transgastric endoscopic primary repair of a ventral hernia in a porcine model. Endoscopy. 2007;39(5):390–3.
15. Fong DG, Ryou M, Pai RD, Tavakkolizadeh A, Rattner DW, et al. Transcolonic ventral wall hernia mesh fixation in a porcine model. Endoscopy. 2007;39(10):865–9.
16. Miedema BW, Bachman SL, Spron E, Astudillo JA, Thaler K. Transgastric placement of biologic mesh to the anterior abdominal wall. Surg Endosc. 2009;23 (6):1212–8.
17. Sporn E, Astudillo JA, Bachman SL, Mayfield TP, Thaler K, et al. Transgastric biologic mesh delivery and abdominal wall hernia repair in a porcine model. Endoscopy. 2009;41(12):1062–8.
18. Sherwinter DA, Eckstein JG. Feasibility study of natural orifice transluminal endoscopic surgery inguinal hernia repair. Gastrointest Endosc. 2009;70 (1):126–30.
19. Sherwinter DA, Gupta A, Eckstein JG. Natural orifice translumenal endoscopic surgery inguinal hernia repair: a survival canine model. J Laparoendosc Adv Surg Tech A. 2011;21(3):209–13.
20. Lomanto D, Dhir U, So JB, Cheah WK, Moe MA, et al. Total transvaginal endoscopic abdominal wall hernia repair: a NOTES survival study. Hernia. 2009;13(4):415–9.
21. Kantsevoy SV, Dray X, Shin EJ, Buscaglia JM, Magno P, et al. Transgastric ventral hernia repair: a controlled study in a live porcine model (with videos). Gastrointest Endosc. 2009;69(1):102–7.
22. Earle DB, Desilets DJ, Romanelli JR. NOTES transgastric abdominal wall hernia repair in a porcine model. Hernia. 2010;14(5):517–22.
23. Mora MC, Kowalski R, Desilets DJ, Romanelli JR, Earle DB. NOTES transgastric ventral hernia repair in a porcine survival model. Hernia [Abstract] 2015; (Suppl2):SI95-S340.
24. Jacobsen GR, Thompson K, Spivack A, Fischer L, Wong B, et al. Initial experience with transvaginal incisional hernia repair. Hernia. 2010;14(1):89–91.
25. Wood SG, Panait L, Bell RL, Duffy AJ, Roberts KE. Pure transvaginal umbilical hernia repair. Surg Endosc. 2013;27(8):2966.
26. Wood SG, Panait L, Duffy AJ, Bell RL, Roberts KE. Pure transvaginal ventral hernia repair in humans. Surg Innov. 2014;21(2):130–6.
27. Bruna M, Noguera J, Martinez I, Oviedo M. Eventroplastia transvaginal hibrida. Cir Esp. 2013;91: 539–41.
28. Kayaalp C, Yagci MA, Soyer V. Hybrid transvaginal incisional hernia repair. J Laparoendosc Adv Surg Tech A. 2014;24(7):497–501.
29. Descloux A, Pohle S, Nocito A, Keerl A. Hybrid NOTES transvaginal intraperitoneal onlay mesh in abdominal wall hernias: an alternative to traditional laparoscopic procedures. Surg Endosc. 2015;29(12):3712–6.
30. Bates AT, Capes T, Krishnan R, LaBombardi V, Pipia G, et al. The prepped vaginal canal may be a sterile conduit for ventral hernia mesh insertion: a prospective comparative study. Surg Endosc. 2014;28(3):886–90.
31. Earle DB, Romanelli JR, McLawhorn T, Omotosho P, Wu P, et al. Prosthetic mesh contamination during NOTES(®) transgastric hernia repair: a randomized controlled trial with swine explants. Hernia. 2012;16(6):689–95.
32. Kantsevoy SV, Jagannath SB, Hideaki N, Isakovich NV, Chung SSC, et al. A novel safe approach to the peritoneal cavity for per-oral transgastric endoscopic procedures. Gastrointest Endosc. 2007;65:497–500.
33. Earle D. A simple and inexpensive technique for closing trocar sites and grasping sutures. J Laparoendosc Adv Surg Tech A. 1999;9(1):81–5.

Flexible Endoscopic Transvaginal Cholecystectomy

16

John R. Romanelli

Abstract

One of the first human NOTES cases reported in the literature was that of transvaginal cholecystectomy. Although early attempts at human NOTES were primarily via the transgastric route, surgeons quickly realized that the transgastric route to the gallbladder was complicated by the need to be in the retroflexed position for the duration of the case. Transvaginal cholecystectomy, on the other hand, presented forward access to the gallbladder, which was technically much simpler to achieve and potentially safer for the patients. While both rigid and flexible endoscopic approaches to the gallbladder are well described, this chapter focuses on flexible endoscopic surgical technique. Transvaginal surgery also had the advantage of facile access to the abdomen without the need for visceral closure. There are multiple published case reports and small series describing good results with flexible endoscopic transvaginal surgery. The author's own series is also detailed. A recent, multicenter, randomized trial comparing transvaginal cholecystectomy with laparoscopic cholecystectomy successfully showed that the transvaginal approach was non-inferior. Although the results show that this approach to gallbladder surgery is safe and effective, issues of time, instrument availability, and cost continue to hinder its widespread adoption.

Keywords

NOTES · Transvaginal · Cholecystectomy · Flexible endoscopy

J.R. Romanelli (✉)
Department of Surgery, Tufts University School of Medicine, Baystate Medical Center, 759 Chestnut Street, S3656, Springfield, MA 01199, USA
e-mail: john.romanelli@baystatehealth.org

J.R. Romanelli et al. (eds.), *NOTES and Endoluminal Surgery*,
Clinical Gastroenterology, DOI 10.1007/978-3-319-50610-4_16

Introduction

One of the first human NOTES cases reported was that of transvaginal cholecystectomy. Within a short time, reports emerged from France [1], Germany [2], the USA [3], and Brazil [4], all describing this new technique. After the video introduction of the NOTES concept in human clinical applications [5] at both the 2005 Society of American Gastrointestinal and Endoscopic Surgeons Annual Meeting and Digestive Disease Week, surgeons around the world raced to their animal laboratories to develop techniques that could be applied clinically with the possibility of few or even no abdominal scars whatsoever. Cholecystectomy was a natural target, not only as a widely performed procedure with relatively minor morbidity, but because peritoneal access to the gallbladder via an endoscopic approach was deemed to be reasonable, and the technical difficulty of an elective cholecystectomy was lower.

Given the initial introduction to NOTES as a transgastric procedure [5], early laboratory work began investigating the transgastric route to cholecystectomy [6–11]. Human case reports appeared soon thereafter [12–14]. While technically feasible, investigators quickly realized that in order to reach the gallbladder to perform transgastric cholecystectomy, the flexible endoscope would have to be retroflexed once located in the abdominal cavity. Thus, the endoscope would have to be locked in this endoscopically unfavorable position. Passage of endoscopic instrumentation became impaired, the view was often disorienting to surgeons, and the overall technical difficulty of the procedure led others to reconsider the approach altogether. Further, the lack of development of a multitasking platform, as suggested in the SAGES/ASGE white paper on NOTES [15], led surgeons away from this technique entirely.

Transvaginal access to the abdomen is not an entirely new approach, even in the hands of general surgeons. A sadly overlooked paper may have foreshowed transvaginal gallbladder surgery: In 1993, Delvaux et al. [16] described transvaginal extraction of gallbladders with large gallstones via a colpotomy. In this paper, the authors cite the need to avoid enlarging the umbilical incision in proposing this technique. Later, another publication [17] discussed extraction of a laparoscopically removed spleen via a posterior colpotomy. In addition, gynecologists had been using the transvaginal route for ovarian and uterine surgery for many years.

An advantage of transvaginal surgery is the forward access to the gallbladder. This allows approaching the target anatomy with the endoscope in the forward position and eliminates much of the difficulty created by trying to perform a procedure in the retroflexed position. It also allows a view that is similar to the laparoscopic view, allowing visual landmarks to remain in similar orientation. Of course with increasing attention on patient safety, specifically in biliary surgery, endoscopic techniques that begin to approach the familiarity of the laparoscopic view make the procedure much more tenable.

There are two different approaches to transvaginal cholecystectomy. While this chapter focuses on using the flexible endoscope as the primary operative platform, there is a separate chapter in this textbook that describes transvaginal cholecystectomy utilizing rigid (laparoscopic) instrumentation and optics. The decision on whether or not to use flexible endoscopic instrumentation is entirely up to the comfort level of the surgeon and/or operating team. In our experience, we employed both a gynecologist to help with the colpotomy (for both safety and credentialing reasons) and a team comprising a gastroenterologist with advanced therapeutic endoscopic skills and a general surgeon with advanced laparoscopic skills. We recognize fully that this luxury of resources is not available at many centers, nor is it realistic if a high volume of cholecystectomies is to be performed.

An interesting factor to consider when deciding to adopt a flexible or rigid platform is the anatomy of the sacrum. A novel study from Japan [18] examined the distance from the vagina, the transverse deviation from the midline, and the sagittal deviation from the "vagina–promontory (V-P)" line. In this study, the authors found that the intra-abdominal length of transvaginal instruments should be at least 35 cm (in Japanese patients); further, they felt that while the gallbladder was generally accessible with rigid instruments, the gastroesophageal junction and spleen were typically not. This speaks to the need to consider a flexible endoscopic approach.

Anatomic Considerations

We have limited transvaginal cholecystectomy to patients with a body mass index ≤35 kg/m^2. Given the propensity for obesity to be a factor in the development of gallstones, a large number of patients are eliminated from consideration due to this limitation. We have found that the increase in visceral fat that comes in morbidly obese patients causes the flexible endoscope to arch high above the viscera after clearing the sacral promontory, thus making it difficult to advance forward toward the gallbladder. In thinner patients with minimal visceral fat, reaching the gallbladder is technically easier. Although we do not have specific experience with rigid instrumentation, one may posit that a rigid endoscopic approach may be preferable in the morbidly obese patient, if a transvaginal approach is considered at all.

We also have not attempted to offer transvaginal surgery to patient with prior pelvic surgery. We have always employed a "hybrid" approach—with at least one laparoscopic trocar at the umbilicus, typically utilizing laparoscopic visualization of the endoscope entering the abdomen. The risk of adhesions and the potential for injuries created by trying to pass a transvaginal endoscope in a patient with prior pelvic surgery have been a limitation in considering transvaginal cholecystectomy. Obviously, pregnant women are also excluded from consideration.

Consent Process

All patients were consented to laparoscopic cholecystectomy with a detailed discussion of the risks, benefits, ramifications, and complications of having the procedure. For the transvaginal approach, all patients agreed to a further discussion of the risks. Although many of the discussed risks were theoretical, and the true incidence of said complications was unknown, included in that discussion was the risks of dyspareunia postoperatively, issues with fertility in the future (when applicable), and risks of injury to the bladder, rectum, uterus, ovaries, or small intestine. It was explained to all patients that abstinence from sexual intercourse was preferred for 30 days postoperatively. All patients must have been under regular gynecologic care and had a pelvic examination in the past year. Those that did not were required to have one by the operating surgeon preoperatively.

Description of Technique

The patient is placed on the operative table in the lithotomy position. After the vagina is prepped using a povidone–iodine solution, a bladder catheter is placed in a sterile fashion. A tenaculum is placed on the cervix, which is elevated anteriorly. Two sutures, typically #0-Vicryl, are placed, one anteriorly in the uterosacral ligaments and the other posteriorly in the posterior fornix. A horizontal colpotomy incision is made between the sutures (which can later be tied together to close the colpotomy). At this point, a 15-mm trocar can be placed directly into the abdominal cavity, or the incision is extended sharply until the peritoneum is entered.

In the meantime, after sterile preparation of the abdominal wall typical for a laparoscopic cholecystectomy, a Veress needle is inserted at the umbilicus. The abdomen is filled with pneumoperitoneum to a pressure of 15 mm Hg. This was typically done by a separate operating team (as previously explained, we employed the help of a gynecologic surgeon with significant transvaginal surgical experience) concurrently with the creation of the colpotomy. In cases where we did not insert a laparoscopic trocar transvaginally, the efflux of gas instituted by the Veress needle confirms entrance into the peritoneal cavity. In most cases, the Veress needle site was converted to a 5-mm laparoscopic trocar. In all cases, a laparoscopic camera was inserted into the abdomen prior to the placement of the transvaginal trocar and/or passage of the endoscope (2T-160 double-channel gastroscope, Olympus America, Center Valley, PA) into the abdominal cavity. Once the endoscope safely entered the abdomen, laparoscopic visualization was discontinued.

Forward access to the gallbladder sounds simple but in fact often is not given the flexibility of the endoscope and the angle of the sacral promontory. Further, the scope has to be positioned to be driven up the right paracolic gutter, to arrive at the right upper quadrant with minimal looping of the scope—which would create paradoxical movement and would further hinder the ability to perform the case. Even with the aid of these maneuvers, reaching the gallbladder can be difficult. We often will reach out with a grasper and will grasp the surface of the gallbladder and will "pull ourselves" up to the gallbladder. One of the two working channels of the endoscope will often be used to hold on to the gallbladder, to keep the endoscope in position to perform the cholecystectomy.

Next, a technique is needed to retract the gallbladder. Much like in single-site surgical approaches to cholecystectomy, creative retraction methods must be employed to lift the liver and elevate the gallbladder to face the endoscope. Our early attempts at transvaginal cholecystectomy involved using a suture placed through the gallbladder wall, with each end of the suture brought out through two separate locations on the abdominal wall (Fig. 16.1). This allowed us to swing the gallbladder back and forth, similar to a pulley, exposing both the medial and lateral surfaces. Later procedures utilized a device called the EndoGrab™ (Virtual Ports, Ltd., Caesarea, Israel) (Fig. 16.2a, b), which is an internal retractor that can be deployed onto the fundus of the gallbladder. The other end of the retractor is then attached to the peritoneum under the rib cage and over the dome of the liver, which elevates the liver and exposes the gallbladder (Fig. 16.3). More recent cases have used another device called the NovaTract™ dynamic retractor

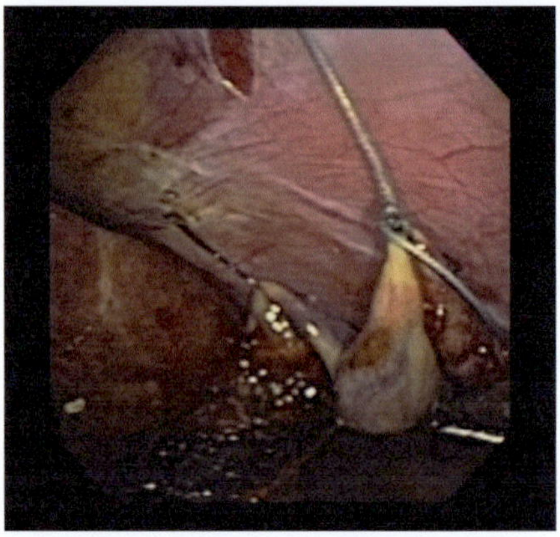

Fig. 16.1 Suture retraction of the gallbladder. Note the use of silk suture (*black*) on the fundus and Ethibond (*green*) on the infundibulum

(NovaTract Surgical, Inc., Madison, CT). The NovaTract™ truly is dynamic as a retractor as it places an anchor into the peritoneum, similar to as described with the EndoGrab™, but it also employs a suture, which can then be manipulated to move the gallbladder to facilitate dissection (Fig. 16.4a, b).

In our early work, once the gallbladder is retracted, we employed a Zimmon® needle knife cautery (Cook Medical, Winston-Salem, NC), with the flexible tip cutoff. Using a hemostat, we gently fashion a hook electrocautery. Important to realize is that the hook cannot be too long, or the knife cannot be passed down the working channel of the endoscope. Also, once the hook is passed down the endoscope, it should not be withdrawn, as it can damage the endoscope with repeated passes. Now that they have become widely available, another option would be to utilize the prefashioned Olympus Hook Knife™ (Olympus America).

Dissection of the hepatocystic triangle is facilitated with laparoscopic instrumentation. We have employed laparoscopic clip appliers on the cystic artery and duct for safety. Although it has been reported that endoscopic clips can be successfully applied on the duct and artery with a slight modification [19], this is not FDA-approved in the USA and may require detailed discussion with the patient in the informed consent process. Further, it has been reported [20]

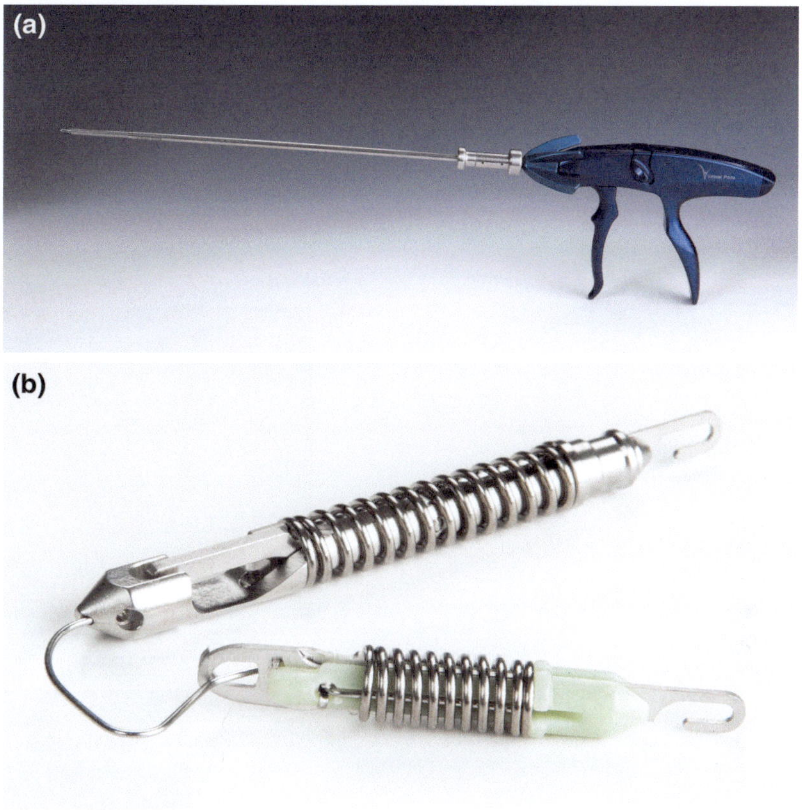

Fig. 16.2 EndoGrab™ laparoscopic applier (**a**) and internal retractor (**b**). Photographs courtesy of Virtual Ports, Ltd.

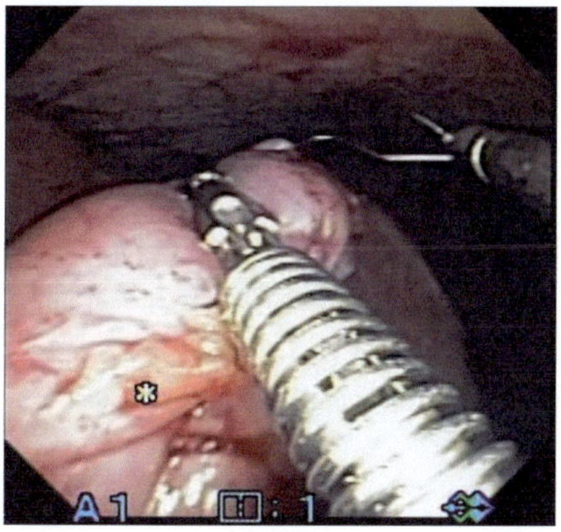

Fig. 16.3 EndoGrab™ attached to the fundus of the gallbladder and being attached to the peritoneum over the liver to retract in a cephalad direction

that endoscopic clips tend to fall off of the cystic duct (in a porcine model), and so we have relied upon laparoscopic instrumentation for this most important task.

The "critical view of safety" is achieved in all cases, although it is important to note that rotational, torque-like maneuvers are often necessary to have the instrumentation reach the target anatomy. This can distort the view such that recognized anatomic landmarks become located in alternate positions (Fig. 16.5), which can disorient the surgeon and lead to injury. It is incumbent on the operating surgeon or surgical team to be knowledgeable about the location of the common bile duct and common hepatic duct at all times when in a "rotated" position. Once the critical view is confirmed, clipping and division of the cystic artery and duct can take place, as it would in a laparoscopic approach. The gallbladder is then divided off of the liver bed using the modified hook electrocautery (Fig. 16.6). Once the gallbladder is free of the liver, the internal retractors (suture, EndoGrab™, or NovaTract™) are released. The gallbladder is then placed above the surface of the right lobe of the liver, and

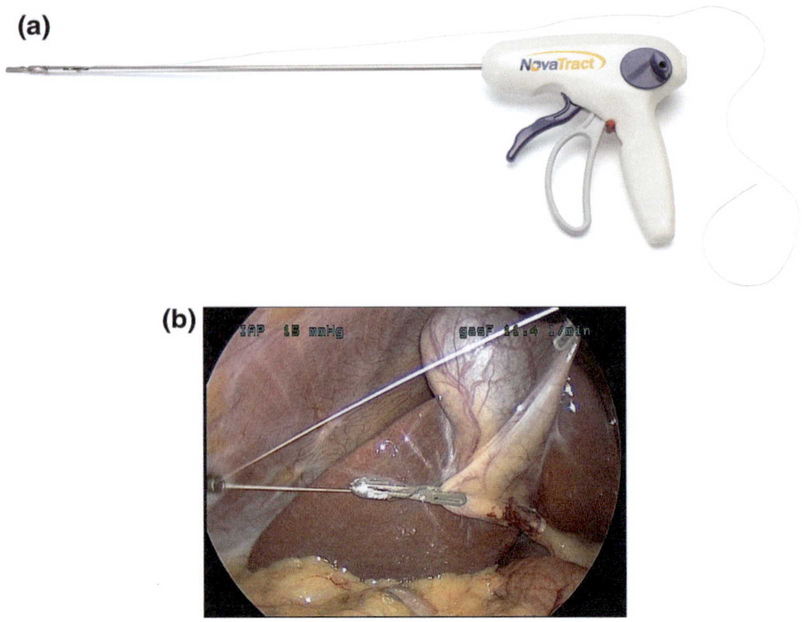

Fig. 16.4 NovaTract™ retractor (**a**) and as seen inside the abdomen attached to gallbladder and abdominal wall (**b**). Photographs courtesy of NovaTract, Inc.

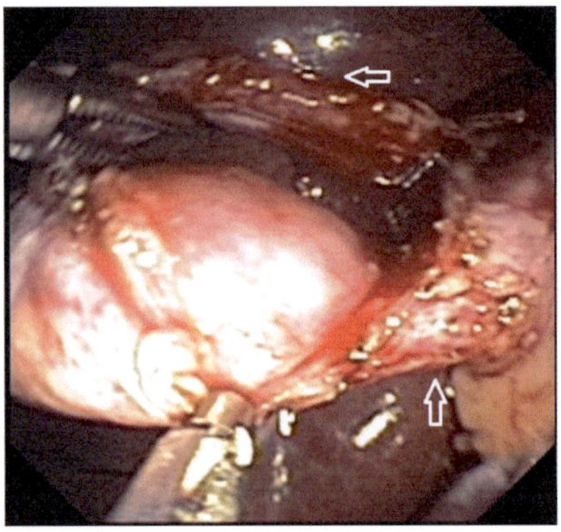

Fig. 16.5 Note the gallbladder anatomy is seen in a rotated view from the endoscope; the *vertical arrow* delineates the cystic duct; the *horizontal arrow* delineates the cystic artery. An endoscopic grasper is seen in the foreground; a laparoscopic grasper is separating the cystic artery from the gallbladder with liver seen in between the structures

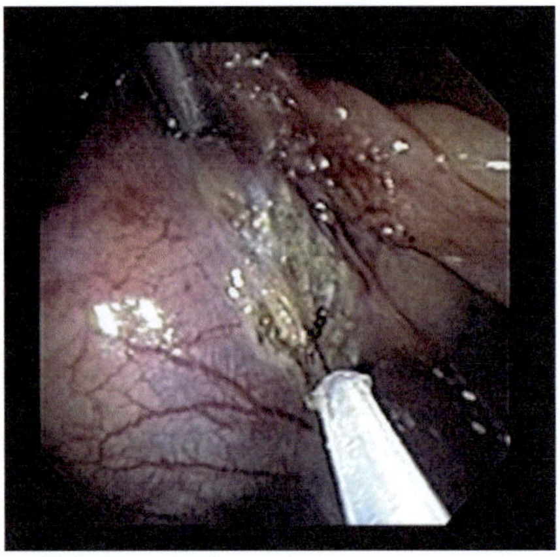

Fig. 16.6 The modified hook electrocautery is an endoscopic instrument used to divide the gallbladder off of the liver bed

irrigation of the liver bed is done through the endoscope. Once this is complete, an endoscopic snare is placed around the gallbladder, which is then brought back to the tip of the endoscope. The specimen is then removed from the patient by removing the endoscope. If gallstones are spilled from the gallbladder during dissection, they can be removed with standard endoscopic stone retrieval tools (Fig. 16.7). The colpotomy is closed by tying the preplaced sutures together.

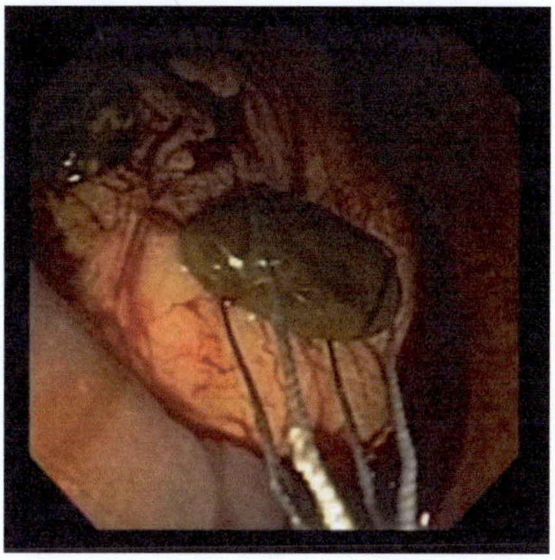

Fig. 16.7 Retrieval of gallstones spilled during dissection with endoscopic stone retrieval basket

Results

Our group performed transvaginal hybrid cholecystectomies using a flexible endoscope in twenty women between 2009 and 2014. Only patients with symptomatic cholelithiasis or biliary dyskinesia were included; patients with acute cholecystitis, gallstone pancreatitis, or suspicion of malignancy were excluded. Women who previously underwent hysterectomy or pelvic surgery or open abdominal surgery were excluded. None of the patients suffered from a major complication. All patients successfully underwent the endoscopic procedure, and all were able to have their gallbladders removed transvaginally (in other words, none were "converted" to laparoscopy). There were no major complications, but there were three minor complications: One woman had an intrauterine device that had been in place at the time of the procedure, which was inadvertently dislodged. A second woman had a metal piece of the EndoGrab™ fracture and fall into the pelvis, which was not found at laparoscopy (even though it was seen on radiograph). It was left in place but never caused symptoms. A third patient had gallstones spill into the abdominal cavity upon retrieval, and we were able to remove these using an endoscopic Roth Net® retrieval device (US Endoscopy, Mentor, OH).

All of the women had at least one laparoscopic trocar utilized, and three patients required a second trocar. Gallbladder retraction methods varied between simple suture retraction, EndoGrab™, and NovaTract™. Mean age of the group was 41 (range 20–66). The median operative time was 163 min (range 110–269). Transvaginal access was generally by direct dissection into the peritoneal cavity, although a 15-mm trocar was placed in five cases. While the trocar does aid in entering the peritoneum, its presence does create a "drag"-like effect, or friction, on the endoscope, which sometimes can be problematic during the procedure.

Thirteen of the patients listed above participated in a randomized clinical trial comparing NOTES transvaginal cholecystectomy with laparoscopic cholecystectomy, which was sponsored by NOSCAR [21]. In this trial, known as the "NOVEL" trial (Natural Orifice VErsus Laparoscopy), transvaginal cholecystectomy was found to be non-inferior to standard laparoscopic approaches in both pain and major complications. There was an unsurprising statistically significant difference in operative time, but no major biliary complications in the study. This study demonstrates both the safety and efficacy of the transvaginal approach.

Of note, during the period of time when the procedure was being offered, five women had consented to the procedure, three of whom were in the NOSCAR trial. One of the three women in the trial went on to develop acute cholecystitis and had to be taken out of the trial and operated on emergently. Two others decided against surgery altogether. One of them later went on to have a cholecystectomy two years later for acute cholecystitis, and the third patient did not return for follow-up. Two more recent patients who consented after the completion of the NOSCAR trial also changed their minds and opted against surgery.

There are several small published series of flexible endoscope transvaginal cholecystectomy in the literature, although the predilection does appear to be toward the use of rigid endoscopic and laparoscopic instrumentation. Palanivelu et al. [22] reported on their initial series of 10 transvaginal cholecystectomies, and although their mean operating time was similar to other studies (148 min), their complication rate was significant, with six of ten cases converted to laparoscopic cholecystectomy—two for hemorrhage—and one cystic duct leak controlled by ERCP and stenting. Forgione et al. [23] published their initial three cases using a flexible endoscope, although this group later adopted a rigid platform for further transvaginal cholecystectomies. Navarra et al. [24] published a series of six hybrid transvaginal cholecystectomies. Similar to our early technique, they reported gallbladder retraction with multiple transabdominal sutures. Salinas et al. [25] published a much larger series of 27 transgastric and 12 transvaginal cholecystectomies using a flexible endoscope and one laparoscopic port. Interestingly, their transvaginal mean operative time of 147 min was 10 min longer than the transgastric route, which has not been reported by other authors. They did, however, present a 25% minor complication rate. Horgan et al. [26] reported on four transvaginal cholecystectomies, among other NOTES procedures, in a series of cases utilizing the Incisionless Operating Platform (USGI Medical, San Clemente, CA). Their mean operating time was 86 min, and they utilized only one additional laparoscopic port. They reported no major complications. Santos et al. [27] reported on a series of seven transvaginal and seven conventional laparoscopic cholecystectomies. Their mean operative time was similar to our group at 162 min; they found less postoperative pain in the immediate postoperative period. Noguera et al. [28] published a randomized trial comparing transumbilical NOTES, transvaginal NOTES, and conventional laparoscopic cholecystectomy. Unsurprisingly, the transvaginal group took the longest in OR time, but it was faster than our series at 64.85 min. There were twenty patients in each group, and no major complications reported in the transvaginal group.

Discussion

Flexible endoscopic transvaginal cholecystectomy has been shown to be feasible. Although early reports from the NOVEL trial [20] showed no difference in pain in the transvaginal group when compared to standard laparoscopic cholecystectomy, it did demonstrate feasibility and safety. Given this, one would think that the procedure would have gained wider acceptance. However, surgeons and gastroenterologists, spurred on by the lead position taken by NOSCAR of slow adoption after appropriate research, took a measured approach to the development of transvaginal cholecystectomy. Although the flexible endoscopic technique has its merits, the fact remains that endoscopic instrumentation was never designed for surgical procedures, and most of the existing products are not that helpful in performing operative maneuvers. For this reason, most authors espouse the use of a hybrid approach with laparoscopic instrumentation as an aid. That has likely also slowed the adoption of transvaginal cholecystectomy. Further, few surgeons have the appropriate experience with advanced therapeutic endoscopy, necessitating either a team approach such as we have adopted, or a conversion to conventional laparoscopic instrumentation (and often using extra long instruments such those designed for bariatric surgery).

A potential drawback to utilizing the flexible technique remains the potential difficulty in performing surgical maneuvers with endoscopic instrumentation. A familiar concept to the advanced endoscopist is the use of torque. Inside the gut lumen, there is less need for anatomic landmarks or specifically to identify geographic directions. In the abdominal cavity, maintenance of anatomy in the standard directions remains a hallmark for safety. For example, if dissection was being done around the cystic duct, and torque was applied to the endoscope to help reach an area of tissue that otherwise may not be reachable, the appearances of the structures on the viewing screen could lead to disorientation and ultimately to patient injury. Concern for this idea was elucidated in the white paper on NOTES [29] where the idea of maintaining spatial orientation was raised. Specifically, there was concern for "access sites creating situations in which the image is upside down… With experience, some of this spatial incongruity may be overcome, though it will prevent complex procedures from being performed with the speed and facility" with which laparoscopic procedures routinely occur. Furthermore, "potential solutions include incorporating visualization systems into platform technology with electronic image stabilization/inversion…" but these have not yet made it to market. In this paper [29], it was acknowledged that the development of "a multitasking platform is critical. Many important maneuvers for manipulating tissue are difficult to perform, even with a two-channel endoscope. For example, aggressive grasping of tissue to set up traction and counter-traction for exposure and division of structures is currently not possible."

Despite the technical difficulties described here, there were no major biliary injuries in our series or the NOVEL trial [20]. Perhaps, this speaks to smart patient selection, much like in the early days of laparoscopic cholecystectomy where acute cholecystitis was considered a contraindication for most early published series. This also speaks to the measured approach taken by surgeons in introducing transvaginal cholecystectomy into their practices. Further, in employing the flexible endoscopic tools, the technical difficulty requires slower speed, and the likelihood of injury may even be less with multiple operators working in concert. Nonetheless, in this era with increasing attention on the prevention of bile duct injuries, one can certainly claim that flexible endoscopic transvaginal cholecystectomy is safe.

Although cost studies have yet to be published, it is undeniable that, at least initially, employing a NOTES approach is much more costly and not cost-effective in the long term. Indeed, our local payer was willing to reimburse us for these procedures, provided that we only billed the cases as a laparoscopic cholecystectomy. Although some of the series described in this chapter have operative times that have begun to approach laparoscopic cholecystectomy [26, 28], for most authors, the operative times are significantly longer and thus more costly. Significant instrumentation development would be needed for surgeons to be able to replicate the speed with which they perform laparoscopic cholecystectomy, and even then, the endoscopic instrumentation tends to be orders of magnitude higher in cost. For example, one need only compare the cost of a laparoscopic clip applier with many clips in it to the individual cost of endoscopic clip appliers which have single clips only. Certainly, cost is a factor which has retarded the growth of flexible endoscopic transvaginal cholecystectomy.

Transvaginal cholecystectomy has been shown to be safe and effective. It is possible that the transvaginal organ extraction may contribute to less postoperative pain. Experience remains limited, especially with the flexible endoscopic approach. The widespread adoption of a technique such as this one remains unlikely unless instrumentation tailored to the performance of these procedures is developed and marketed.

References

1. Marescaux J, Dallemagne B, Perretta S, Wattiez A, Mutter D, Coumaros D. Surgery without scars: report of transluminal cholecystectomy in a human being. Arch Surg. 2007;142(9): 823–6; discussion 826–7.
2. Zornig C, Emmermann A, von Waldenfels HA, Mofid H. Laparoscopic cholecystectomy without visible scar: combined transvaginal and transumbilical approach. Endoscopy. 2007;39(10):913–5.
3. Bessler M, Stevens PD, Milone L, Parikh M, Fowler D. Transvaginal laparoscopically assisted endoscopic cholecystectomy: a hybrid approach to natural orifice surgery. Gastrointest Endosc. 2007;66 (6):1243–5.
4. Zorrón R, Filgueiras M, Maggioni LC, Pombo L, Lopes Carvalho G, Lacerda Oliveira A. NOTES. Transvaginal cholecystectomy: report of the first case. Surg Innov. 2007; 14(4): 279–83.
5. Rao GV, Reddy DN. Personal communication.

6. Park PO, Bergström M, Ikeda K, Fritscher-Ravens A, Swain P. Experimental studies of transgastric gallbladder surgery: cholecystectomy and cholecystogastric anastomosis (videos). Gastrointest Endosc. 2005;61(4):601–6.
7. Swanstrom LL, Kozarek R, Pasricha PJ, Gross S, Birkett D, et al. Development of a new access device for transgastric surgery. J Gastrointest Surg. 2005; 9 (8): 1129–36; discussion 1136–7.
8. Rolanda C, Lima E, Pêgo JM, Henriques-Coelho T, Silva D, et al. Third-generation cholecystectomy by natural orifices: transgastric and transvesical combined approach (with video). Gastrointest Endosc. 2007;65(1):111–7.
9. Feretis C, Kalantzopoulos D, Koulouris P, Kolettas C, Archontovasilis F, et al. Endoscopic transgastric procedures in anesthetized pigs: technical challenges, complications, and survival. Endoscopy. 2007;39 (5):394–400.
10. Sumiyama K, Gostout CJ, Rajan E, Bakken TA, Knipschield MA, et al. Transgastric cholecystectomy: transgastric accessibility to the gallbladder improved with the SEMF method and a novel multibending therapeutic endoscope. Gastrointest Endosc. 2007;65(7):1028–34.
11. Perretta S, Dallemagne B, Coumaros D, Marescaux J. Natural orifice transluminal endoscopic surgery: transgastric cholecystectomy in a survival porcine model. Surg Endosc. 2008;22(4):1126–30.
12. Auyang ED, Hungness ES, Vaziri K, Martin JA, Soper NJ. Human NOTES cholecystectomy: transgastric hybrid technique. J Gastrointest Surg. 2009;13(6):1149–50.
13. Asakuma M, Perretta S, Allemann P, Cahill R, Con SA, et al. Challenges and lessons learned from NOTES cholecystectomy initial experience: a stepwise approach from the laboratory to clinical application. J Hepatobiliary Pancreat Surg. 2009;16 (3):249–54.
14. Dallemagne B, Perretta S, Allemann P, Asakuma M, Marescaux J. Transgastric hybrid cholecystectomy. Br J Surg. 2009;96(10):1162–6.
15. Rattner D, Kalloo, A, and the SAGES/ASGE Working Group on Natural Orifice Translumenal Endoscopic Surgery. ASGE/SAGES working group on natural orifice translumenal endoscopic surgery. Surg Endosc. 2006;20:329–33.
16. Delvaux G, Devroey P, De Waele B, Willems G. Transvaginal removal of gallbladders with large stones after laparoscopic cholecystectomy. Surg Laparosc Endosc. 1993;3(4):307–9.
17. Vereczkei A, Illenyi L, Arany A, Szabo Z, Toth L, et al. Transvaginal extraction of the laparoscopically removed spleen. Surg Endosc. 2003;17(1):157.
18. Nakajima K, Souma Y, Takahashi T, Yamasaki M, Miyazaki Y, et al. Anatomical measurements to optimize instrumentation for transvaginal surgery. Surg Endosc. 2013;27(6):2052–7.
19. Gumbs AA, Fowler D, Milone L, Evanko JC, Ude AO, et al. Transvaginal natural orifice translumenal endoscopic surgery cholecystectomy: early evolution of the technique. Ann Surg. 2009;249 (6):908–12.
20. Perretta S. Personal communication.
21. Schwaitzberg SD, Kochman ML. Prospective randomized trial of NOTES® cholecystectomy versus laparoscopic cholecystectomy. Presented as an Oral Presentation, SAGES Annual Meeting Nashville, TN, 15–18 Apr 2015.
22. Palanivelu C, Rajan PS, Rangarajan M, Parthasarathi R, Senthilnathan P, et al. Transumbilical flexible endoscopic cholecystectomy in humans: first feasibility study using a hybrid technique. Endoscopy. 2008;40(5):428–31.
23. Forgione A, Maggioni D, Sansonna F, Ferrari C, Di Lernia S, et al. Transvaginal endoscopic cholecystectomy in human beings: preliminary results. J Laparoendosc Adv Surg Tech A. 2008;18 (3):345–51.
24. Navarra G, Rando L, La Malfa G, Bartolotta G, Pracanica G. Hybrid transvaginal cholecystectomy: a novel approach. Am J Surg. 2009;197(6):e69–72.
25. Salinas G, Saavedra L, Agurto H, Quispe R, Ramírez E, et al. Early experience in human hybrid transgastric and transvaginal endoscopic cholecystectomy. Surg Endosc. 2010;24(5):1092–8.
26. Horgan S, Thompson K, Talamini M, Ferreres A, Jacobsen G, et al. Clinical experience with a multifunctional, flexible surgery system for endolumenal, single-port, and NOTES procedures. Surg Endosc. 2011;25(2):586–92.
27. Santos BF, Teitelbaum EN, Arafat FO, Milad MP, Soper NJ, et al. Comparison of short-term outcomes between transvaginal hybrid NOTES cholecystectomy and laparoscopic cholecystectomy. Surg Endosc. 2012;26(11):3058–66.
28. Noguera JF, Cuadrado A, Dolz C, Olea JM, García JC. Prospective randomized clinical trial comparing laparoscopic cholecystectomy and hybrid natural orifice transluminal endoscopic surgery (NOTES) (NCT00835250). Surg Endosc. 2012;26(12): 3435–41.
29. Rattner D, Kalloo A, and the SAGES/ASGE Working Group on Natural Orifice Translumenal Endoscopic Surgery. ASGE/SAGES working group on natural orifice translumenal endoscopic surgery: white paper. Surg Endosc. 2006; 20:329–33.

NOTES Rigid Transvaginal Cholecystectomy

17

Karl-Hermann Fuchs, Carsten Zornig, Benjamin Babic and Gabor Varga

Abstract

Cholecystectomy is one of the most frequently performed operative procedures in gastrointestinal abdominal surgery. The concept of NOTES moves the reduction in access trauma one step further by using a natural orifice as an access route to the intra-abdominal cavity. NOTES stands for a reduction in access trauma by approaching the abdominal cavity by natural orifices as much as possible for a safe performance of the necessary procedure. Based on their previous experience with colpotomy and surgical procedures, transvaginal hybrid NOTES technique with rigid standard instruments for cholecystectomy was developed. On the contrary to the method with flexible endoscopy, this technique was comprehensible to surgeons. The most common techniques of NOTES cholecystectomy have been the hybrid transvaginal with the aid of rigid laparoscope. The need to convert to laparoscopy was absolutely minimal. The overall incidence of postoperative complication was extremely low and similar between the two most frequently used techniques. First comparative trials have been published demonstrating the only possible advantage of these NOTES Hybrid procedures over classic laparoscopic cholecystectomy regarding the cosmetic result.

Keywords

Cholecystectomy · Transvaginal cholecystectomy · NOTES · Transvaginal surgery

K.-H. Fuchs (✉) · B. Babic · G. Varga
Agaplesion Markus Krankenhaus,
Frankfurt am Main, Germany
e-mail: Karl-Hermann.Fuchs@fdk.info

B. Babic
e-mail: Benjamin.Babic@fkd.info

G. Varga
e-mail: Gabor.Varga@fdk.info

C. Zornig
Israelitisches Krankenhaus, Hamburg, Germany
e-mail: info@ik-h.de

K.-H. Fuchs
Department of Surgery, Agaplesion
Markus-Krankenhaus, Wilhelm-Epstein-Straße 4,
60431 Frankfurt am Main, Germany

J.R. Romanelli et al. (eds.), *NOTES and Endoluminal Surgery*,
Clinical Gastroenterology, DOI 10.1007/978-3-319-50610-4_17

Introduction

Cholecystectomy is one of the most frequently performed operative procedures in gastrointestinal abdominal surgery, and the introduction of minimal-access surgery was mainly pushed by the success of laparoscopic cholecystectomy among patients [1, 2]. With the advent of the NOTES concept into the endoscopic and surgical world, some anticipated that NOTES cholecystectomy could repeat a similar success story, facilitating the introduction of transgastric cholecystectomy [3–8].

The principle of minimal-access surgery is the reduction in access size and trauma, aiming for a shorter patient recovery, improved postoperative well-being, better cosmesis, fewer postoperative restrictions in order to get the patient quickly back to full physical and psychological abilities, and possibly an improved long-term outcome [9]. The latter could be achieved by a lower wound infection rate and by fewer incisional hernias over time.

The advantage of this concept of minimal-access surgery over conventional open surgery has been clearly shown in the past decades [10, 11]. It must be emphasized that the improvements in patient care 20 years ago with the advent of minimal-access surgery were not only caused by the reduction in abdominal incisions, but also caused by conceptual changes that came along with rethinking perioperative care [12].

The concept of NOTES follows that line of thinking and moves the reduction in access trauma one step further by using a natural orifice as an access route to the intra-abdominal cavity [7, 8, 13]. NOTES represents a reduction in access trauma by approaching the abdominal cavity by natural orifices as much as possible for a safe performance of the necessary procedure. The "hybrid" solution uses a natural orifice and limits access via the abdominal wall by reducing number and size of ports. Further minimizing access trauma at the abdominal wall could possibly lead to less postoperative pain, improved recovery from surgery, fewer postoperative complications, including wound infection and incisional hernia [8, 13].

However, initial experimental and clinical experience quickly revealed the technical difficulties posed by the use of a flexible endoscope for complex intra-abdominal operative procedures, along with the shortcomings in training and experience in flexible endoscopy by most surgeons [8, 13, 14].

The Transvaginal Technique of Laparoscopic Hybrid Cholecystectomy

Facing these difficulties, the transvaginal approach quickly came to the mind of surgeons, as this route has been used for many decades by gynecologists and for more than 10 years by general and GI surgeons for larger specimen retrieval such as spleens and colon segments [15–20].

In the spring 2007, Bessler and Marescaux were the first to remove a gallbladder transvaginally with flexible endoscopes. Both used several additional mini-trocars or instruments to assist the flexible endoscopic instrumentation [21, 22]. The technical difficulties of using insufficient instruments made it very difficult for the average GI surgeon to perform the procedure safely and to get through the learning curve quickly.

In June 2007, based on their previous experience with colpotomy, Zornig et al. [23] developed the transvaginal hybrid NOTES technique with standard, rigid laparoscopic instruments for cholecystectomy. Contrary to the method with flexible endoscopy, this technique was easier for surgeons to understand, and it could more readily be put into practice by surgeons with experience in advanced minimal-access surgery.

Zornig et al. describe their original technique as follows [23, 24]: The patients are placed in the lithotomy position. The vagina is prepped around the introitus and inside with an antiseptic fluid which is appropriate for mucosa. The operation starts with an incision of 5 mm inside the umbilicus for insufflation with a Veress needle, which is subsequently replaced by a 5-mm port through which a 5-mm rigid laparoscope is inserted. Diagnostic laparoscopy is performed, and the patient is put in a steep Trendelenburg position. The cervix is fixed by a clamp, and a metal bar is inserted into the uterus to lift it up. From the umbilical trocar, a good view can be had of the pouch of Douglas (Fig. 17.1). This allows for the inspection of all important anatomical landmarks and the "triangle of safety" as mentioned by Roberts [25].

A 5-mm extra-long dissector is inserted through the posterior fornix of the vagina, and beside that an extra-long 10-mm port is inserted for the laparoscope (Fig. 17.2). The camera is moved to the transvaginal port, and a 5-mm dissector is inserted through the umbilicus.

The gallbladder is retracted by the transvaginal instrument, and the dissection of the triangle of Calot is performed by the umbilical instrument (Fig. 17.3). The cystic artery and duct are identified and clipped with a multi-fire clip applier placed through the umbilical port. The gallbladder is removed from the liver bed with a monopolar hook. The scope is then moved back to the umbilical port, and the gallbladder is

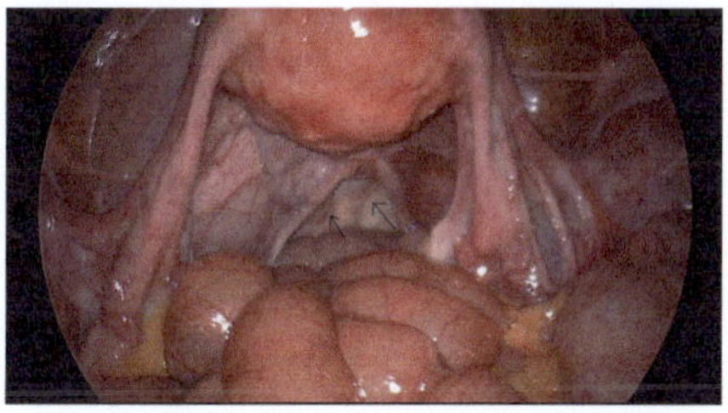

Fig. 17.1 Laparoscopic view in the pelvic region and vaginal area for penetration of the transvaginal trocars and instruments

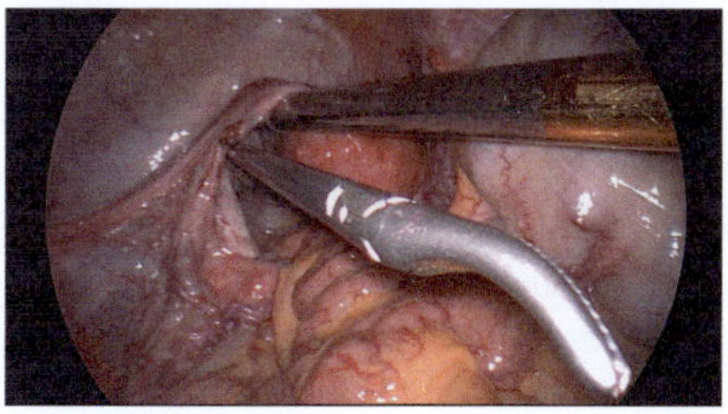

Fig. 17.2 Insertion of the 10-mm camera and one grasper

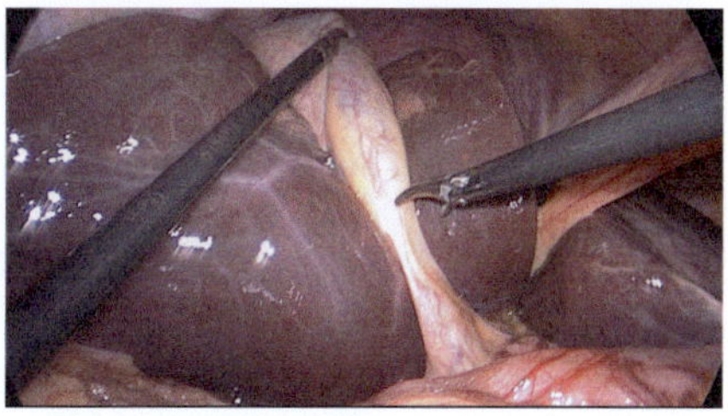

Fig. 17.3 Gallbladder is exposed along with the cystic duct and the hepatoduodenal ligament, to check all necessary anatomical landmarks

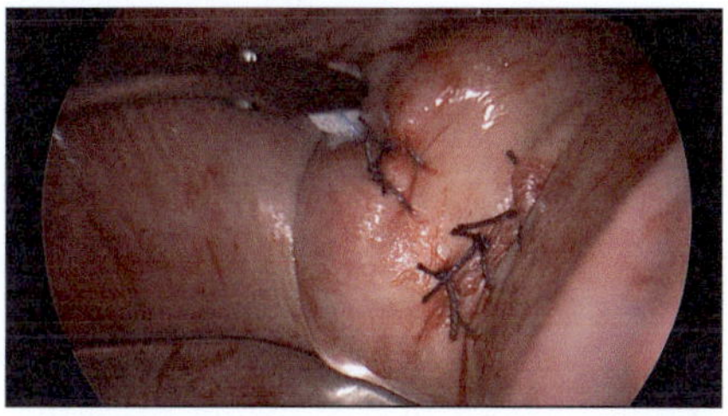

Fig. 17.4 Closure of the vagina with a colposcope under direct vision

removed through the 10-mm port site in the vagina. If required, the port site can be widened with a blunt clamp. After releasing the pneumoperitoneum, the incisions in the posterior fornix are closed with absorbable suture (Fig. 17.4).

A single dose of prophylactic antibiotics with cefuroxime and metronidazole is administered. Postmenopausal patients receive estrogen suppositories for 5 days for better wound healing. Sexual intercourse should be avoided for 2 weeks, as originally described by Zornig [23].

Results

1. **The Hamburg Results**:

The group in Hamburg, Germany, summarizes their results as follows [24]: All operations ($n = 204$) could be successfully performed in the described method except one case (0.5%). The latter case was converted to a traditional laparoscopic cholecystectomy due to severe acute inflammation. In 9 cases (4.5%), an additional abdominal port was used for larger clips, drainage, or a linear stapler.

The average operation time was 50 (23–110) minutes. In 9 cases (4.5%), the transvaginal approach was abandoned and no instruments were inserted through the vagina due to difficulties of the inspection of the pouch of Douglas. The most common reason for this decision was adhesions in the pelvis. These patients were not included in the group of the 204 patients.

There was one (0.5%) intraoperative and two postoperative (1.0%) complications. During the insertion of the transvaginal port, the urinary bladder was perforated with a 5-mm dissector in a patient with a previous hysterectomy. A transurethral catheter was placed for 3 days, and the injury healed spontaneously as was shown using contrast radiography. One patient (0.5%) developed a biliary fistula from the liver parenchyma and a laparoscopic closure with a suture on postoperative day 3 was performed. The other (0.5%) postoperative complication was an abscess in the pouch of Douglas 3 weeks after surgery, which was drained laparoscopically. No other complications occurred. The average length of the hospital stay was 2.1 [1–7] days.

Zornig et al. asked their patients to be examined by the associated gynecologists within one week after hospital discharge, and 183 (90%) of the patients underwent this examination. Interestingly, the patient with the abscess in the pouch of Douglas was one of the patients who did not follow this recommendation. They were asked about discomfort or pain in the lower abdomen/pelvis or vagina, and the wounds in the vagina were inspected. A transvaginal ultrasound was performed. None of the examinations presented pathological findings. In another study, Zornig et al. compared the results of matched pairs, investigating transvaginal cholecystectomy with traditional laparoscopic cholecystectomy, and found no differences in all analyzed parameters with the exception of duration of the procedures and cosmesis [26]. The latter was based on subjective patient opinion after transvaginal procedures.

2. **Results of the EuroNOTES Clinical Registry**:

The EuroNOTES Clinical Registry (ECR) was created as a European database to monitor the clinical application of Natural Orifice Translumenal Endoscopic Surgery™ (NOTES®) [27]. The ECR was sponsored by the EuroNOTES Foundation, founded in 2008 as a joint initiative of the European Society for Gastrointestinal Endoscopy (ESGE) and the European Association for Endoscopic Surgery (EAES). The concept of a NOTES clinical registry was announced at several congresses, and all members of ESGE and EAES performing (or intending to perform) NOTES procedures were asked to participate to the ECR.

Data were collected between May 2010 and April 2014, and are visible in an anonymous way online (http://www.euronotes.world.it). Although 62 accounts were created, indicating the number of centers that were interested in participating, only 14 centers participated in data collection. Procedures were included in the ECR retrospectively, so the ECR includes cases performed between April 2007 and April 2014.

At the time of publication in 2014, a total of 571 patients had been entered into the registry [27]. The most frequent procedure in the ECR was cholecystectomy, performed in 442 cases (78.5%). Cholecystectomy was performed in 4 different techniques:

1. A hybrid technique consisting of a transvaginal and transumbilical access, with the aid of a flexible endoscope [14], reported by 9 different centers
2. A hybrid technique consisting of a transvaginal and transumbilical access, with the aid of a rigid laparoscope [15], reported by 2 different centers
3. A hybrid technique consisting of a transgastric and transumbilical access, with the aid of a flexible endoscope [16, 17], reported by 2 different centers
4. A hybrid NOTES transvaginal technique, by means of modified transanal endoscopic

microsurgery (TEM) equipment combined with a transumbilical access, reported by one center.

Table 17.1 demonstrates patient characteristics, showing an average age of 45.3 years and a BMI of 25.3 kg/m. The mean operative time of transvaginal cholecystectomy was 60.5 min (15–270). Age and BMI did not differ significantly among the groups. In all cases, optics were introduced through the transmural access, i.e., transvaginal or transgastric technique.

The transvaginal approach was chosen in 430 of 442 cholecystectomies (97.2%), and only 12 patients underwent a transgastric hybrid approach. Analyzing the transvaginal approach, 145 cases were performed with the support of a flexible endoscope, 279 cases with the aid of a rigid laparoscope, and the remaining 6 cases were conducted with modified TEM equipment. In 406 cases, the transvaginal access was created with a direct surgical opening after a stable pneumoperitoneum was established via transumbilical access. In the remaining 24 cases, the access to the abdominal cavity was obtained by direct insertion of a 12-mm trocar transvaginally, without a previous pneumoperitoneum. The transvaginal access was sutured closed in all cases via a standard colposcope.

In most hybrid NOTES procedures, the transabdominal trocar was used for introducing instruments for dissection, with the exception of the transvaginal approach, which used modified TEM instrumentation with the transabdominal trocar only used to obtain a safe and clear transvaginal access. The TEM instrumentation consists of a 50-cm-long and 33-mm diameter dedicated colposcope through which four dedicated extra-long instruments were used for tissue manipulation, dissection, and suturing.

Conversion to traditional laparoscopy was needed in only 3 cases during any of the transvaginal cholecystectomy procedures, not related to the use of flexible or rigid instruments. The reasons for adding one or more trocarswere for better manipulation in 21 cases, while in 2 cases it was to control bleeding, in 2 additional cases it was due to unclear anatomy, and in 1 case because of a large cystic duct.

Overall, transvaginal procedures were faster than transgastric procedures (58.7 min vs. 125.4 min, $P < 0.001$). Among transvaginal techniques, operative time was significantly shorter in the group with rigid laparoscopes compared to each of the other techniques ($P < 0.001$).

Table 17.2 summarizes complications and hospital stay for the different cholecystectomy techniques. Eight complications (2.5%) were observed post-operatively. Two complications (1.4%) occurred after transvaginal and transumbilical access with a flexible endoscope. One intra-abdominal hematoma was probably due to the dislodgement of the endoscopic clip on the cystic artery. One complication consisted of minimal vaginal bleeding which was controlled by suture. Five complications (1.8%) occurred post-operatively after transvaginal and transumbilical access with a rigid laparoscope. Two required additional surgery due to a bile leak and a pelvic abscess. Another 2 patients needed postoperative ERCP for a bile leak.

Table 17.1 EuroNOTES clinical registry: NOTES cholecystectomies with different access techniques Arezzo et al. [27]

Procedure	*n*	Center	Age	BMI	Add Trocard %	OR time
TV flexible endoscope	145	9	46	27	5.5	76
TV rigid laparoscope	279	2	45	25	4.7	49
TG flexible endoscope	12	2	48	25	25	125
TV with TEM device	6	1	37	–	–	80
Total	442	12	46	25	5.4	61

Table 17.2 EuroNOTES clinical registry: NOTES cholecystectomy with different access techniques: complications Arezzo et al. [27]

Procedure	*n*	Intraop	Postop %	Overall %	Hospital stay
TV flexible endoscope	145	0	1.4	1.4	2.1
TV rigid laparoscope	279	0.7%	1.8	2.5	2.0
TG flexible endoscope	12	0	0	0	2.4
TV with TEM device	6	0	16.7	16.7	2.5
Total	442	0.5%	1.8	2.3	2.1

The mean hospital stay was 2.1 days and ranged from 0 to 11 days. The transvaginal hybrid technique with a rigid laparoscope showed a significantly shorter hospital stay compared to access techniques with a flexible endoscope ($P = 0.02$).

3. **Results of the German DGAV Registry**:

The German Society of General and GI-Surgery (Deutsche Gesellschaft für Allgemein- und Visceralchirurgie, Berlin, Germany) started a NOTES registry in 2007, in which every member was welcome to register their NOTES and hybrid cases. Results were published, and continuous reports were presented in several meetings [28]. Table 17.3 demonstrates the results of the comparative data presented at the D-NOTES meeting in 2014 [24, 27, 28]. In total, 3239 patients were at that time registered, out of which 2708 were transvaginal cholecystectomies. There was a 1.5% conversion rate, with 34 to laparoscopy and 12 to laparotomy. There were 48 intraoperative complications (1.6%) and 116 postoperative complications (3.8%). The complication rate did not differ between low-volume hospitals and high-volume (>100 cases) hospitals.

Discussion

The available data around transvaginal rigid cholecystectomy indicate it is a safe approach in selected patients at centers with adequate training. Similar to the introduction of laparoscopic surgery, cholecystectomy is generally considered the target procedure for developing and testing a novel surgical technique such as NOTES. For this reason, cholecystectomy represents almost 80% of the procedures documented in European registries.

The 2 most common techniques of NOTES cholecystectomy, i.e., hybrid transvaginal with the aid of either a flexible endoscope or a rigid laparoscope, both required a further transabdominal trocar in about 5% each. The need to convert to laparoscopy was minimal. The overall

Table 17.3 Overview on transvaginal cholecystectomy series

	DGAV registry	EuroNOTES registry	Zornig et al.
TV CE n	2411	442	100
Age years	48	45	49
BMI	27	25	26
OR time min	57	60 (15–270)	52 (23–100)
Intraoperative complications	1.4%	1.8%	0
Postoperative complications (%)	2.6	1.8	1–2

incidence of postoperative complications was extremely low and similar between the two most frequently used techniques. The shorter operative time in the hybrid transvaginal techniques with a rigid laparoscope might reflect the similarity to the standard multiport laparoscopic technique, as well as the standardization of a consistent series of only two centers compared to the fragmentation of data reported by many different centers. This has probably increased confidence and reduced the duration of the learning curve.

Rigid transvaginal cholecystectomies were well established in Europe by 2010. There is an experience of several thousand cases. The safety record of the published series is remarkable, with less than 3% complications. Comparative trials have been published demonstrating a possible cosmetic advantage of NOTES hybrid procedures over classic laparoscopic cholecystectomy [26].

The concept of hybrid transvaginal cholecystectomy is comprehensible to surgeons and can be quickly introduced in clinical practice with a steep (rapid) learning curve [16–24]. As with many hybrid techniques, primary abdominal access is performed via a safe standard laparoscopic approach, with establishment of a capnoperitoneum and a transumbilical camera port, preferably 5 mm in size. This allows for a safe introduction of a larger access via the vagina with several ports and/or instruments. Technical maneuvers to dissect and remove the gallbladder are similar to established laparoscopy.

In addition to cholecystectomy, transvaginal appendectomy and colon resections were introduced into clinical practice with a remarkable safety record [29–33].

Although concern remains about possible side effects of postoperative dyspareunia after transvaginal procedures, the transvaginal technique has a good safety record and is well established [25, 26, 28, 33]. Several working groups recommended that transvaginal NOTES procedures should be performed initially in cooperation with gynecologists until surgeons have gained enough experience to perform this technique safely [18, 23, 26].

Contraindications for transvaginal access are recto-vaginal endometriosis, pregnancy, and malignant tumors of the cervix and vagina. Previous gynecologic operations can cause severe adhesions. Therefore, it is advisable to use extra caution in these cases, such as a preliminary capnoperitoneum and intraperitoneal visual control, when penetrating the vagina. It is advised to perform a suture closure of the access route of the posterior vaginal wall. Also, a gynecologic postoperative check is advised.

In the USA, NOSCAR has finished a randomized trial comparing various methods of cholecystectomy, one of which is the transvaginal procedure. Schwaitzberg [34] presented the data at the 2015 NOTES annual summit, showing a low complication rate.

Despite the above-mentioned results, the attractiveness of this technique has not persisted, since the frequency of applications, especially in Germany, has decreased after the initial hype. Table 17.4 shows the number of registered patients and the number of actively participating centers in the German DGAV-NOTES Registry has substantially decreased after 2010. The proposed and anticipated benefits of transvaginal surgery are less postoperative pain, fewer wound-related complications (including wound infections and hernias), shorter length of hospital stay, shorter convalescence, and superior cosmesis. Several series in the literature have supported these benefits. However, these benefits have not yet been confirmed in prospective, randomized trials.

The overall penetrance of transvaginal cholecystectomy as a mainstream operation is limited.

Table 17.4 Overview on case development in German DGAV-NOTES registry D Bulian & K Lehmann (May 2014) (3239 patients, 58 hospitals)

Year	2008	2009	2010	2011	2012	2013
Cases	318	584	662	707	488	391
Active centers	22	36	31	22	17	11

A survey of 409 women revealed that only 41% would consider the transvaginal approach for cholecystectomy [25]. Patients expressed concern over pain, infection, recovery time, and technical aspects of the technique. These concerns do not seem to be supported by the data published to date.

Nobody can predict what the future will bring regarding transvaginal procedures in gastrointestinal surgery, but it is not imaginable that many cholecystectomies will be performed by NOTES techniques. Without any doubt, this is even more valid for the more complex procedures such as colectomies. Traditional standard laparoscopic procedures, and especially laparoscopic cholecystectomy, are excellent and safe operative techniques which will be difficult to be surpassed by other approaches. As of now, better cosmesis will be the main driver for NOTES. Whether surgeons will ultimately accept longer operative times and more difficult techniques just to achieve better cosmesis remains an open question.

References

1. Deziel DJ, Milikan KW, Economou SG. Complications of laparoscopic cholecystectomy: a national survey of 4292 hospitals and an analysis of 77,604 cases. Am J Surg. 1993;165:9–14.
2. Härkki-Siren P, Sjöberg J, Kurki T. Major complications of laparoscopy: a Finnish study. Obstet Gynecol. 1999;94(1):94–8.
3. Kalloo AN, Singh VK, Jagannath SB, Niiyama H, Hill SL, Vaughn CA, Magee CA, Kantsevoy SV. Flexible transgastric peritoneoscopy: a novel approach to diagnostic and therapeutic interventions. Gastrointest Endosc. 2004;60:114–7.
4. Jagannath SB, Kantsevoy SV, Vaughn CA, Chung SSC, Cotton PB, Gostout CJ, et al. Peroral transgastric endoscopic ligation of fallopian tubes with long-term survival in a porcine model. Gastrointest Endosc. 2005;61:449–53.
5. Park PO, Bergstrom M, Ikeda K, Fritscher-Ravens A, Swain P. Experimental studies of transgastric gallbladder surgery: cholecystectomy and cholecystogastric anastomosis. Gastrointest Endosc. 2005;61:601–6.
6. Kantsevoy SV, Jagannath SB, Niiyama H, Vaughn CA, Chung SSC, Cotton PB, et al. Endoscopic gastrojejunostomy with survival in a porcine model. Gastrointest Endosc. 2005;62:287–92.
7. Rattner D, Kalloo AN. ASGE/SAGES working group white paper on natural orifice translumenal endoscopic surgery. Surg Endosc 2006;20(2):329–33.
8. Rattner D, Hawes R, Schwaitzberg S, Kochman M, Swanstrom L. The second SAGES/ASGE white paper on natural orifice translumenal endoscopic surgery: 5 years of progress. Surg Endosc. 2011; 25:2441–8.
9. Cuschieri A. Minimal access surgery and the future of interventional laparoscopy. Am J Surg. 1991; 161:404–7.
10. Olsen MF, Josefson K, Dalenback J, Lundell L, Lonroth H. Respiratory function after laparoscopic and open fundoplication. Eur J Surg. 1997;163(9): 667–72.
11. Abraham NS, Young JM, Solomon MJ. Meta-analysis of short-term outcomes after laparoscopic resection for colorectal cancer. Br J Surg. 2004;91:1111–24.
12. Kehlet H, Whilmore DW. Evidence-based surgical care and the evolution of fast-track surgery. Ann Surg. 2008;248:189–98.
13. Fuchs KH, Meining A, von Renteln D, Fernandez-Esparrach G, Breithaupt W, Zornig C, et al. The EuroNOTES Status paper—NOTES from the concept to clinical practice. Surg Endosc. 2013;27:1456–67.
14. Meining A, Feussner H, Swain P, Yang GZ, Lehmann K, Zorron R, et al. Natural-orifice transluminal endoscopic surgery (NOTES) in Europe: summary of the working group reports of the Euro-NOTES meeting 2010. Endoscopy. 2011;43(2):140–3.
15. Decker A, Cherry TH. Culdoscopy—a new method in the diagnosis of pelvic disease—preliminary report. Am J Surg. 1944;64:40–4.
16. Tsin DA, Colombero LT, Mahmood D, Padouvas J, Manolas P. Operative culdolaparoscopy: a new approach combining operative culdoscopy and mini-laparoscopy. J Am Assoc Gyn Laparosc. 2001; 8:438–41.
17. Gordts S, Puttemans P, Brosens I, Campo R. Transvaginal laparoscopy. Best Pract Res Clin Obstet Gynaecol 2005;19(5):757–67.
18. Zornig C, Emmermann A, von Waldenfels HA, Felixmüller C. Colpotomy for specimen removal in laparoscopic surgery. Chirurg. 1994;65:883–5.
19. Vereczkei A, Illenyi L, Arany A, Szabo Z, Toth L, Horvath OP. Transvaginal extraction of laparoscopically removed spleen. Surg Endosc. 2003;17:157.
20. Tsin DA, Sequeria RJ, Giannikas G. Culdolaparoscopic cholecystectomy during vaginal hysterectomy. J Soc Lap Surg. 2003;7:171–2.
21. Bessler M, Stevens PD, Milone L, Parikh M, Fowler D. Transvaginal laparoscopically assisted endoscopic cholecystectomy: a hybrid approach to natural orifice surgery. Gastrointest Endosc. 2007; 66:1243–5.
22. Marescaux J, Dallemagne B, Perretta S, Wattiez A, Mutter D, Coumaros D. Surgery without scars: report of transluminal cholecystectomy in a human being. Arch Surg. 2007;142:823–6.

23. Zornig C, Mofid H, Siemssen L, Emmermann A, Alm M, von Waldenfels HA, Felixmuller C. Transvaginal NOTES hybrid cholecystectomy: feasibility results in 68 cases with mid-term follow-up. Endoscopy. 2009;41:391–4.
24. Mofid H, Zornig C. The transvaginal hybrid cholecystectomy: an enduring alternative to the laparoscopic cholecystectomy—experience with 204 cases. In: Fuchs KH, Breithaupt W, editors. Natural orifice surgery in training and clinical practice. Winterburg: MedeServ GbR; 2014. p. 217–23.
25. Roberts K, Park K. The potential of transvaginal NOTES procedures. In: Fuchs KH, Breithaupt W, editors. Natural orifice surgery in training and clinical practice. Winterburg: MedeServ GbR; 2014. p. 202–9.
26. Zornig C, Siemssen L, Emmermann A, Alm M, von Waldenfels HA, Felixmüller C, Mofid H. NOTES cholecystectomy: matched pair analysis comparing the transvaginal hybrid and conventional laparoscopic techniques in a series of 216 patients. Surg Endosc. 2001;25(6):1822–6.
27. Arezzo A, Zornig C, MofidH, Noguera J, Kaehler G, Magdeburg H, et al. In: Fuchs KH, Breithaupt W, editors. Natural orifice surgery in training and clinical practice. Winterburg: MedeServ GbR; 2014. p. 157–74.
28. Lehmann KS, Ritz JP, Wibmer A, Gellert K, Zornig K, Burghardt J, et al. The German registry for natural orifice translumenal endoscopic surgery: report of the first 551 patients. Ann Surg. 2010;252(2):263–70.
29. Bernhardt J, Gerber B, Schober HC, Kahler G, Ludwig K. NOTES-case report of a unidirectional flexible appendectomy. Int J Colorectal Dis. 2008;23:547–50.
30. Roberts KE, Solomon D, Mirensky T, Silasi DA, Duffy AJ, Rutherford T, Longo WE, Bell RL. Pure transvaginal appendectomy versus traditional laparoscopic appendectomy for acute appendicitis: a prospective cohort study. Ann Surg. 2012;255:266–9.
31. Lacy AM, Delgado S, Rojas OA, Almenara R, Blasi A, Llach J. MA-NOS radical sigmoidectomy: report of a transvaginal resection in the human. Surg Endosc. 2008;22(7):1717–23.
32. Tarantino L, Linke GR, Lange J, Siercks I, Warschkow R, Zerz A. Transvaginal rigid-hybrid natural orifice transluminal endoscopic surgery technique for anterior resection treatment of diverticulitis: a feasibility study. Surg Endosc. 2011;25(9):3034–42.
33. Linke GR, Luz S, Janczak J, Zerz A, Schmied BM, Siercks I, Warschkow R, Beutner U, Taratino I. Evaluation of sexual function in sexual active women 1 year after transvaginal NOTES: a prospective cohort study of 106 patients. Langenbecks Arch Surg. 2013;398(1):139–45.
34. Schwaitzberg S. The NOSCAR cholecystectomy trial; presentation at the 2015 10th International NOTES Summit, Downers Grove, USA, July 2015.

NOTES Transvaginal Appendectomy 18

Kurt E. Roberts

Abstract

This chapter discusses the history and the different techniques of transvaginal appendectomy, which may consist of "pure NOTES" or "hybrid NOTES." The two main technical differences including rigid and flexible approaches are explained in detail. All these techniques are described from the positioning of the patient to the closure of the colpotomy. Next to the indications, contraindications and complications are discussed as well. In summary, it appears that no specific transvaginal approach, pure or hybrid, using endoscopic or laparoscopic instruments, has been shown to be superior. Yet, the hybrid approach may be technically easier and therefore safer over the pure transvaginal approach for most surgeons. Several studies of transvaginal appendectomy suggest that there is a faster recovery to normal activities and improved cosmetic results compared to conventional laparoscopic appendectomy. Overall, transvaginal appendectomy in the management of acute appendicitis is a viable option for patients.

Keywords

Transvaginal appendectomy · NOTES appendectomy · Transvaginal access

Abbreviations

NOTES Natural orifice translumenal endoscopic surgery

K.E. Roberts (✉)
Department of Surgery, Yale Gastrointestinal Surgery, 40 Temple Street Suite 7B, New Haven CT 06510, USA
e-mail: kurt.roberts@yale.edu

J.R. Romanelli et al. (eds.), *NOTES and Endoluminal Surgery*, Clinical Gastroenterology, DOI 10.1007/978-3-319-50610-4_18

Introduction

Acute appendicitis is the most common acute surgical condition of the abdomen, with an overall incidence of approximately 7%, and an overall mortality of 0.2–0.8% [1]. The surgical treatment of acute appendicitis has evolved significantly from the initial open appendectomy pioneered by McBurney [2] in the nineteenth century to the first laparoscopic appendectomy performed by Semm [3] in 1980. The latest advancement in surgical technique is natural orifice translumenal endoscopic surgery or NOTES. The first human transgastric appendectomy was performed by Rao et al. [4] in 2004. Transvaginal access for cholecystectomy and incidental appendectomy during hysterectomy has been reported as safe and effective in the gynecological literature.

The transition from open to laparoscopic surgery has been associated with a marked reduction in the degree of invasiveness, and NOTES may represent the next step in the evolution of surgery [5, 6]. The potential benefits of NOTES include reduction of postoperative pain, shorter convalescence, avoidance of wound infections, and abdominal wall hernias, as well as the absence of visible scars on the abdomen.

The treatment of choice for acute appendicitis is appendectomy. Currently, these are the following surgical techniques to perform an appendectomy:

- Open appendectomy,
- Laparoscopic appendectomy,
- Transgastric appendectomy, and
- Transvaginal appendectomy, which may consist of "pure NOTES" or "hybrid NOTES" (combined laparoscopic and NOTES techniques, which usually means that one port is placed transabdominally through the umbilicus and the remaining port or trocars are placed through the vagina).

History of Transvaginal Appendectomy

Initial reports of transvaginal appendectomies were published in the gynecological literature. The first incidental transvaginal appendectomy was performed during a transvaginal hysterectomy in 1949 [7]. More recently, Palanivelu et al. [8] were recognized as the first to publish a transvaginal appendectomy for appendicitis in 2008. Yet already in 2001 Tsin et al. [9] had published the initial transvaginal appendectomy on 3 patients prior to the advent of NOTES. Also in 2008, Bernhardt et al. [10] reported a pure transvaginal appendectomy using endoscopic instruments. Tabutsadze and Kipshidze [11] followed with a report of two transvaginal appendectomies using a single-channel gastroscope. Nezhat et al. [12] described 42 patients who underwent incidental appendectomy at the time of total laparoscopic or laparoscopic-assisted hysterectomies, where the appendix was transected with a stapler and removed transvaginally. It should also be noted that a specific anatomical landmark for transvaginal appendectomies, "the triangle of safety," has been described by Roberts et al. [13] in 2013.

Since the early reports of transvaginal appendectomies, the two main established approaches include pure transvaginal appendectomy and hybrid transvaginal appendectomy, utilizing endoscopic or laparoscopic instruments, or a combination of both.

Indications

Female patients 18 years and older are candidates for transvaginal appendectomy, if they have one of the following:

- Acute appendicitis,
- Subacute appendicitis, and
- Chronic appendicitis

Contraindications

Absolute and relative contraindications to transvaginal appendectomy include the following:

- Evidence of perforation,
- Pregnancy,
- Recent delivery (within the preceding 2 months),
- American Society of Anesthesiologists (ASA) classification 3 or 4,
- History of pelvic inflammatory disease,
- History of endometriosis,
- History of inflammatory bowel disease, and
- History of retroflexed uterus.

Presently, a traditional laparoscopic appendectomy or open appendectomy may be the better surgical approach for the contraindications mentioned above.

However, the list of contraindications is likely to decrease as transvaginal appendectomy advances and surgeon expertise increases.

Patient Positioning

After general anesthesia, the patient is placed in the low lithotomy (Lloyd-Davies) position in Allen stirrups. The arms are tucked to the patient's sides. The shoulders need to be padded and protected as there is a tendency for the

Fig. 18.1 Positioning of surgeon and assistant for pure transvaginal appendectomy

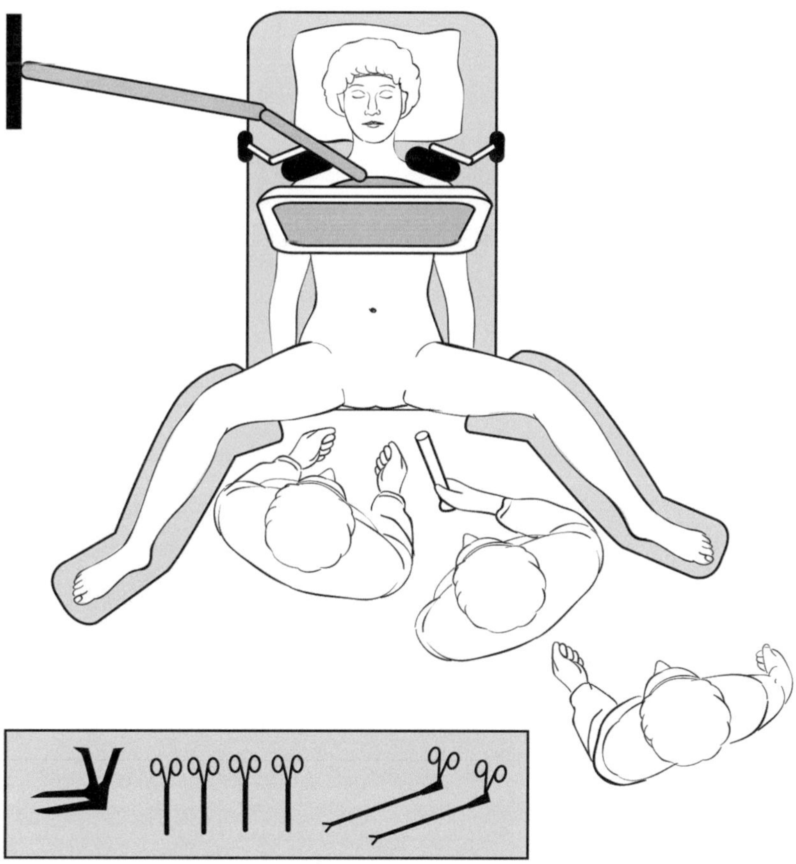

patient to slide during the necessary steep Trendelenburg position during the case. The vagina is disinfected with a topical antiseptic solution, usually povidone-iodine, and a urinary catheter is placed. The abdomen is also prepped and draped. Antibiotic prophylaxis is typically given unless the patient was placed on antibiotics for an acute infection. The operating surgeon is positioned between the patient's legs, and when hybrid laparoscopic procedures are performed, a first assistant is on the patient's left (Fig. 18.1).

Operative Approaches

Currently, most transvaginal appendectomies are performed using the pure transvaginal technique or the hybrid transvaginal technique with either flexible or rigid instruments.

Pure Transvaginal Appendectomy

Access to the peritoneal cavity during pure transvaginal appendectomy is obtained by incising the mucosa of the posterior fornix of the vagina with entry into the peritoneum in the cul-de-sac, with or without assistance from a gynecologist depending on the comfort level of the general surgeon with transvaginal anatomy. A weighted speculum is introduced to the vagina, and a uterine retractor is used to lift the uterus anteriorly to expose the posterior vaginal fornix. The cervix is grasped with a single-toothed tenaculum and retracted anteriorly. The colpotomy is created transversely in the posterior fornix using electrocautery or, alternatively, using scissors. Specific landmarks have been described to identify "the triangle of safety" within the posterior fornix [13], using the base of the cervix and the rectovaginal fold (Figs. 18.2 and 18.3).

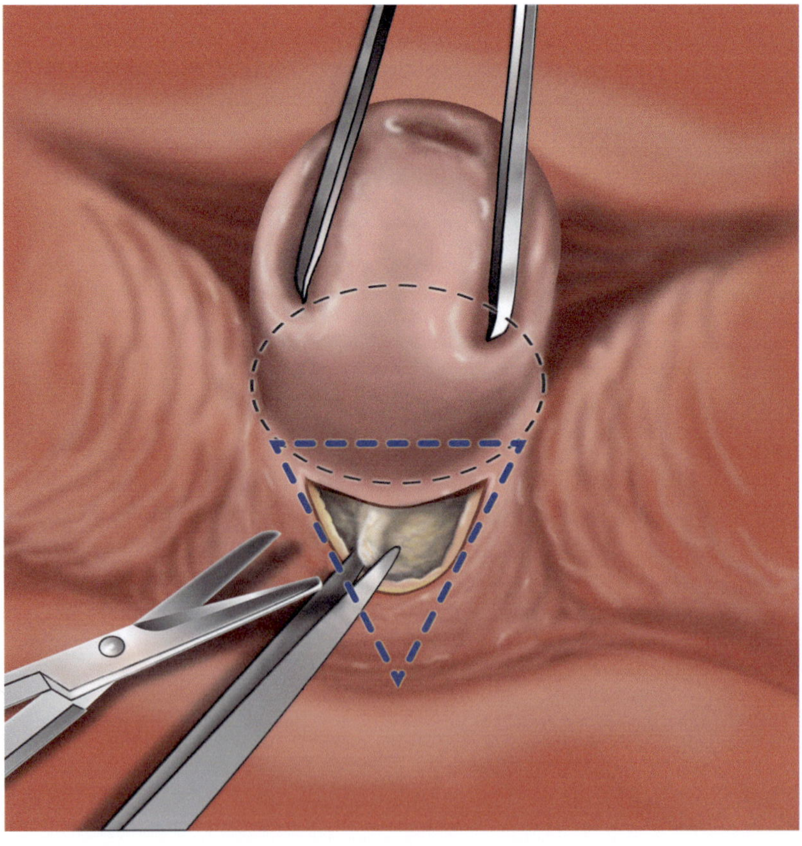

Fig. 18.2 Triangle of safety allows safe entry into the abdominal cavity when the access is angled upward toward the umbilicus. The *circle* is the base of the cervix. The *upper corners of the triangle* are at the 4 and 8 o'clock of the cervix and the *lower corner in the middle* of the rectovaginal fold

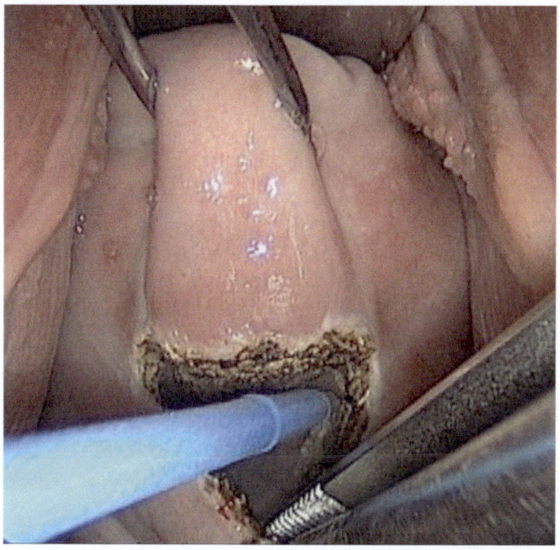

Fig. 18.3 Transvaginal abdominal access obtained with electrocautery

Pure Rigid Laparoscopic Approach

The pure rigid laparoscopic appendectomy technique employs the use of a SILS™ port (Covidien, Mansfield, MA) that is inserted into the colpotomy site (Fig. 18.4) [14]. Two 5-mm ports and one 12-mm port are used. The right lower quadrant of the abdomen is inspected, and the appendix is identified (Fig. 18.5). A flexible endograsper may be used to elevate the appendix medially and superiorly, so that the mesoappendix and base can be adequately visualized.

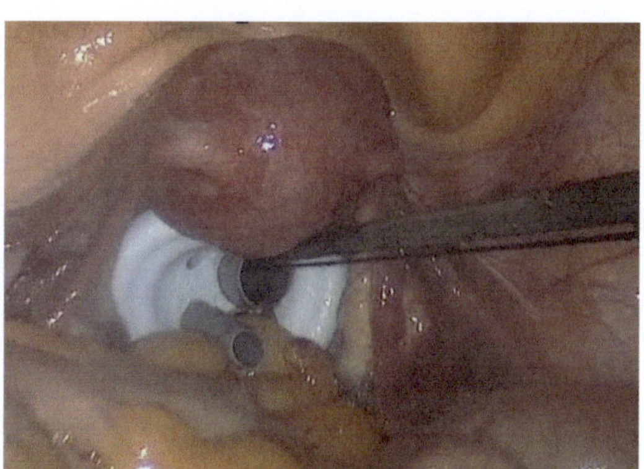

Fig. 18.4 Transumbilical view of SILS port within the colpotomy

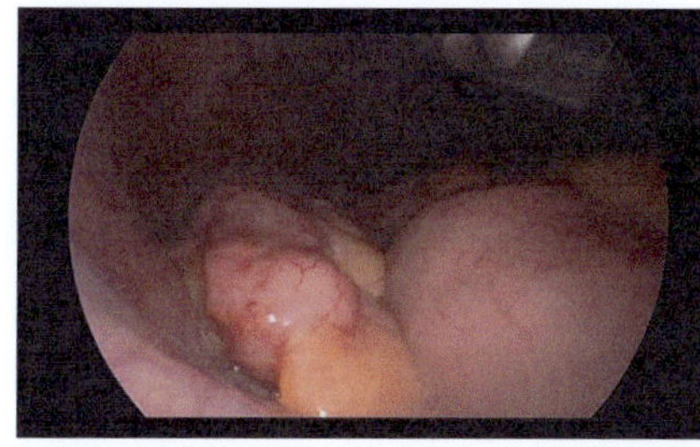

Fig. 18.5 First transvaginal view of appendix

A Maryland dissector is passed through the port and used to dissect the appendix at its base of the mesoappendix. The appendix is divided at the ceco-appendiceal junction with a stapler (Fig. 18.6). The mesoappendix is divided using an ultrasonic dissector, a ligating cautery device, or a stapler (Fig. 18.7). Then, the appendix is placed in a retrieval bag and removed (Fig. 18.8). The staple lines are inspected for completeness and hemostasis (Fig. 18.9).

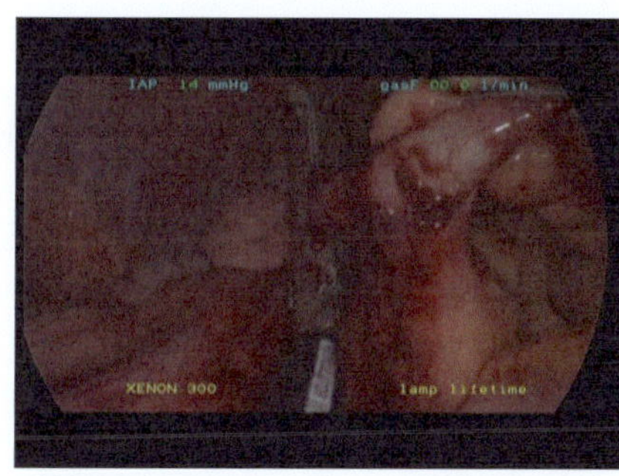

Fig. 18.6 Stapling of the appendix at the ceco-appendiceal junction

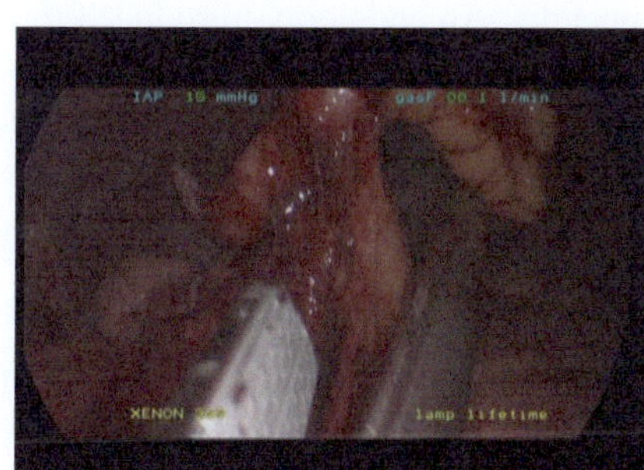

Fig. 18.7 Stapling of the mesoappendix

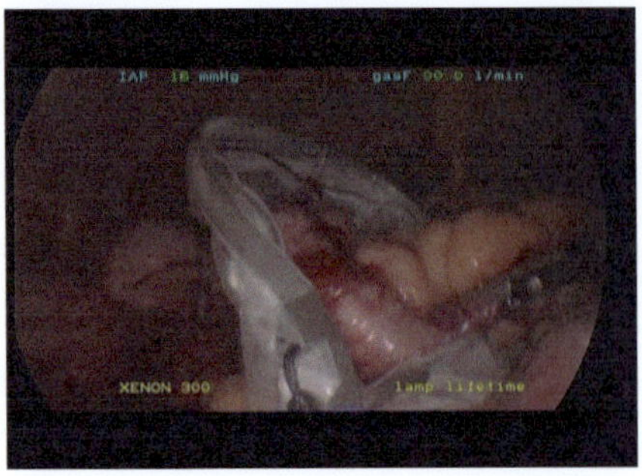

Fig. 18.8 Placement of appendix into specimen retrieval bag

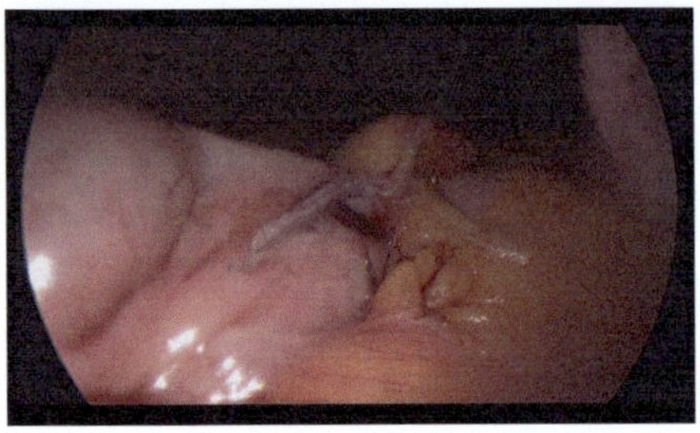

Fig. 18.9 Inspection of staple lines

Pure Flexible Endoscopic Approach

A single-channel endoscope (gastroscope or colonoscope) is introduced after the colpotomy is made. Carbon dioxide insufflation can be achieved through the endoscope, or alternatively, a Veress needle introduced at the umbilicus can be used. Endoscopic instruments passed through the working endoscope channels are used for dissection of the appendix. The endoscopic needle-knife cautery is used to dissect the mesoappendix. An endoloop, introduced through the channel, is used for ligation of the base of the appendix. A second endoloop is placed slightly distal to the first, and the appendix is sharply transected between the endoloops with endoscopic scissors or needle-knife cautery. Grasping the free end of the endoloop with an endoscopic grasper, the appendix can be retrieved from the abdominal cavity [10, 11].

Hybrid Transvaginal Appendectomy

In hybrid transvaginal appendectomy, access to the peritoneal cavity is first obtained transumbilically with a Veress needle. Capnoperitoneum is established to a pressure of 15 mm Hg, and a 5-mm trocar is placed through the umbilical incision. The patient is placed in steep Trendelenburg position, and the pelvis is inspected for adhesions that obliterate the pouch of Douglas. In the absence of these findings, the uterus is elevated with a uterine retractor (Humi retractor). Once the "triangle of safety" is exposed, the colpotomy is performed with simultaneous direct laparoscopic visualization of the cul-de-sac by penetrating the posterior fornix of the vagina with a trocar. Alternatively, scissors or electrocautery may be used.

Hybrid Rigid Laparoscopic Approach

Knuth et al. [5] placed a transvaginal 5-mm trocar followed by an adjacent 13-mm trocar for the camera and stapler. Standard, rigid laparoscopic instruments are used. The laparoscope can alternate between the transvaginal or transumbilical port as needed for optimal visualization. A transvaginal, rigid, curved, grasper forceps is introduced to retract the appendix. The mesoappendix can be divided with a stapler, coagulation, clips, or a combination of these. The specimen is retrieved transvaginally through the 13-mm port.

Hybrid Flexible Endoscopic Approach

The working ports of the transvaginal endoscope are used to proceed with appendiceal dissection similar to the pure endoscopic approach described above. The umbilical port acts as an added working port for a grasper to retract the appendix. Endoscopic coagulation forceps are used to dissect the mesoappendix, and the appendiceal artery is coagulated [15, 16]. Alternatively, the endoscopic graspers are used to retract or lift the tip of appendix, and the mesoappendix is dissected free using an ultrasonic dissector introduced through the umbilical port [17]. Endoscopic graspers retract the appendix, and a laparoscopic snaring device is introduced via the umbilical port to ligate the base of the appendix. Transection of the appendix is made with laparoscopic scissors or the ultrasonic scalpel. The specimen is recovered transvaginally.

The addition of a transvaginal 12-mm trocar parallel to the endoscope can allow the use of a laparoscopic linear stapler when encountering difficulty with ligating the base of appendix [16]. Jacobsen et al. [6] described placing a dual-lumen, 15-mm trocar through the colpotomy to accommodate both the endoscope and additional operating instruments. The appendix is retracted using a percutaneous endoloop, and the mesoappendix is ligated with the ultrasonic dissector placed through the umbilical port. The appendiceal base is transected with a transvaginally placed articulating laparoscopic linear stapler, and the appendix is retrieved within an endoscopic retrieval bag.

Closure

At the completion of both pure and hybrid transvaginal appendectomy techniques, pneumoperitoneum is released and primary closure of the colpotomy is performed with a running, braided, absorbable suture under direct visualization (Fig. 18.10). Postoperatively, most surgeons recommend 2–4 weeks of pelvic rest before resuming vaginal intercourse. Some surgeons elect to perform a routine gynecological pelvic examination at 2–4 weeks postoperatively, although the necessity and benefit remain unclear.

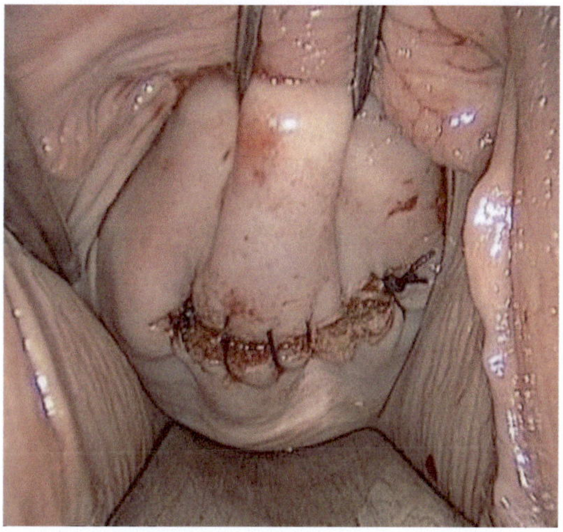

Fig. 18.10 Colpotomy closure

Complications

Potential complications of transvaginal appendectomies may be extrapolated from the gynecologic literature, namely the complications of culdoscopy (accessing the abdominal cavity through the posterior fornix), which is performed as an office procedure for the evaluation of infertility, for the treatment of polycystic ovarian disease, or for the harvest of oocytes. One potential complication described is bowel or rectal injury, which occurs in approximately 0.25% of cases [18]. Other potential adverse effects from a gynecologic perspective include the formation of adhesions and spread of preexisting endometriosis.

Although the potential for infertility or dyspareunia was once a concern, the uterus is only passed by and uninjured on the way to the posterior fornix, so any effect on potential childbearing is highly unlikely and has never been shown in the literature.

Also extrapolated from the gynecologic literature is that preservation of sexual function with transvaginal access for hysterectomy is similar to that associated with transabdominal access [19]. However, patients commonly are recommended to refrain from vaginal intercourse for a period of 2 weeks.

Surgical Instruments

The following equipment and instruments are used for the transvaginal pure NOTES appendectomy approach:

- Vaginal retractor kit,
- Standard laparoscopic kit,
- Electrocautery,
- SILS™ port (Covidien, Mansfield, MA),
- Laparoscope (30°, 5 mm),
- Flexible endograsper, and
- Endoscopic stapler.

Recent Outcome Reports

Roberts et al. [14] compared pure transvaginal appendectomy as described above to conventional laparoscopic appendectomy. The transvaginal mean operating room time was 44 min. Length of stay and operative times between conventional laparoscopic and transvaginal appendectomy patients were similar. The transvaginal appendectomy patients reported a faster recovery compared to the laparoscopic patients. Of note, there was a decreased need for postoperative analgesia, and faster return to work or normal activity for the transvaginal appendectomy patients.

Bernhardt et al. [16] compared 10 laparoscopic appendectomy patients to 10 hybrid transvaginal endoscopic appendectomy patients. The median operating time in the transvaginal group was 75 min compared to 40 min for the laparoscopy group. A shorter hospital stay was noted for the transvaginal compared to the laparoscopic patients. The transvaginal patients reported a more rapid postoperative recovery to normal activities, health, and wellness compared to the laparoscopic group.

Transvaginal Versus Conventional Laparoscopic Appendectomy

In the few studies comparing transvaginal to laparoscopic appendectomy to date, the operative time was shown to be significantly greater for transvaginal appendectomy compared to laparoscopic appendectomy [14, 20].

Postoperatively, transvaginal appendectomy patients were shown to have shorter length of hospital stay, less opioid requirement, and faster recovery to normal activities. Albrecht et al. [20] noted higher cosmetic satisfaction in the transvaginal group compared to laparoscopic group. Two studies assessing female sexual function noted that the female sexual function scores were unaffected by the transvaginal approach [16, 21].

Rigid Versus Flexible Endoscopic Transvaginal Appendectomy

To date, there are no studies directly comparing endoscopic to laparoscopic transvaginal appendectomy. However, the employment of standard laparoscopic instruments for transvaginal appendectomy may shorten the overall operative time compared to endoscopic instruments [5, 14]. The lack of a standard endoscopic platform creates a barrier to application for intra-abdominal surgery. Both techniques appear to have similar complication rates.

Hybrid Versus Pure Transvaginal Approach

The hybrid transvaginal appendectomy is a more common approach. This is likely due to visualization of safe entry of the transvaginal port and adds a working port optimizing triangulation of the appendix [22]. This approach may be technically easier and may shorten the learning curve. However, there are no studies yet comparing outcomes of pure to hybrid transvaginal appendectomy.

Summary

The application of NOTES transvaginal appendectomy for acute appendicitis seems to be favorable. In the setting of uncomplicated appendicitis, the transvaginal appendectomy has been shown to be safe and efficacious. No specific transvaginal approach, pure or hybrid, using endoscopic or laparoscopic instruments, has been shown to be superior. Yet, the hybrid approach may be technically easier and therefore safer over the pure transvaginal approach for most surgeons. Several studies of transvaginal appendectomy suggest that there is a faster recovery to normal activities and improved cosmetic results compared to conventional laparoscopic appendectomy. It is important to mention that as of today there are no randomized controlled trials, and therefore, the accumulated knowledge about the risks and benefits of a transvaginal appendectomy has to be viewed with caution. Overall, transvaginal appendectomy in the management of acute appendicitis is a viable option for patients.

References

1. Addiss DG, Shaffer N, Fowler BS, Tauxe RV. The epidemiology of appendicitis and appendectomy in the United States. Am J Epidemiol. 1990;132 (5):910–25.
2. McBurney C II. The indications for early laparotomy in appendicitis. Ann Surg. 1891;13(4):233–54.
3. Semm K. Endoscopic appendectomy. Endoscopy. 1983;15(2):59–64.
4. Rao GV, Reddy DN, Banerjee R. NOTES: human experience. Gastrointestinal endoscopy clinics of North America. 2008;18(2):361–70; x.
5. Knuth J, Heiss MM, Bulian DR. Transvaginal hybrid-NOTES appendectomy in routine clinical use: prospective analysis of 13 cases and description of the procedure. Surg Endosc. 2014;28(9):2661–5.
6. Jacobsen GR, Barajas-Gamboa JS, Coker AM, Cheverie J, Macias CA, et al. Transvaginal organ extraction: potential for broad clinical application. Surg Endosc. 2014;28(2):484–91.
7. Bueno B. Primer caso de apendicectomia por via vaginal. Tokoginecol Pract. 1949;8(72):152–8.
8. Palanivelu C, Rajan PS, Rangarajan M, Parthasarathi R, Senthilnathan P, et al. Transvaginal endoscopic appendectomy in humans: a unique approach to NOTES–world's first report. Surg Endosc. 2008;22(5):1343–7.
9. Tsin DA, Colombero LT, Mahmood D, Padouvas J, Manolas P. Operative culdolaparoscopy: a new approach combining operative culdoscopy and minilaparoscopy. J Am Assoc Gynecol Laparosc. 2001;8 (3):438–41.
10. Bernhardt J, Gerber B, Schober HC, Kahler G, Ludwig K. NOTES—case report of a unidirectional flexible appendectomy. Int J Colorectal Dis. 2008;23 (5):547–50.
11. Tabutsadze T, Kipshidze N. New trend in endoscopic surgery: transvaginal appendectomy NOTES (Natural Orifice Transluminal Endoscopic Surgery). Georgian Med News. 2009;168:7–10.
12. Nezhat C, Datta MS, Defazio A, Nezhat F, Nezhat C. Natural orifice-assisted laparoscopic appendectomy. JSLS. 2009;13(1):14–8.
13. Roberts K, Solomon D, Bell R, Duffy A. "Triangle of safety": anatomic considerations in transvaginal natural orifice surgery. Surg Endosc. 2013;27 (8):2963–5.
14. Roberts KE, Solomon D, Mirensky T, Silasi DA, Duffy AJ, et al. Pure transvaginal appendectomy versus traditional laparoscopic appendectomy for acute appendicitis: a prospective cohort study. Ann Surg. 2012;255(2):266–9.
15. Noguera JF, Cuadrado A, Sanchez-Margallo FM, Dolz C, Asencio JM, et al. Emergency transvaginal hybrid natural orifice transluminal endoscopic surgery. Endoscopy. 2011;43(5):442–4.
16. Bernhardt J, Steffen H, Schneider-Koriath S, Ludwig K. Clinical NOTES appendectomy study: comparison of transvaginal NOTES appendectomy in hybrid technique with laparoscopic appendectomy. Int J Colorectal Dis. 2015;30(2):259–67.
17. Shin EJ, Jeong GA, Jung JC, Cho GS, Lim CW, Kim HC, et al. Transvaginal endoscopic appendectomy. J Korean Soc Coloproctol. 2010;26(6):429–32.
18. Gordts S, Watrelot A, Campo R, Brosens I. Risk and outcome of bowel injury during transvaginal pelvic endoscopy. Fertil Steril. 2001;76(6):1238–41.
19. Mokate T, Wright C, Mander T. Hysterectomy and sexual function. J Br Menopause Soc. 2006;12 (4):153–7.
20. Albrecht R, Bochmann C, Susse A, Jablonski L, Settmacher U. Hybrid NOS appendectomy (NA): clinical assessment of a new surgical technique. Zentralbl Chir. 2013;138(4):449–55.

21. Solomon D, Lentz R, Duffy AJ, Bell RL, Roberts KE. Female sexual function after pure transvaginal appendectomy: a cohort study. J Gastrointest Surg. 2012;16(1):183–6; discussion 6–7.

22. Yagci MA, Kayaalp C. Transvaginal appendectomy: a systematic review. Minim Invasive Surg. 2014;2014:384706.

NOTES Transvaginal Sleeve Gastrectomy

19

Shanglei Liu, Santiago Horgan and Garth R. Jacobsen

Abstract

Sleeve gastrectomy has become one of the most commonly performed operations in the world. Given the difficulties with incisions in morbidly obese patients, strategies to reduce the number of incisions (and thus potential complications) could be beneficial. NOTES has gained the interest of surgeons as the next evolution in minimally invasive surgery. Using a NOTES approach for sleeve gastrectomy, specifically for organ extraction, has the potential to reduce postoperative pain and incisional hernias after sleeve gastrectomy.

Keywords

Sleeve gastrectomy · NOTES · Transvaginal · Organ extraction

Abbreviations

NOTES	Natural orifice translumenal endoscopic surgery
TE	Transesophageal
TG	Transgastric
TR	Transrectal
TV	Transvaginal

S. Liu (✉)
Department of Surgery, UCSD Healthcare Systems, 200 West Arbor Drive, San Diego, CA 92103, USA
e-mail: s5liu@ucsd.edu

S. Horgan · G.R. Jacobsen
Center for the Future of Surgery, Department of Surgery, University of California at San Diego, San Diego, CA, USA
e-mail: SHorgan@ucsd.edu

G.R. Jacobsen
e-mail: GJacobsen@ucsd.edu

J.R. Romanelli et al. (eds.), *NOTES and Endoluminal Surgery*, Clinical Gastroenterology, DOI 10.1007/978-3-319-50610-4_19

Background

The adoption of minimally invasive surgical techniques in the past 20 years has made special advances in the weight loss surgery arena. The advantages of minimally invasive surgery include fewer wound complications, shorter hospital stays, less postoperative pain, and better cosmetic results [1]. Laparoscopic sleeve gastrectomy has become the most common surgical treatment for morbid obesity over the last decade [2]. In the last 5 years, natural orifice transluminal endoscopic surgery (NOTES) has quickly gained the interest of surgeons as the next natural evolution of minimally invasive surgery. NOTES access routes that have been utilized include transgastric (TG), transrectal (TR), transvaginal (TV), and transesophageal (TE) [3]. Small organ extractions (cholecystectomy) were first reported in two small series with no complications in the late 2000s [4, 5]. Since then, the application of NOTES has expanded to the realm of weight loss surgery, specifically sleeve gastrectomy [6]. In this chapter, we will review the operative techniques used at our institution for transvaginal sleeve gastrectomy.

Justification for a NOTES Approach

A basic principle of NOTES is to minimize abdominal incisions by utilizing a natural orifice such as the vagina as a viable route for intra-abdominal access. In addition to the obvious benefit of better cosmesis with fewer external scars, the advantages of NOTES over laparoscopic operations may be decreased incision-related complications such as postoperative pain and incisional hernias, although published data are lacking.

Incisional hernias specifically are of major consideration after surgery for the obese patient. The incidence of postoperative incisional hernias after midline laparotomy reaches as high as 24% for obese and 51% for the super-obese patients [7]. Even with laparoscopic techniques, obese patients experience hernia rates of 1.9% when using 12-mm trocars, and approaching 6% when patients' BMI exceed 30 [8]. This hernia rate is likely to be increased at the port site where the excised stomach is extracted because blunt spreading of the fascia is often needed for organ extraction.

NOTES is postulated to be beneficial for several reasons. Given the high BMI of patients typically requiring sleeve gastrectomy, they stand to benefit from decreasing abdominal trocar insertions due to higher surgical site complications. This is one of the greatest benefits of NOTES. Additionally, in transvaginal sleeve gastrectomy the gastric remnant is removed through the colpotomy. This avoids additional stretching of the abdominal fascia where the remnant is removed in the pure laparoscopic approach. Hernia occurrence at the wall of the colpotomy is an event that should be much rarer compared to abdominal incisional hernias. Finally, the usage of a flexible endoscopy through the vaginal trocar may allow a more diverse viewing angle not offered by the top-down view of traditional laparoscope.

Preoperative Workup/Patient Selection

The patient undergoing preoperative planning for transvaginal sleeve gastrectomy must undergo the same selection process as that of laparoscopic sleeve gastrectomy, with a few additional selection criteria. Briefly, the preoperative workup for weight loss surgery should include the following:

1. Medical evaluation for underlying metabolic conditions as well as optimal medical management of comorbidities,
2. Psychological evaluation for underlying psychological disorders and the ability to undergo dramatic dietary change,
3. Dietician evaluation and teaching to optimized nutritional support before and after the surgery,
4. Trial weight loss on regimented medical weight loss program before surgery,
5. Anesthesia evaluation for perioperative morbidity,

6. Surgical evaluation, and
7. Patient understanding and commitment to a strict, small-volume, progressive liquid diet postoperatively, and close dietician follow-up.

Additionally, the inclusion criteria for the consideration for transvaginal sleeve gastrectomy would include the following:

1. Female gender,
2. Age 18–65,
3. ASA Classification 1 or 2,
4. Morbid obesity per NIH criteria for weight loss surgery,
5. Normal pap smear within 12 months to rule out malignancy,
6. Normal OB-GYN exam within 12 months, and
7. Desire for surgical treatment for obesity.

Exclusion criteria would include the following:

1. Pregnancy,
2. Evidence of intra-abdominal abscess or mass,
3. Sepsis or peritonitis,
4. Prior major abdominal surgery (previous cesarean section is a relative contraindication),
5. History of ectopic pregnancy,
6. Pelvic inflammatory disease,
7. Severe endometriosis,
8. Previous perineal trauma, and
9. Pelvic or abdominal malignancy.

Equipment List

Endoscopic Equipment

Two standard single- or double-channel endoscopes (Olympus America, Center Valley, PA) are used in this procedure. These scopes will be separated during the procedure to prevent cross-contamination, as one will used for intraluminal evaluation while the other is used for transvaginal intra-abdominal visualization. This also requires the use of two separate endoscopic towers, although it is feasible to use only one tower and switch between the two devices as long as sterility is maintained for the transvaginal scope. Endoscopic graspers or endoscopic snares will also be needed. Because of the larger than average amount of tissue expected to be handled by the endoscope, a larger-toothed grasper should be employed.

Laparoscopic Equipment

Standard bariatric laparoscopic equipment will be needed. Laparoscopic linear staplers will also be used to create the tubularized stomach. Though devices may vary, stapler loads able to accommodate up to 4.5 mm in tissue thickness should be used and adjusted on a case-by-case basis during the operation. Finally, an advanced energy tissue sealer device is needed for dissection. Our experience has been using the ultrasound dissector (Harmonic Scalpel™, Ethicon Endosurgery Inc., Cincinnati, OH), but it may be up to surgeon preference to use bipolar energy division.

Technique

Patient Positioning/OR Planning

Patients are placed in a split leg position with hips lying flat in neutral position (Fig. 19.1). This minimizes any interference between the patient's legs and the laparoscopic instruments. Both arms can be extended. A urinary catheter should be placed and the vagina prepared with iodine-based surgical prep solution. Extra foam padding is placed under the knees and ankles by the surgical team in order prevent compressive tissue and nerve injuries.

The head of the patient's bed should have a laparoscopic monitor and enough room for a surgeon to perform upper endoscopy at the beginning of the case. We typically place our first endoscopy tower to the left of the patient, at the head of the operating table. A second endoscopy tower is placed just next to the patient's left foot.

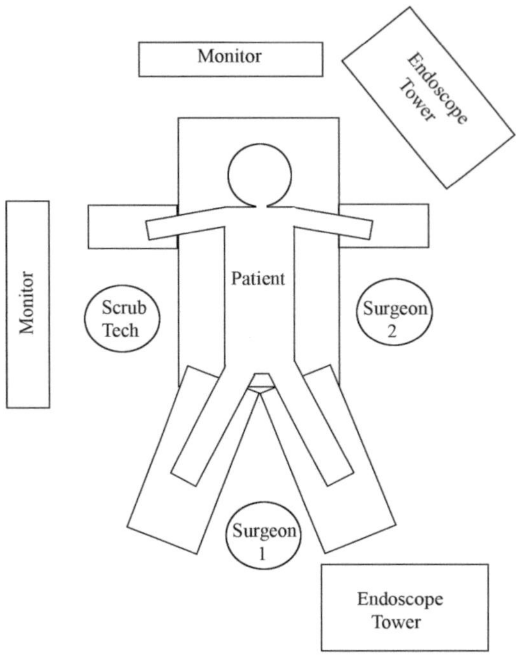

Fig. 19.1 Patient positioning along with layout of the operating room

There should be enough room between the patient's legs for the main operating surgeon to stand and operate. The assistant surgeon should be positioned on the patient's left and the scrub technician to the right of the assistant surgeon. The right side of the patient is reserved for surgical towers, an additional monitor facing the assisting surgeon, suction, and other equipment (Fig. 19.1). There should also be enough space to access the right side of the operating table at the beginning of the case to secure a liver retractor such as a Nathanson.

Perioperative Endoscopy

After intubation and initiation of general anesthesia, an upper endoscopy is first performed to evaluate the intraluminal health of the stomach and esophagus. We advocate only proceeding if there is no evidence of gastritis, ulcer, or other pathologies of the stomach or esophagus. If an abnormality is detected, then the operation should be aborted until a later time when optimal medical management is complete. After evaluation, either the scope or a separate sizing device such as a bougie can be left in the stomach as a guide for resection later.

Transvaginal Access/Colpotomy

The first step in performing a transvaginal sleeve gastrectomy is to obtain transvaginal access. Sterile surgical draping should be donned over the patient's abdomen and perineal area. The vagina is examined for any inflammation or infections, which would be a contraindication to proceeding. Early on in our learning curve, this examination should be done by a gynecologist experienced in vaginal surgery, who would assist for the colpotomy access as well. After several procedures, the bariatric surgeon should be comfortable performing the colpotomy access independently, although they may need to get separate operative privileges for this from their institution.

A 5-mm trocar is placed through the umbilicus under direct visualization and pneumoperitoneum is established via CO_2 through this trocar. An exploratory laparoscopy is then performed via a 5-mm laparoscope before proceeding with the colpotomy. The abdomen is examined for any aberrant anatomy, adhesions, and mobility of the uterus. Once complete, we proceed with the colpotomy.

A speculum is placed into the vagina for visualization. Either a uterine manipulator or a surgical clamp is placed on the cervix. This is used in order to elevate the uterus into an anteverted position. At this point, the patient is placed in steep Trendelenburg position. The posterior vaginal mucosa is exposed, and an incision is made through the cul-de-sac just anterior to the rectum but posterior to the cervix. A 15-mm dilating trocar is then inserted through the colpotomy under direct visualization both externally as well as intra-abdominally (Fig. 19.2).

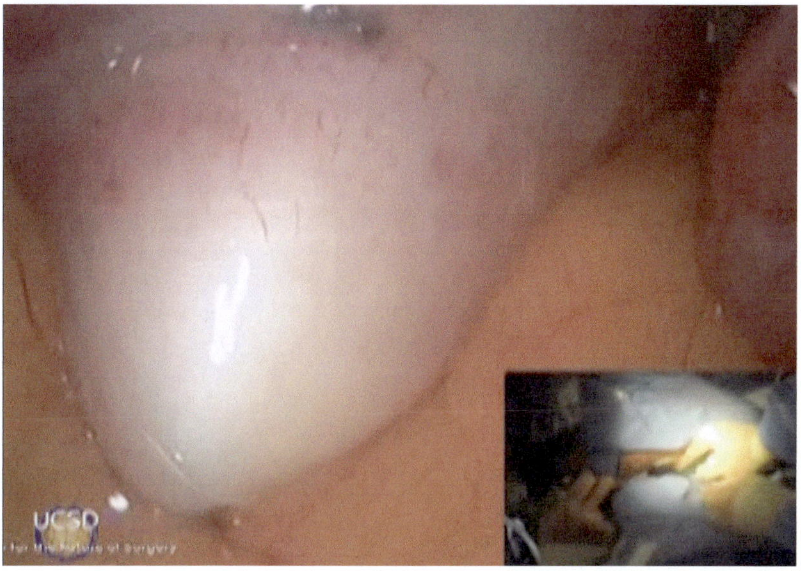

Fig. 19.2 Laparoscopic view of the posterior colpotomy trocar being inserted

Sleeve Gastrectomy

After establishing transvaginal access, a liver retractor can be placed (though not required) through the subxiphoid region to elevate the left lobe of the liver in order for adequate visualization of the crus and gastroesophageal junction. A 5-mm transabdominal trocar is placed in the right upper quadrant of the abdomen to assist in the procedure. Finally, a 12-mm transabdominal trocar is placed in the left upper quadrant to accommodate the passage of a linear laparoscopic stapler. The insufflation throughout the case will be provided through this trocar via standard CO_2 laparoscopic insufflator. [9] At this point, visualization is switched to the 15-mm transvaginal port via the flexible endoscope.

The gastrocolic ligament and short gastric vessels are divided with the ultrasonic dissector or similar advanced energy dissector starting 8 cm from the pylorus, and extending cranially to the left crus. The posterior aspect of the fundus is cleared of its attachments until the decussation of the left crus is identified as well to ensure adequate mobilization.

A laparoscopic stapler is then placed through the 12-mm transabdominal port to perform a vertical gastrectomy and create a tubular gastric remnant (Fig. 19.3). Sequential staple firings are used with thicker staplers toward the antrum (Fig. 19.4). The endoscope used at the beginning of the case now serves as a bougie for the gastric sleeve. If one is to use this method rather than a larger bougie, care needs to be taken not to hug the endoscope as this would result in a narrow caliber sleeve, predisposing the patient to leak. One must be extremely mindful of over-narrowing the sleeve at the level of the incisura, the result of which can be problematic.

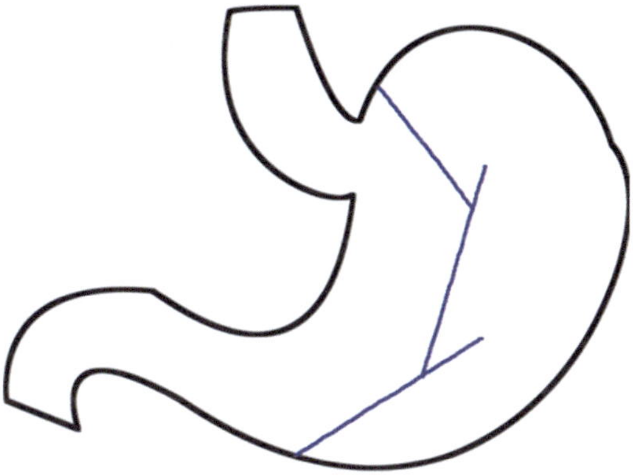

Fig. 19.3 Planned stapler routes for sleeve gastrectomy

Alternatively, the surgeon can use the bougie they usually would employ for a sleeve gastrectomy. It would be nice to completely remove the larger abdominal trocars in favor of placement of

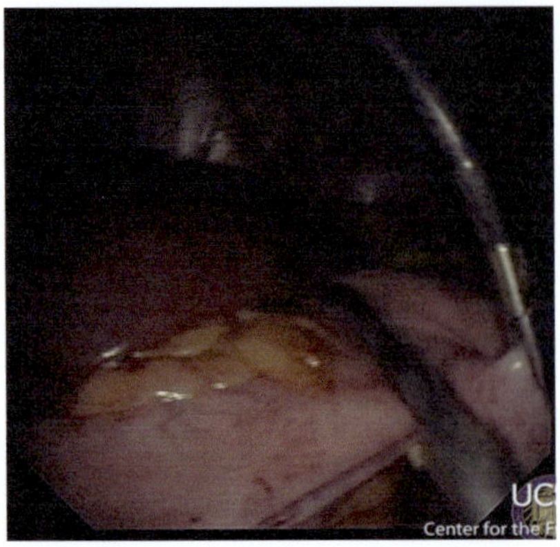

Fig. 19.4 Placing staples along the greater curvature using the endoscope as camera

the stapler through the larger transvaginal port. However, without the aid of a flexible linear stapler, the angle that the rigid stapler approaches the stomach from the transvaginal trocar tends to be prohibitive. The sacral promontory puts the stapler on a trajectory toward the anterior abdominal wall precluding adequate stapling of the stomach. We have been unable to overcome this limitation with standard staplers. This limitation of reaching upper abdominal viscera with rigid instrumentation from a transvaginal approach has been noted before [10].

Once complete, the staple line is inspected for leaks. Some surgeons advocate leak testing intraoperatively, although it is of unclear benefit

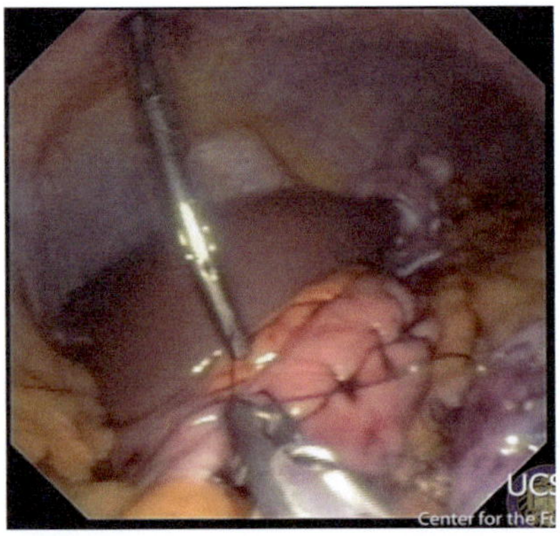

Fig. 19.5 Final evaluation of the cut edge of stomach after imbrication

as postoperative leaks tend to occur well after discharge from the hospital. In our series, we have imbricated the staple line with a running suture, and this is all performed with laparoscopic suturing techniques (Fig. 19.5).

Organ Extraction

The resected stomach is grasped with a snare from the transvaginal endoscope and removed with the vaginal trocar (Fig. 19.6). The orientation of the excised stomach for extraction is key in facilitating an easy extraction. Often times the excised stomach has a jagged appearance on the staple line side due to efforts taken to create a smooth and rounded gastric remnant. Because of this, extraction is greatly facilitated by grasping the anatomical proximal portion (fundus) of the excised stomach and removing it first with the vaginal trocar. Large surgical clamps can be used externally for traction during this process.

Closure

At the end of the procedure, pneumoperitoneum is deflated and all the trocars are removed. Although not all surgeons routinely leave a drain after sleeve gastrectomy, we still prefer to do so. A Jackson-Pratt drain is thus left through the right upper quadrant 5-mm trocar site, with the end terminating at the angle of His. The colpotomy is sutured closed in figure-of-eight stitches under direct visualization using absorbable suture material such as 0-Vicryl (Fig. 19.7). The rest of the abdominal trocar sites are closed with subcutaneous closure only using absorbable suture such as 4-0 Monocryl, and wound adhesive is applied to the skin. In our experience, it is not necessary to apply transfascial sutures to trocar sites as long as the trocar used is no greater than 12 mm. Given that transfascial sutures tend to cause the most postoperative discomfort, we see this approach as one that may reduce postoperative pain and discomfort.

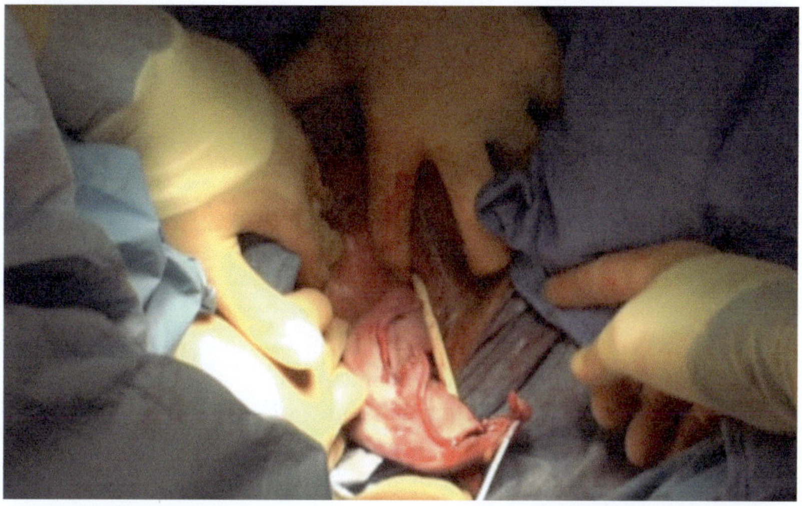

Fig. 19.6 Vaginal extraction of resected stomach

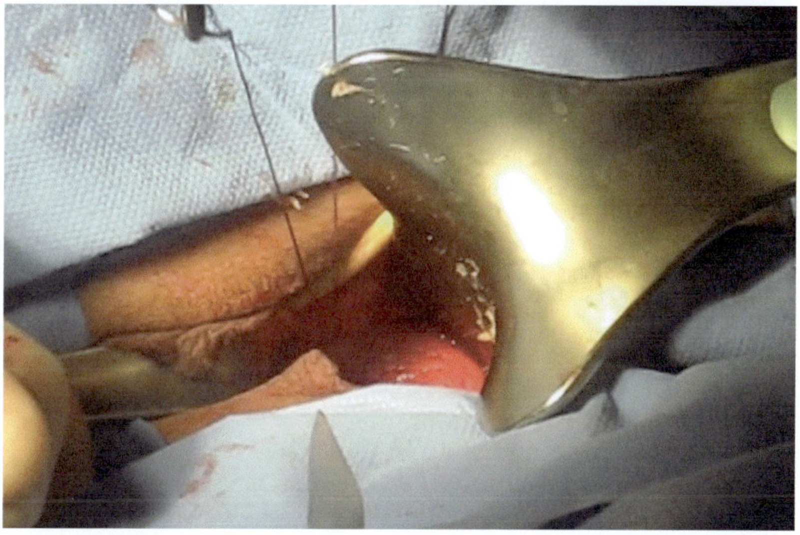

Fig. 19.7 Repair of the colpotomy under direct visualization

Postoperative Care

The postoperative care of transvaginal sleeve gastrectomy is identical to that of laparoscopic sleeve gastrectomy. It is acceptable to place the patients on a limited clear liquid diet postoperatively. Patients are expected to complete a Gastrografin swallow study on postoperative day 1 to demonstrate passage of contrast without extravasation. After this, patients are placed on a strictly regimented small-volume progressive liquid diet as per the preoperative discussion. The surgical drain can also be removed at this point if output is clear and minimal. Patients are typically discharged on postoperative day 1 or 2.

Surgical port pain after this procedure tends to be minimal and should be controlled adequately with acetaminophen or an oral narcotic as long as the medication can be given in liquid form for the first several days. Most patients do not complain of perineal or vaginal discomfort; however, mild spotting is to be expected. Patients should be advised to avoid tampon insertion or intercourse for at least 4 weeks to allow healing. They should also be instructed to call immediately or come to the emergency room if they experience any of symptoms of infection at the colpotomy site including: heavy bleeding (>1 pad per hour), foul smelling vaginal discharge, or erythema involving the entire perineal area.

Results

Transvaginal solid organ extraction has been previously described in 2012 in a series of 34 women [11]. In this study, 34 women underwent transvaginal organ extraction over the course of 5 years, with mean follow-up of 24 months. All patients were ASA classification of 2 or below. Average time of sleeve gastrectomy was 135 min with no conversions to open operations or intraoperative complications. The mean hospital stay of all cases was two days. In follow-up, there were two pregnancies and two successful vaginal deliveries. Six patients reported heavy menses immediately following the operation. There were no long-term complications and no mortalities.

Conclusion

The transvaginal approach to sleeve gastrectomy is an effective method to perform the operation. It poses few complications from the vaginal wall incision. The biggest benefit is that it avoids additional abdominal incisions for trocar placement and stomach extraction, which should decrease the rates of hernia and may possibly reduce postoperative pain. Other complications due to the sleeve gastrectomy itself (leak, fistula, stricture, gastric outlet obstruction, etc.) are not reduced or eliminated by the transvaginal approach and are presumed to occur at roughly the same rate as in laparoscopic sleeve gastrectomy.

References

1. Pelligrini C, Wetter LA, Patti M, LeichterR Mussan G, et al. Thoracopscopic esophagomyotomy: initial experience with a new approach for the treatment of achalasia. Ann Surg. 1992;216 (3):291–6.
2. ASMBS. Estimate of bariatric surgery numbers. www.asmbs.org. 2014;1. http://asmbs.org/2014/03/estimate-of-bariatric-surgery-numbers/.
3. Mintz Y, Horgan S, Cullen J, Ramamoorthy S, Chock A, et al. NOTES: the hybrid technique. J Laparoendosc Adv Surg Tech A. 2007;17(4): 402–6.
4. Zorron R, Soldan M, Filgueiras M, Maggioni LC, Pombo L, et al. NOTES: transvaginal for cancer diagnostic staging: preliminary clinical application. Surg Innov. 2008;15(3):161–5.
5. Zornig C, Mofid H, Siemssen L, Emmermann A, Alm M, et al. Transvaginal NOTES hybrid cholecystectomy: feasibility results in 68 cases with mid-term follow-up. Endoscopy. 2009;41(5):391–4.
6. Fischer LJ, Jacobsen G, Wong B, Thompson K, Bosia J, et al. NOTES laparoscopic-assisted transvaginal sleeve gastrectomy in humans-description of preliminary experience in the United States. Surg Obes Relat Dis. 2009; 5(5):633–6.
7. Arribas D, Elía M, Artigas C, Jiménez A, Anguilella V, et al. Incidence of incisional hernia following vertical banded gastroplasty. Hernia. 2004;8(2):135–7.
8. Mintz Y, Horgan S, Savu MK, Cullen J, Chock A, et al. Hybrid natural orifice translumenal surgery (NOTES) sleeve gastrectomy: a feasibility study using an animal model. Surg Endosc. 2008;22 (8):1798–802.
9. Meireles O, Kantsevoy SV, Kalloo AN, Jagannath SB, Giday SA, et al. Comparison of intraabdominal pressures using the gastroscope and laparoscope for transgastric surgery. Surg Endosc. 2007;21(6):998–1001.
10. Nakajima K, Souma Y, Takahashi T, Yamasaki M, Miyazaki Y, et al. Anatomical measurements to optimize instrumentation for transvaginal surgery. Surg Endosc. 2013;27(6):2052–7.
11. Jacobsen GR, Barajas-Gamboa JS, Coker AM, Cheverie J, Macias CA, et al. Transvaginal organ extraction: potential for broad clinical application. Surg Endosc. 2014;28(2):484–91.

Transvaginal Tubal Sterilization and Hysterectomy

20

Oz Harmanli

Abstract

In the growing world of ever less invasive surgery, minimalist approaches to hysterectomy have begun to proliferate. Vaginal hysterectomy (VH) is an old operation—dating to antiquity—that was widely used until the advent of laparoscopic surgery, although its use has declined as minimally invasive efforts, including the robotic approach, have grown in popularity. A thorough knowledge of pelvic anatomy and positioning is required to safely perform VH. This understanding of anatomy also allows for the performance of posterior colpotomy, which can be utilized for transvaginal approaches to other abdominal operations, as described in NOTES transvaginal surgery. Other transvaginal procedures, such as culdocentesis, culdotomy, and culdoscopy, are performed in a similar manner. Strategies for employing these techniques and potential complications to avoid are discussed in detail. Transvaginal sterilization, or tubal ligation, is also described, as are the complications of the procedure.

Keywords

Hysterectomy · Transvaginal surgery · Culdocentesis · Culdotomy · Culdoscopy · Tubal ligation

Abbreviations

LH	Laparoscopic hysterectomy
TAH	Total abdominal hysterectomy
THL	Transvaginal hydrolaparoscopy
VH	Vaginal hysterectomy

Oz. Harmanli (✉)
Chief, Yale Urogynecology & Reconstructive Pelvic Surgery, Professor, OB/GYN/RS, Department of OB/GYN/RS, Yale Medical School, 330 Cedar Street, Suite FMB 329B, New Haven, CT 06510, USA
e-mail: oz.harmanli@yale.edu

J.R. Romanelli et al. (eds.), *NOTES and Endoluminal Surgery*, Clinical Gastroenterology, DOI 10.1007/978-3-319-50610-4_20

Introduction

In any surgical discipline, the objective has always been to develop the least invasive, fastest, least complicated, and least expensive operative technique, with the shortest hospital stay. The motivation to achieve this goal has led to the birth of minimally invasive surgery, primarily with the advances in endoscopic instrumentation. In this age of minimally invasive surgery and growing interest in avoiding visible incisions, it is intuitive to think that in the field of gynecology, this would be best accomplished through the vagina, the natural orifice to the female genital system. Vaginal hysterectomy (VH), which has unfortunately been eclipsed by today's laparoscopic and robotic approaches, fits this definition very well. Transvaginal intraperitoneal access has a few other applications including tubal sterilization, infertility assessment, and ovarian and uterine surgery.

Vaginal Hysterectomy

If every hysterectomy candidate were made aware of an approach which offers no abdominal incision, i.e., vaginal hysterectomy (VH), she would undoubtedly not choose another route. If she were also told that this least invasive approach has been shown to minimize the complications, decrease operative and recovery times, and shorten hospital stay, there would probably be very few hysterectomies performed by any other technique (1). Systematic analysis provided by the Cochrane group has established that VH offers the lowest morbidity, least pain, fastest recovery, and quickest return to normal activities at a lower cost (2). Unfortunately, without the glamour of modern technology and support from the industry, VH is becoming a lost art.

The only contraindications to VH are advanced malignancy, pelvic mass of undetermined origin, and tubo-ovarian abscess (3). However, advanced skills may be required for certain conditions such as uterine size greater than 12 weeks' pregnancy, prior pelvic surgery such as cesarean delivery and myomectomy, nulliparity, suspected severe endometriosis, and suspected obliteration of cul-de-sac (3).

VH is typically performed for benign uterine conditions such as uterine leiomyoma, abnormal uterine bleeding, pelvic organ prolapse, and chronic pelvic pain. However, after consultation with gynecologic oncology, VH may also be suitable for precancerous or early-stage cancer of the cervix or endometrium, including severe cervical intraepithelial neoplasia, *in situ* or stage Ia1 cervical cancer, endometrial hyperplasia, and stage I, grade I endometrial cancer.

VH should not be attempted without good knowledge of fundamental pelvic anatomy. The major blood supply to the uterus is provided by the uterine arteries which reside in the cardinal ligaments. They communicate with ovarian arteries through their ascending branches on both sides. The ovarian arteries must also be occluded before removal of the uterus. The bladder is attached to the cervix with 1–2-cm-long supravaginal septum. Once it is incised, an avascular vesicouterine plane is entered. Placement of a retractor between the uterus and the bladder in this area protects not only the bladder but also the ureters. Although the ureters are just 1–1.5 cm lateral to the uterus at the level of uterine artery insertion, traction on the cervix with tenacula and deflection of the bladder by the retractor almost always prevent injury to the ureters. It is important to know that the rectum is not attached to the apical vagina. Under normal circumstances, the proximal posterior vagina is free by about 4 cm.

The informed consent process, for any type of hysterectomy, must cover alternative treatment options such as nonsurgical and uterine-sparing modalities. As there is growing circumstantial evidence associating fallopian tubes with the development of ovarian cancer, opportunistic salpingectomy is often recommended. While elective oophorectomy in women with average risk of ovarian cancer is not recommended before menopause, it can be offered to those remotely postmenopausal and with family history of hereditary and genital cancers. In addition to the general risks of surgery, those specific to hysterectomy must also be reviewed, including its association with future childbearing. Every hysterectomy candidate must be made aware that open or laparoscopic routes may be used if VH does not appear feasible intraoperatively.

In cases of anemia, it is a common practice to transfuse women until preoperative hemoglobin level is 10 g/L or greater and cross-matching blood products for them if there is not enough time for transfusion. Storing autologous blood for most hysterectomy procedures was not shown to be cost-effective in a large study. Preoperative Pap smear and endometrial sampling are indicated in women who have abnormal uterine bleeding, cervical intraepithelial neoplasia, or endometrial hyperplasia. In the event of suspicious pelvic masses and/or any abnormal uterine bleeding, preoperative transvaginal ultrasound is crucial. More invasive procedures such as dilatation and curettage and hysteroscopy are needed only in the presence of an inadequate office biopsy or, in the postmenopausal stage, or when endometrial thickness is greater than 4 mm on transvaginal ultrasound. Mechanical bowel preparation is not necessary.

Among all hysterectomy approaches, VH is the only one amenable to spinal or epidural anesthesia. Sequential compression boots and, when indicated, chemoprophylaxis for the prevention of venous thromboembolism are standard. Routine use of single-dose antibiotics has effectively reduced postoperative infectious complications.

Even though outpatient VH is possible when stringent criteria are used and close telephone follow-up is available, most gynecologists admit their patients for an overnight stay. Women should be advised to refrain from strenuous physical activity and intercourse for approximately 6 weeks.

History

It is not surprising that utilization of the vaginal route for gynecologic problems can be traced back to ancient Greek history. Vaginal excision of prolapsed uteri with urinary fistula formation was reported as early as 50 B.C. (4). VH in the modern world predates introduction of anesthesia. The German surgeon, Conrad Langenbeck, performed the first successful planned VH in 1813. It was not until 1843 that the first abdominal hysterectomy was performed by Charles Clay of England. He opened the abdomen hoping to remove an ovarian tumor, but ran into a leiomyomatous uterus instead. Unfortunately, the patient did not survive. Johann Nepomuk Sauter and Joseph Claude Recamier performed VH successfully in 1822 and 1824, respectively, and are also considered among the pioneers of VH in the German literature (5).

Alexander Freund, Vinzenz Czerny, and Jules Pean helped standardize VH in the ensuing years. Radical hysterectomy for gynecologic cancer was later introduced and popularized by Schuchardt and Ernst Wertheim for the abdominal approach, and by Friedrich Schauta for the vaginal route (6). Mortality from VH, which was at around 10–15% just before the turn of twentieth century, was reduced to 2.5% with the new improvements in instrumentation, anesthesia, and antisepsis. However, mortality from abdominal hysterectomy, which remained as high as 70% in 1880, started to decrease in the early twentieth century so dramatically that the abdominal route became more widely preferred (6).

Until the first total abdominal hysterectomy (TAH) performed by Richardson in 1929 in the USA, abdominal supracervical hysterectomy was a more common practice (5). TAH was widely adapted to prevent cervical cancer in the following decades. The morbidity and mortality of hysterectomy was further reduced with the advent of antibiotics and the availability of blood transfusion after World War II. Hysterectomy became one of the most common major surgical procedures performed by gynecologists, second only to cesarean deliveries. The abdominal route was chosen in approximately three quarters of hysterectomies until the first laparoscopically assisted hysterectomy by Harry Reich in 1988. The rate of laparoscopic hysterectomy (LH) has increased dramatically from 0.3% in 1990 to 14% in 2005, predominantly at the expense of abdominal hysterectomy rate which was reduced to 64%. Unfortunately, this enthusiasm for laparoscopy resulted in a small drop in the VH rate from 24 to 22% (7). As the laparoscopic approach became more popular, interest in supracervical hysterectomy resurfaced and gained increasing acceptability. Despite some new efforts to increase interest and skills for VH, gynecologists have been adapting to the robotic trend very quickly in recent years. The effects of more recent trends such as single-port laparoscopy remain to be seen.

Procedure

Possibly the most important factor for success in VH is positioning (Fig. 20.1a, b). The dorsal lithotomy position must allow enough space for the surgeon and two assistants between the patient's lower extremities. The thighs should be elevated to provide at least a 60° angle between the thigh and the torso, and at least 90° at the knee. Stirrups supporting the entire leg or "candy cane stirrups" are both appropriate. It is critical to extend the patient's buttocks slightly over the edge of the table. Trendelenburg position may improve access but it should not be too steep. Today, most vaginal surgeons stand during this procedure but those who sit prefer to elevate the chair/stool so that the assistants do not have to bend down.

Essential instruments for VH include weighted specula, retractors, tenacula, scissors, and clamps with special design and length. Some vaginal surgeons prefer a self-retaining vaginal retractor system. Lighting is also critically important, which can be improved with a headlight, lighted retractor, or suction/irrigation devices with lighting option.

The use of an indwelling urinary catheter is optional. Leaving some urine in the bladder may help the surgeon recognize cystotomy in a timely fashion. The procedure is initiated by grasping the cervix with tenacula anteriorly and posteriorly. Some may choose to inject vasoconstricting agents into the cervix before making an incision. This initial incision should be made outside the cervical transformation zone, at point of decreased vaginal rugae. Electrocautery can be used to make this incision.

To make the posterior colpotomy (Fig. 20.2a, b), one should first palpate the uterosacral ligaments and posterior fornix to identify the

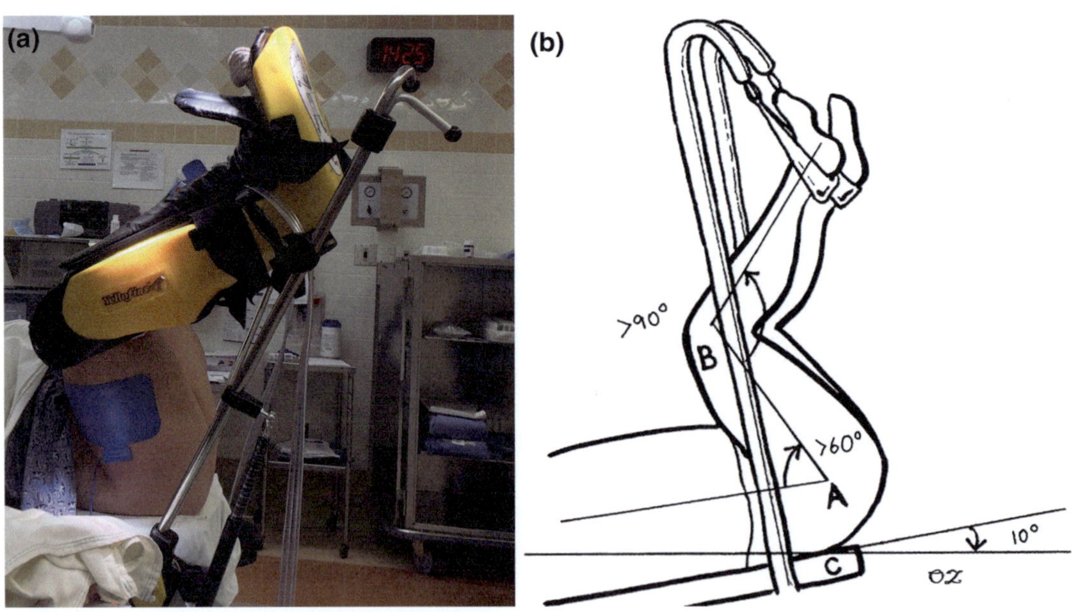

Fig. 20.1 Positioning for vaginal hysterectomy: both **a** stirrups supporting the entire leg and **b** candy cane stirrups are appropriate

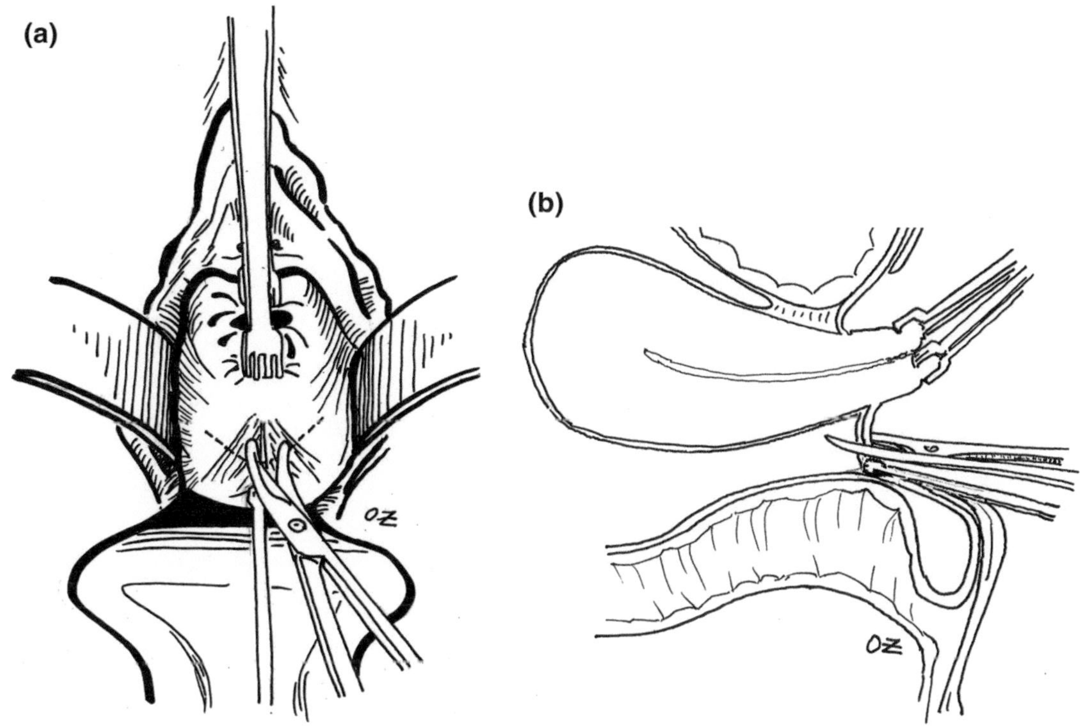

Fig. 20.2 Posterior colpotomy: Cul-de-sac is entered at a perpendicular angle with sharp dissection at about 1 cm from the uterosacral ligamentous attachments. This step is facilitated by downward traction provided with an Allis clamp placed about 2 cm from cervico-vaginal reflection. **a** Front view and **b** sagittal view

cervix–vagina border. The cul-de-sac is entered at a perpendicular angle with sharp dissection at about 1 cm from the uterosacral ligamentous attachments. This step is facilitated by downward traction provided with an Allis clamp placed about 2 cm from cervico-vaginal reflection. Pediatric laparotomy sponges may be used to pack the bowels and omentum as needed. The location of the anterior part of the colpotomy incision is critical. The bladder location can be determined by the appearance of the rugae in the anterior vagina.

The anterior incision can be made exactly where the rugae ends. However, it may be safer (especially for less experienced surgeons to make the incision at about 5-mm cephalad to the anterior cervical tenaculum. It is essential to hold the scissors parallel to the cervical axis and press them against the firm surface of the cervix and lower uterine segment. After the so-called vesicouterine septum, a 1.5–2 cm connective tissue band which firmly attaches the bladder to the lower uterine segment, is divided, the avascular vesicouterine space opens leaving only a thin sheet of peritoneum intact (Fig. 20.3a, b). An expert vaginal surgeon may be able to determine the vesicouterine plane precisely and may prefer to complete the anterior colpotomy by identifying the peritoneum floating freely over the lower uterine segment. This may not be necessary, as it is safe to start clamping the uterosacral and cardinal ligaments as long as a retractor is deflecting the bladder, and down and outward traction is applied to the cervix. In many cases anterior entry into the peritoneal cavity may be deferred until after the division and ligation of the uterosacral and cardinal ligaments. Once the cardinal ligaments are transected, the uterus will descend more (Fig. 20.4). Before any attempt for delivery of the uterus, the abdomen must be entered both anteriorly and posteriorly. If the uterus is small, it can be delivered through an anterior or posterior

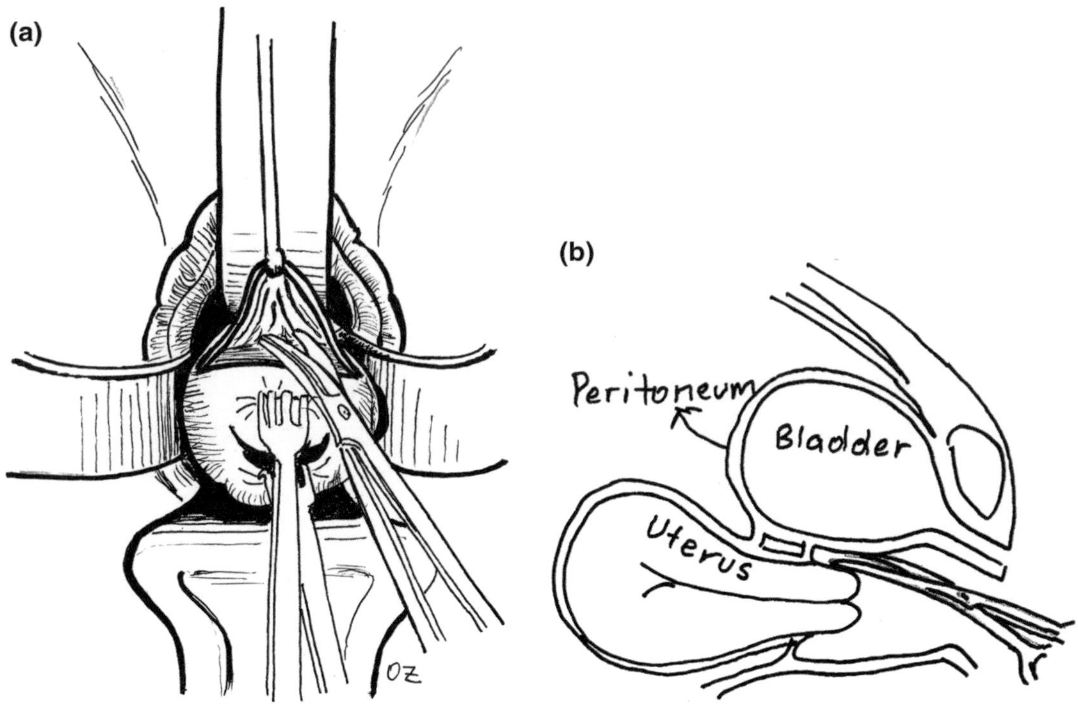

Fig. 20.3 Anterior colpotomy: After the so-called vesicouterine septum, a 1.5–2 cm connective tissue band which firmly attaches the bladder to the lower uterine segment, is divided, the avascular vesicouterine space opens leaving only a thin sheet of peritoneum intact. **a** Front view and **b** sagittal view

colpotomy, but when it is large, it may have to be removed in several pieces with manual morcellation techniques. It is safe to do this after the uterine arteries are ligated bilaterally.

After the cornual end of the fallopian tubes, round ligaments, and utero-ovarian ligaments are clamped and divided altogether and ligated in one pedicle bilaterally, the uterine specimen can be removed. Confirmation of hemostasis by inspecting the pedicles in a clockwise fashion using sponge on ring forceps and irrigation is a necessary step. After ensuring hemostasis systematically, the vaginal cuff is closed with full-thickness sutures including the peritoneal edge on the posterior side, usually in a transverse fashion. Peritoneal closure is typically not necessary. Optionally, the cuff can be closed sagittally to prevent shortening of the vagina. Ovaries and tubes can also be removed at the time of hysterectomy if so desired. Clamping the round ligament separately may facilitate oophorectomy.

At the end of the procedure, many recommend cystoscopy to confirm ureteral integrity, but this may not be needed routinely, as ureteral injury is least likely with VH. Vigorous jets confirm ureteral patency. Vaginal packing is typically not necessary. Leaving an indwelling Foley catheter is not standard unless indicated for a concomitant procedure. Oral intake may start as tolerated. Same-day discharge may be possible in some cases if pain control is appropriate.

One should consider utilizing laparoscopy if it is unsafe to complete the procedure due to uterine size, adhesions, or unexpected pathology. Even though most cases can be accomplished with traditional surgical instruments, vessel sealing bipolar devices have been well-tested and are appropriate to use in difficult, if not all, cases of VH. Endoloops, hemostatic clips, and other hemostatic devices should also be made available for complicated cases.

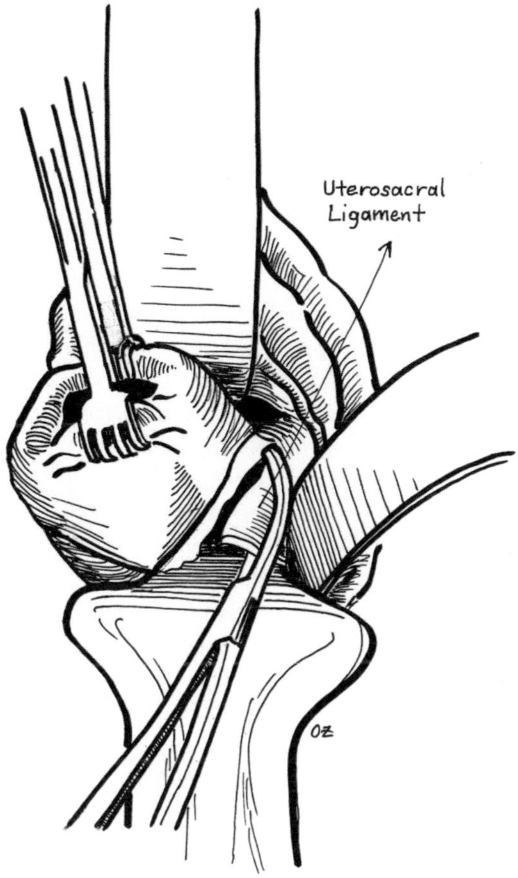

Fig. 20.4 Once the uterosacral and especially cardinal ligaments are clamped and transected, the uterus will descend

Complications

When hysterectomies performed for malignancies and perinatal indications are excluded, the mortality rate of hysterectomy is estimated to be in the range of 1–3 in 10,000. A recently updated meta-analysis on hysterectomy approaches by the Cochrane Library included 34 trials with 4495 women (2). This analysis showed that VH is the least complicated and the shortest hysterectomy approach. The most frequent complications of VH are infections and bleeding. Hematoma formation from contained bleeding, if not relieved, may eventually lead to an infectious process. Most bleeding complications arise from the area between the utero-ovarian and uterine artery pedicles, and sometimes from the posterior vaginal cuff. Among the other less common complications, bladder injury usually occurs well above the trigone, therefore, not near the ureters. One must avoid blunt dissection of the bladder, especially in women with a history of previous cesarean delivery. While gynecologists are responsible for most ureteral injuries, the majority of which occur during hysterectomies, this occurs less commonly in VH. Vaginal cuff dehiscence with or without evisceration, a serious complication unique to hysterectomy, occurs less frequently in VH (0.2–0.3%) vs. LH (>1%) (8). The risk of bowel injury is small (0.15–0.7%) and statistically similar in all hysterectomy approaches.

Conversion to laparotomy should not be considered a complication, as a prudent surgeon will use the safest method when unexpected conditions are encountered during any surgery. Most studies including this meta-analysis were underpowered for many outcome measures (2). Importantly, the information regarding the long-term effects of hysterectomy routes is sparse.

Other Transvaginal Procedures

The shortest distance to the abdominal cavity is through the posterior vaginal fornix, where the full-thickness vaginal wall has very few fibromuscular elements. Combined thickness of the vaginal wall and adjacent peritoneal lining is about 5 mm. All vaginal surgeons are well aware that the area immediately distal to the attachment of the uterosacral ligaments is safe for approximately 3–4 cm, as the rectum is not attached there, and changes its direction toward the left side of the pelvic cavity. In recent years, interest in exploring even less invasive approaches has resulted in reappraisal of transvaginal surgery by both gynecologic surgeons and general surgeons (9).

Historically, transvaginal access to the abdominal cavity has been used in several ways for a variety of indications:

Culdocentesis, aspiration of fluid collected in the cul-de-sac via needle puncture of the posterior fornix, used to be a key step in the differential diagnosis of ruptured ectopic pregnancy before sensitive pregnancy tests and pelvic ultrasonography (Fig. 20.5).

Culdotomy is the entry into the cul-de-sac by means of an incision in the posterior vaginal fornix. When this is performed as the first step of VH, it is often called **colpotomy**. This access can be used with traditional surgical or laparoscopic instruments to perform tubal sterilization, salpingectomy, oophorectomy, abscess drainage, and myomectomy. Most recently, this route has been used by pioneers of the NOTES movement to perform procedures such as nephrectomy, appendectomy, and cholecystectomy, which are detailed elsewhere in this textbook.

In **culdoscopy,** an endoscope is inserted into the abdominal cavity through the culdotomy incision for the evaluation of pelvic structures or tubal sterilization. When this access is combined with laparoscopy as a port site for instrumentation or specimen retrieval, it is considered **culdolaparoscopy**. Advocates of the latter technique suggest that making the entry under laparoscopic visualization may reduce the risk of visceral injury (10).

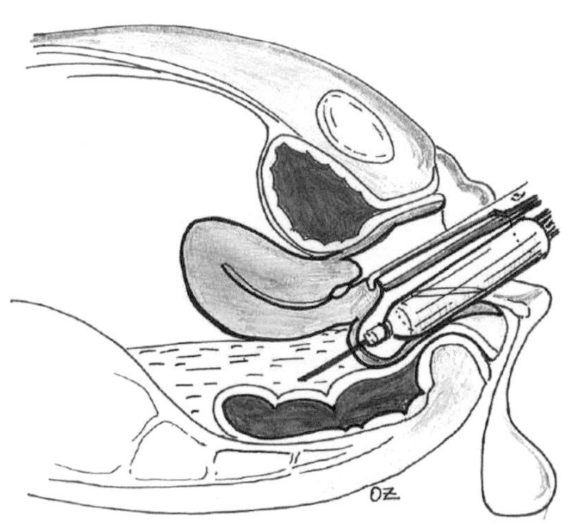

Fig. 20.5 Culdocentesis: Aspiration of fluid collected in the cul-de-sac via needle puncture of the posterior fornix, which used to be a key step in the differential diagnosis of ruptured ectopic pregnancy

History

The first reported procedure via colpotomy was drainage of a tubo-ovarian abscess by Pelleton in 1835 (9). In 1896, Howard Kelly published his experience with 10 cases of ectopic pregnancy managed transvaginally (9). This route continued to be used by some with advanced skills in vaginal surgery in the industrialized countries, and by many others in the developing world due to limited resources (9, 11–16). Culdotomy never gained widespread acceptance until it was combined recently with laparoscopic techniques mainly for specimen retrieval.

Culdoscopy was first performed by a Russian surgeon, Dimitri Oskarovic von Ott, in St. Petersburg in 1891 (5). In 1903, he reported on more than 606 gynecological operations using normal light with a reflector, which he named "ventroscopy". Albert Decker, who started with laparoscopy in 1928, but "gave it up because it required general anesthesia," is responsible for increasing popularity of culdoscopy in the USA in the 1940s and 1950s. He thought culdoscopy performed in knee-chest position, which allows "air to enter the abdomen … as a result of negative pressure", was more suitable for the evaluation of gynecologic conditions (Fig. 20.6). With his influence, culdoscopy was preferred over laparoscopy for over 20 years in the USA. However, with the introduction of CO_2 for pneumoperitoneum in late fifties, and cold light through fiberoptic systems in the early sixties by Frangenheim, laparoscopy began to be preferred not only in Europe but also in the USA (5). More recently, a growing interest in natural orifice transluminal endoscopic surgery (NOTES) brought culdoscopy back into favor.

Procedure

The patient is placed in a dorsal lithotomy position as described for VH. The vaginal apex is exposed with a speculum and/or retractors. Because a previous history of a pelvic infection or severe endometriosis may be considered as relative contraindications to culdotomy, it may be prudent to combine this approach with

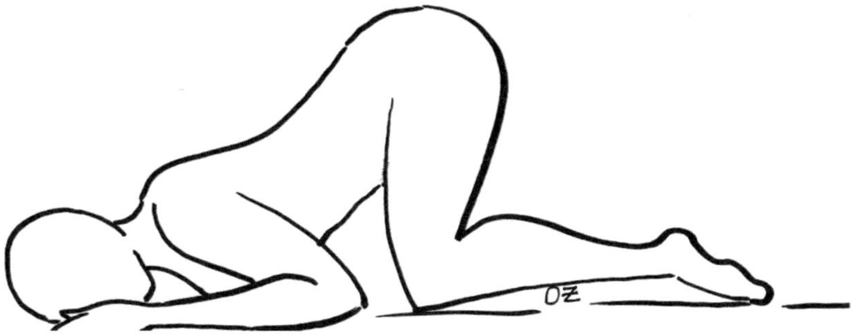

Fig. 20.6 Knee-chest position for culdoscopy performed by Decker

intraoperative ultrasonographic guidance when these conditions are suspected. The posterior portion of the cervix is grasped with a tenaculum and pulled anteriorly and distally. It is then moved up and down and in and out to visualize the creases forming in this area. This delineates the exact location of the bilateral uterosacral ligaments as well as the dimple forming immediately at the edge of posterior cervix. This area represents the part of the cul-de-sac where the only structures separating the vaginal and abdominal cavities are the peritoneum and the vaginal wall. Location of this free area can also be confirmed by palpation of the posterior fornix or by pressing a blunt surgical instrument against the posterior cervix and moving it down and visualizing a drop-off effect where the cervix ends (Fig. 20.7). The full-thickness vaginal wall is held with an Allis clamp at approximately 2 cm from the demarcation signifying where the cervix ends. If grasped appropriately, the peritoneum is also included in this grip. Using traction and counter-traction between the Allis clamp and the tenaculum holding the cervix, a vertical line is formed in the most apical portion of the posterior fornix. Mayo scissors are then used to cut the full-thickness vaginal wall firmly in the middle of and perpendicular to this line. This typically allows direct entry into the cul-de-sac between the uterosacral ligaments. It is important not to make this incision too close to the cervix in an effort to avoid entry into the uterine serosa instead. Even though bleeding from the cut edge of the posterior cuff is typically not significant, some surgeons choose to suture this edge at this time. This incision can be extended to up to 3 cm for removal of larger specimens. The incision is often closed with a figure-of-eight absorbable suture. Peritoneal closure is not necessary.

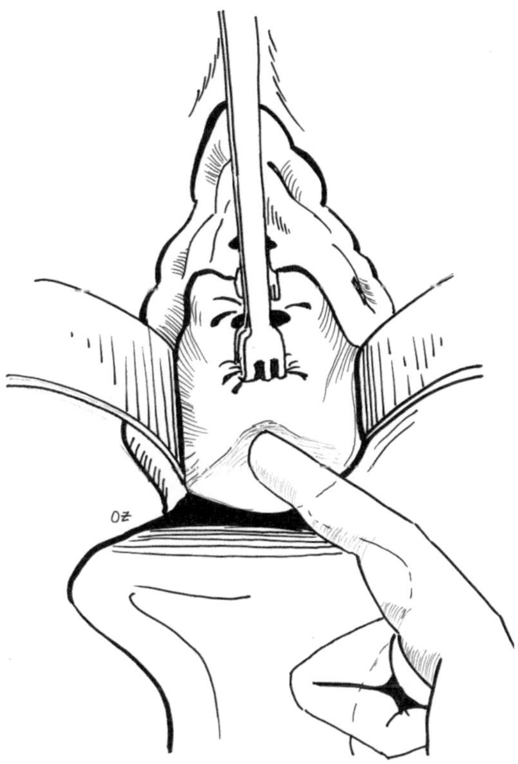

Fig. 20.7 Culdoscopy site can also be determined by palpation of this the posterior fornix or pressing a blunt surgical instrument against the posterior cervix and moving it down and visualizing a drop-off effect where the cervix ends

For culdoscopy, a laparoscopic port can be inserted through the culdotomy incision created with the aforementioned technique. Alternatively, a laparoscopic trocar can be pushed into make the incision as in laparoscopy after delineation of the safe entry point and stabilization of the posterior fornix between a tenaculum and an Allis clamp (11).

Diagnostic Culdoscopy

Culdoscopy, originally introduced by Decker in the USA, recently gained renewed interest with the new advances in endoscopic technology (12). In the late 1990s, transvaginal hydrolaparoscopy (THL) was proposed as an outpatient procedure and successfully used for diagnostic purposes mainly in infertility evaluation (13–15). This procedure is generally performed in the dorsal lithotomy position, in most cases under local anesthesia, using isotonic solution as a distention medium. The choice of endoscope varied from 0 to 30º rigid to flexible, often with 3-mm instruments. This approach was used for ovarian drilling as well (12). The risk of bowel injury was less than 1% and is expected to decrease with more experience and improved technique. When compared to laparoscopy, accuracy of this approach was found to be over 90%.

Transvaginal Sterilization

Female sterilization can be achieved with partial or complete removal, interruption, occlusion, and destruction of the bilateral tubes using traditional surgical instruments, silastic bands, clips, and unipolar or bipolar cauterization. Today, this is commonly performed with laparoscopy or in the immediate postpartum stage via mini-laparotomy. Transvaginal sterilization via culdotomy was frequent until the 1970s but, with the introduction of CO_2 insufflation and fiberoptic lighting, laparoscopy became more popular later. There has not been a randomized trial between transvaginal and laparoscopic sterilization methods; however, transvaginal sterilization has been shown to be a safe option in the hands of skilled vaginal surgeons in numerous reports.

In 1971, Yuzpe published 1383 cases of transvaginal sterilization via culdotomy. They excluded women who underwent concomitant pregnancy termination (16). They performed either fimbriectomy or removed the mid-segment of the tubes as in the Pomeroy technique. In 40 women, they used local anesthesia only. In only one case (1/1383) was laparoscopy needed due to adhesions in the cul-de-sac. One patient who was started under local anesthesia had to be given general anesthesia. During their up to 24-month follow-up period, they did not identify any pregnancy in 1010 tubal sterilization procedures with either laparoscopy or laparotomy, but there were 4 (0.21%) pregnancies in the group who had transvaginal sterilization.

Whitaker in 1979 reviewed his experience with 585 transvaginal tubal sterilization cases using the Pomeroy method (17). Operative time ranged from 15 to 60 min, with a mean of 26 min. Thirteen percent had pregnancy termination with the sterilization procedure. Conversion to laparotomy was necessary for sterilization in 8 (1.4%) cases. In 1980, Miesfeld et al. reported a high pregnancy rate of 2.4% after 329 transvaginal sterilization procedures (18). This rate was even higher (4.2%) when sterilization was combined with pregnancy termination. In 1991, Smith reported his outcomes after performing transvaginal sterilization with unipolar cautery (19). Over half of the patients were followed for over 5 years. He was able to complete half of his 240 transvaginal operations in 12 min or less, with an average time of 14.5 min. Median estimated blood loss was 20 mL. Two women required laparotomy for dense adhesions during culdotomy attempt. There were one intrauterine and two ectopic pregnancies in this series.

The most contemporary report came from Mayo Clinic in 2012 (9). Tolcher et al. compiled 219 transvaginal sterilization procedures performed using the total salpingectomy method between 1995 and 2005. Of these procedures, 97 (44%) underwent additional procedures (73% of them were dilatation and curettage), leaving 122 for analysis specific to transvaginal sterilization. Their operative time ranged from 13 to 98 min (mean: 33 min). Culdotomy attempt failed in 10/219 (4.6%) women. Older age and higher BMI were associated with failure of culdotomy.

Complications

In Yuzpe's study, 36 patients (1.9%) among the women who underwent posterior colpotomy had infectious complications treated as outpatients with antibiotics, 6 (0.32%) were readmitted for postoperative infections or bleeding and recovered with medical management, and only 10 (0.53%) required surgery for treatment of bleeding and infectious complications (16). Whitaker noted 9 (1.5%) patients had prolonged hospital stay due to minor infections or bleeding-related complications, none of which led to more serious entities such as hematoma and abscess requiring intervention (17). Miesfeld stressed that the risk of infection associated with transvaginal sterilization is very low, contrary to the findings of previous studies (18). In his series, only 6 (1.8%) patients needed antibiotic treatment for presumed infections, and none needed hospitalization. Bleeding-related complications were also low and were often managed as outpatients, in 8 (2.4%) patients. Brenner compared sterilizations performed via 401 culdoscopies, 799 culdotomies, 482 laparoscopies, and 279 laparotomies in 1981 (20). His conclusion favored the laparoscopic route due to lower pelvic infection rates than with culdoscopy and culdotomy. All four approaches had similar and acceptable technical failure rates. Tubal visualization was significantly more difficult with endoscopic techniques as compared to the open techniques. Intraoperative complications were significantly more common with culdoscopy as compared to the other approaches. Smith reported no infectious complications and attributed this to routine antibiotic prophylaxis and shorter operative time. Tolcher et al. reported no intraoperative complications, but 6 (2.7%) postoperative infections and 1 (0.9%) hemorrhage (9). All 11 women with no prior vaginal deliveries had successful transvaginal sterilization but sustained significantly more complications compared to patients with prior vaginal delivery (18.2% vs. 2.5%, $p = 0.045$). It appears that transvaginal sterilization may be a safe option when today's preoperative precautions such as preoperative antibiotic prophylaxis are taken, but this approach is not ready for the main stream.

Conclusion

Transvaginal surgery is not new. In fact, it is one of the oldest surgical approaches. Strong evidence favoring VH over other approaches attests to the merits of transvaginal intraperitoneal access. With the advances in endoscopic technology and more interest in utilizing natural orifices, there is no doubt that the vaginal route will be more widely utilized. One only hopes that gynecologists who pioneered this approach do not fall behind the innovative surgeons from other fields.

References

1. American College of Obstetricians and Gynecologists. ACOG Committee Opinion No. 444: choosing the route of hysterectomy for benign disease. Obstet Gynecol. 2009;114:1156–8.
2. Johnson N, Barlow D, Lethaby A, et al. Surgical approach to hysterectomy for benign gynaecological disease. Cochrane Database Syst Rev. 2006;2: CD003677.
3. Cornella J, Gala R, Harmanli O, Moen M, Nihira M, Zimmerman C. The Council on Resident Education in Obstetrics and Gynecology (CREOG), the American College of Obstetricians and Gynecologists (ACOG), Surgical Curriculum in Obstetrics and Gynecology, Vaginal hysterectomy module. http://cfweb.acog.org/scog/scog008. Accessed 8 Jan 2016.
4. Sutton C. Past, present, and future of hysterectomy. J Minim Invasive Gynecol. 2010;17:421–35.
5. Litynski GS. Hans Frangenheim–culdoscopy vs. laparoscopy, the first book on gynecological endoscopy, and "cold light". JSLS. 1997;1:357–61.
6. Graham H. Eternal eve: the history of gynaecology and obstetrics. Garden City, NY: Doubleday; 1951.
7. Whiteman MK, Hillis SD, Jamieson DJ, et al. Inpatient hysterectomy surveillance in the United States, 2000-2004. Am J Obstet Gynecol. 2008;198:34.e1–7.
8. Hur HC, Guido RS, Mansuria SM, et al. Incidence and patient characteristics of vaginal cuff dehiscence

after different modes of hysterectomies. J Minim Invasive Gynecol. 2007;14:311–7.

9. Tolcher MC, Kalogera E, Hopkins MR, Weaver AL, Bingener J, Dowdy SC. Safety of culdotomy as a surgical approach: implications for natural orifice transluminal endoscopic surgery. JSLS. 2012;16: 413–20.
10. Tsin DA, Colombero LT, Lambeck J, Manolas P. Minilaparoscopy-assisted natural orifice surgery. J Soc Laparoendosc Surg. 2007;11:24–9.
11. Tsin DA. Culdolaparoscopy: a preliminary report. JSLS. 2001;5(1):69–71.
12. Escobar PF, Starks D, Fader AN, Catenacci M, Falcone T. Laparoendoscopic single-site and natural orifice surgery in gynecology. Fertil Steril. 2010;94: 2497–502.
13. Gordts S, Campo R, Rombauts L, Brosens I. Transvaginal hydrolaparoscopy as an outpatient procedure for infertility investigation. Hum Reprod. 1998;13(1):99–103.
14. Darai E, Dessolle L, Lecuru F, Soriano D. Transvaginal hydrolaparoscopy compared with laparoscopy for the evaluation of infertile women: a prospective comparative blind study. Hum Reprod. 2000;15 (11):2379–82.
15. Cicinelli E, Matteo M, Causio F, Schonauer LM, Pinto V, Galantino P. Tolerability of the mini-pan-endoscopic approach (transvaginal hydrolaparoscopy and minihysteroscopy) versus hysterosalpingography in an outpatient infertility investigation. Fertil Steril. 2001;76(5):1048–51.
16. Yuzpe AA, Allen HH, Collins JA. Tubal sterilization: methodology, postoperative management and follow-up of 2934 cases. Can Med Assoc J. 1972;107:115–7.
17. Whitaker CF Jr. Tubal ligation by colpotomy incision. Am J Obstet Gynecol. 1979;134:885–8.
18. Miesfeld RR, Giarratano RC, Moyers TG. Vaginal tubal ligation–is infection a significant risk? Am J Obstet Gynecol. 1980;137:183–8.
19. Smith RP, Maggi CS, Nolan TE. Morbidity and vaginal tubal cautery: a report and review. Obstet Gynecol. 1991;78:209–12.
20. Brenner WE. Evaluation of contemporary female sterilization methods. J Reprod Med. 1981;26:439–53.

NOTES Transanal Colorectal Resection

21

Anthony P. D'Andrea and Patricia Sylla

Abstract

The transanal natural orifice translumenal endoscopic surgery (NOTES) approach for rectal cancer is one of the few NOTES applications that has successfully transitioned from experimental model to clinical practice. Transanal NOTES total mesorectal excision (taTME) facilitates the completion of minimally invasive, sphincter-preserving, total mesorectal excision (TME) in patients with distal rectal tumors who would otherwise require abdominoperineal resection (APR) or conversion from laparoscopic to open TME. This chapter reviews the evolution of transanal NOTES applied to colorectal surgery, as well as the most recent published outcomes of taTME to date, for both benign and malignant indications. A detailed description of laparoscopic-assisted taTME for a low rectal tumor is provided, with description of instrumentation, team, and operative setup and related technical pearls. The chapter emphasizes appropriate patient and tumor selection, a stepwise approach during transanal dissection, troubleshooting, and the recommended training pathway for taTME, all of which are critical to achieve an adequate oncologic resection and favorable perioperative outcomes in patients with rectal cancer.

A.P. D'Andrea · P. Sylla (✉)
Department of Surgery, Division of Colon and Rectal Surgery, Icahn School of Medicine at Mount Sinai, 5 East 98th Street, Box 1259, New York, NY 10029, USA
e-mail: patricia.sylla@mountsinai.org

A.P. D'Andrea
e-mail: anthony.dandrea@mountsinai.org

J.R. Romanelli et al. (eds.), *NOTES and Endoluminal Surgery*, Clinical Gastroenterology, DOI 10.1007/978-3-319-50610-4_21

Keywords
Transanal endoscopic surgery (TES) · Transanal endoscopic microsurgery (TEM) · Transanal endoscopic operating system (TEO) · Transanal minimally invasive surgery (TAMIS) · Natural orifice translumenal endoscopic surgery (NOTES) · Total mesorectal excision (TME) · Transanal total mesorectal excision (taTME) · Proctectomy

Abbreviations

ACOSOG	American College of Surgeons Oncology Group
ALaCaRT	Australasian laparoscopic cancer of the rectum trial
APR	Abdominoperineal resection
CLASSICC trial	Conventional versus laparoscopic-assisted surgery in colorectal cancer
COLOR II trial	Colorectal cancer laparoscopic or open resection
COREAN trial	Comparison of open versus laparoscopic surgery for mid- and low rectal cancer after neoadjuvant chemoradiotherapy
CRM	Circumferential radial margin
CT	Computed tomography
DRE	Digital rectal examination
ELAPE	Extralevator abdominoperineal excision
FAP	Familial adenomatous polyposis
ICG	Indocyanine green
IPAA	Ileal pouch-anal anastomosis
IRB	Institutional review board
ISR	Intersphincteric resection
LOREC	Low rectal cancer (pertains to an international tumor registry)
MRI	Magnetic resonance imaging
NOSE	Natural orifice specimen extraction
NOTES	Natural orifice translumenal endoscopic surgery
PPH	Procedure for prolapsed hemorrhoid
ROLARR	Robotic versus laparoscopic resection for rectal cancer
TAMIS	Transanal minimally invasive surgery
TAP	Transversus abdominis plane
TATA	Transanal transabdominal
taTME	Transanal NOTES total mesorectal excision
TEM	Transanal endoscopic microsurgery
TEO	Transanal endoscopic operating system
TES	Transanal endoscopic surgery
TME	Total mesorectal excision

Introduction

Since the advent of laparoscopy with the first colectomy performed in the early 1990s, surgical approaches for colon and rectal disease have continued to evolve, with increased adoption of laparoscopy and robotics. Alongside these minimally invasive transabdominal approaches, transanal techniques for the resection of rectal lesions have also progressed. Through improvements in platforms and instrumentation, transanal endoscopic surgery (TES) provides excellent local control for proximal benign rectal lesions and low-risk, early-stage, rectal cancer. Relative to traditional transanal techniques, submucosal or full-thickness resection can be performed using TES with improved visualization and reduced incidence of specimen fragmentation and margin positivity. TES also provides a minimally invasive alternative to radical rectal resection for select mid- and upper rectal lesions that are not otherwise amenable either to endoscopic polypectomy, mucosal resection or to conventional transanal excision.

Currently, locally invasive rectal cancers are not eligible for local excision and require radical oncologic resection with total mesorectal excision (TME). Rectal tumors located in the distal third of the rectum, 6 cm or less from the anal verge, remain a major surgical challenge when using transabdominal techniques. This is due to difficulty achieving a complete TME with negative margins, especially in male patients with a narrow pelvis. Technical challenges in these cases include distal rectal transection below tumors with adequate resection margins while preserving the anal sphincters and autonomic nerves, and providing adequate coloanal reconstruction.

While the use of laparoscopy in rectal cancer has been shown to be oncologically safe, and associated with reduced blood loss, length of hospital stay, and faster recovery relative to open surgery, conversion rates remain high, and overall adoption low [1–4]. Robotic TME has been suggested as an enabling technology to facilitate completion of these complex procedures and to lower conversion rates, but the recent Robotic versus Laparoscopic Resection for Rectal Cancer (ROLARR) trial results have not demonstrated a significant difference in conversion rates between robotic and non-robotic laparoscopic TME [5]. In light of the technical difficulties with transabdominal approaches, there has been significant interest in transanal natural orifice translumenal endoscopic surgery (NOTES) applied to colorectal diseases and rectal cancer in particular.

To date, the transanal NOTES approach for rectal cancer is one of the few NOTES applications that has successfully transitioned from experimental model to clinical practice. Transanal NOTES TME (taTME) has been found to facilitate completion of minimally invasive sphincter-preserving TME in patients with distal rectal tumors who would otherwise require abdominoperineal resection (APR) or conversion from laparoscopic to open TME. This chapter briefly reviews the evolution of transanal NOTES applied to colorectal surgery and the most recent published outcomes of taTME. A detailed description on how to perform laparoscopic-assisted taTME for a low rectal tumor is then provided, with description of instrumentation, team, and operative setup, all with related technical pearls. The chapter emphasizes appropriate patient and tumor selection, a stepwise approach during transanal dissection, troubleshooting, and issues related to appropriate training in taTME, all of which are critical for the successful adoption of taTME.

Evolution of NOTES for Colorectal Surgery

The benefits of laparoscopy in colon resection have been demonstrated in prospective clinical trials. It is now widely accepted that laparoscopy offers comparable oncologic outcomes for patients with colon cancer while providing improved postoperative recovery from pain, wound-related complications, and return of bowel function [1–4]. Despite these benefits, the laparoscopic approach still requires port sizes of 10–15 mm for stapler applications and extraction sites of variable length, depending on the size of the specimen, which are susceptible to infection and herniation in up to 22% of patients [6].

To avoid painful and potentially morbid abdominal wounds, transanal natural orifice specimen extraction (NOSE) was described as early as 1993 by Franklin, demonstrating a 0% trocar-site hernia rate [7]. Similarly, Cheung [8] demonstrated transanal NOSE for resection of left-sided colonic tumors but with use of a combined laparoscopic and transluminal technique. While Franklin used the natural orifice purely for specimen retrieval, Cheung and colleagues employed a transanal endoscopic operating system (TEO) to use the natural orifice for specimen extraction as well as anvil delivery and creation of the transanal stapled anastomosis [8]. Since then, it has been accepted that there is no higher risk of peritoneal contamination, and there have been no significant reports of clinical anal incontinence or extraction site metastasis in oncologic cases after colorectal NOSE [8–10]. The recognition that NOSE was safe, feasible, and could bypass some of the comorbidity associated with laparoscopy served as a bridge toward transanal NOTES.

With regard to TME and laparoscopic versus open surgery for rectal cancer, there have been multiple, randomized, controlled trials, including the COLOR II, CLASICC, and COREAN trials that show superiority in short-term postoperative outcomes as well as non-inferiority of short- and long-term oncologic outcomes for laparoscopic TME [2, 11–17]. More recently, the ACOSOG Z6051 and ALaCaRT trials failed to show non-inferiority for laparoscopic TME when compared to open surgery [18, 19]. Despite there being comparable oncologic outcomes with open surgery for rectal cancer, laparoscopic TME has not been widely adopted due to the technical difficulty of the pelvic dissection, long operative times, and minimal impact on functional outcomes [20]. The rates of morbidity for laparoscopic and open TME are similar (30–50%) and include urinary dysfunction (5–12%), sexual dysfunction (10–35%), fecal incontinence (20–30%), wound complications, pain, and long recovery [21, 22]. Even in the hands of experienced surgeons, laparoscopic TME is associated with conversion to laparotomy in up to one-third of patients, as demonstrated in each of the randomized trials (1% in the COREAN trial, 9% in ALaCaRT, 11% in ACOSOG Z6051, 17% in COLOR II, 30% in the Hong Kong study by Ng et al., and 34% in CLASICC) [2, 3, 11, 14, 17–19]. It was also noted that the patients who suffered the most complications were the ones whose surgery was converted from a laparoscopic to an open approach [2, 15, 23].

To circumvent the difficulty of the deep pelvis, studies for robotic-assisted laparoscopic TME were performed, demonstrating safety in accordance with current oncologic principle, with lower rates of conversion to open operation [5, 24]. That being said, the impact of robotic assistance on long-term oncologic outcomes remains to be seen. A recently completed randomized clinical trial (ROLARR) comparing laparoscopic and robotic-assisted laparoscopic TME preliminarily indicated similar perioperative outcomes and a lower conversion rate with robotic-assisted TME, although this was not statistically significant (unpublished results).

The resection of rectal cancer in the deep pelvis has been a technical challenge with both open and laparoscopic techniques. This is significant because, excluding patients who underwent preoperative neoadjuvant therapy, the strongest predictor of long-term oncologic outcomes in rectal cancer besides tumor stage is the adequacy of the TME performed. Distal and circumferential radial margins (CRM) and the completeness of the mesorectal excision strongly influence the likelihood of local and distant recurrence after rectal cancer surgery [25–28].

In search of a better way to ensure clear distal margins and sphincter preservation for low rectal tumors that would otherwise require APR, Gerald Marks and subsequently John Marks described the transanal transabdominal (TATA) method [29, 30]. This technique initially was performed without laparoscopy, and later was modified to be performed laparoscopically. The unique aspect of this operation was to begin with a transanal approach to achieve a negative distal margin [30]. When combined with open or laparoscopic TME, acceptable local recurrence and survival rates can be achieved for tumors less than 3 cm from the anal verge [30]. The TATA approach has demonstrated that much of the distal portion of the TME can be performed from a transanal approach, although it is limited by difficulties with exposure using a special self-retaining retractor (Lone Star Medical Products Inc., Houston TX) and a standard transanal instrument tray.

The advantages of TATA, which has also been referred to as intersphincteric resection (ISR), include definition of the distal margin from below, external anal sphincter muscle preservation, and avoiding the need for stapling devices for distal rectal transection, which do not comply with the bony constraints of the pelvis [31]. Unfortunately, despite the appropriate rationale behind TATA, its widespread adoption has been limited by the difficulty mastering the technique and achieving an R0 resection, as well as the concerns for poor functional outcomes following partial and especially complete en bloc resection of the internal anal sphincter. This has largely favored APR over TATA, especially in the USA [31].

In parallel with TATA, in the early 1980s, Buess [32] described the first single multiport platform to perform transanal endoscopic microsurgery (TEM) of sessile polyps of the mid- and upper rectum not otherwise resectable using endoscopic polypectomy. This was the first instance where full-thickness local resection of a rectal cancer was performed in a minimally invasive transanal endoscopic fashion with low morbidity. Unfortunately, TEM involves the use of a rigid endoscopic platform, and its adoption remained limited due to cost and the complexity of the operating platform [31]. It was not until 2010, with the introduction of alternative disposable platforms named transanal minimally invasive surgery (TAMIS), that TES became popularized worldwide [33]. TAMIS employs versatile, low cost, disposable, multiport channels that are compatible with standard laparoscopic towers and equipment. TAMIS was used initially for local excision of rectal tumors, but led to a surge of interest in transanal access and minimally invasive surgery via the transanal route.

Today as the field of minimally invasive colorectal surgery continues to mature, transanal NOTES represents the next step in the evolution of endoluminal approaches. The ultimate goal of transanal NOTES is to employ a natural orifice to access the abdominal cavity to perform complex procedures without the need for abdominal incisions. The theoretical advantages include better cosmesis, reduced incisional complications of pain, infections and hernia, and faster patient recovery compared to open surgery and laparoscopy [6, 34, 35]. The transanal approach can also improve distal and circumferential margins for a distal rectal cancer and is not limited by patients' gender. It is also technically advantageous in obese patients and those with a narrow pelvis [20, 36].

Transanal Colectomy: Results and Published Outcomes

The final step on the path of transanal NOTES colorectal surgery would be to perform a segmental colectomy and rectal resection via a transanal endoscopic platform without requiring access through the abdominal wall. Whiteford et al. [37] described in 2007 the first pure NOTES technique for transanal rectosigmoidectomy in three human cadavers using the TEM platform. Radical sigmoid colectomy with en bloc lymphadenectomy was achieved entirely transanally with standard laparoscopic and TEM instrumentation [37]. Quoted advantages for this approach included the excellent visualization provided by the TEM system, the ability to achieve tissue retraction and manipulation using TEM instrumentation, and to replicate all essential steps of an oncologic rectal dissection using this approach. The technical limitations included difficulties overcoming the acute angle at the sacral promontory and ability to reach deeper into the pelvis with standard TEM instrumentation. The extent of sigmoid colon that could be mobilized with this approach was therefore limited.

With regard to clinical application, Lacy et al. [38] were the first to report a laparoscopic-assisted, transanal, total colectomy in a 36-year-old man with medically refractory ulcerative colitis without complication. Fuchs et al. [39] performed 15 transanal hybrid colon resections for indications such as recurrent diverticulitis, rectal prolapse, internal rectal intussusception, and slow-transit constipation. The extent of their resections varied from rectosigmoid resection to subtotal colectomy. They reported no significant intraoperative and postoperative complications and no anal functional deficit after 6-month follow-up [39]. Since then, however, the clinical experience with transanal colectomy has been limited to the rectosigmoid. Transanal resection for the proximal colon thus far has only been demonstrated in cadaver studies [40]. Because of the anatomical limitation of the sacral promontory and available instrumentation, the vast and rapidly growing experience with transanal NOTES has been for rectosigmoid dissection in a hybrid, laparoscopic-assisted fashion.

Transanal Total Mesorectal Excision: Results and Published Outcomes

Since the first published case report of laparoscopic-assisted taTME in 2010 for a mid-rectal T2N1 cancer treated with neoadjuvant therapy, a number of case series have published their preliminary perioperative and oncologic results with taTME performed either with open, laparoscopic, robotic or with no abdominal assistance [41–53]. Currently, the most common transanal device used is the GelPoint Path TAMIS platform (Applied Medical, Inc., Rancho Santa Margarita, CA), but other platforms commonly used include the TEO rigid platform (Karl Storz, Tuttlingen, Germany), TEM, and the SILS platform (Covidien, USA).

Cumulatively, the published data from case series on taTME demonstrate technical feasibility and preliminary oncologic safety in carefully selected patients with resectable upper, mid-, and low rectal cancers. Overall good-quality TME, adequate lymph node harvest, adequate distal margins and circumferential resection margins, as well as morbidity comparable to that following laparoscopic TME has repeatedly been demonstrated [41, 43–54]. The majority of reports describes the use of taTME for mid- and lower rectal tumors, although taTME can be used for tumors throughout the rectum. The quoted benefits of a transanal endoscopic approach for very low rectal cancers in particular include the ability to expand the upper limit of ISR under much improved visualization and exposure, and the facilitation of a complete rectal and mesorectal dissection. This is especially helpful in male patients with visceral obesity and narrow pelvises in whom a laparoscopic approach poses substantial technical difficulty, with a high risk of conversion and of an incomplete mesorectal excision. Additional benefits of taTME build upon those from TATA and NOSE and include superior visualization and retraction of perirectal tissue planes provided by transanal endoscopic platforms, early identification of the distal resection margins that may reduce the incidence of margin positivity, and avoidance of an abdominal extraction site when transanal specimen extraction is feasible.

All published case series with an experience of at least 15 patients are included in Tables 21.1 and 21.2. Out of the 13 series, 577 patients underwent taTME, with 6% (37/577) of taTME cases performed as part of an APR and 94% as part of sphincter-preserving restorative proctectomy. With respect to tumor selection for taTME, the majority of studies performed taTME for non-obstructing, resectable tumors including preoperatively staged T1, T2, and T3, and N0 or N1 tumors. When studies were performed early in their operative experience, most authors specifically excluded T4 and metastatic tumors, local recurrences, and tumors with threatened circumferential resection margins based on preoperative staging MRI. Cumulatively, across the 13 published series with sample size ranging from 16 to 140 patients, the mesorectal resection was complete in 89% and near complete in 9% of patients, with negative resection margins achieved in 96%, and average harvests of 10–23 lymph nodes. The intraoperative complication rate for taTME was 3% and included eight cases of significant intraoperative bleeding, three perforations, four urethral injuries, one ureteral

Table 21.1 Patient characteristics of published clinical series of taTME for rectal cancer

Series	*N*	Age (year)	Gender	BMI (kg/m^2)	Tumor location	Neoadjuvant CRT	Operative technique
Veltcamp Helbach et al. [41]	80	66.5 (42–86)	M (48), F (32)	27.5 (19.5–40)	5.3 (1–10) cm from DL	Yes (65) No (15)	LA, SILS
Lacy et al. [43]	140	65.5 ± 12.7	M (89), F (51)	25.2 ± 3.9	7.6 ± 3.6 cm from AV	Yes (94) No (46)	LA
Tuech et al. [44]	56	65 (39–83)	M (41), F (15)	27 (20–42)	4.0 (0–5) cm from AV	Yes (47) No (9)	LA (41), SILS (8), laparotomy (4), RA (1)
Muratore et al. [45]	26	66 (38–84)	M (16), F (10)	26.2 (16.9–38.2)	4.4 (3–6) cm from AV	Yes (19) No (7)	LA, SILS
Serra-Aracil et al. [46]	32	68 (39–88)	M (24), F (8)	25 (20–35)	8.0 (5–10) cm from AV	Yes (16) No (16)	LA
Rouanet et al. [47]	30	65 (43–82)	M (30)	26.0 (21.0–32.4)	<5 cm from AV (20), 5–10 cm from AV (10)	Yes (29) No (1)	LA
Atallah et al. [71]	50	56.5 (50.0–65.0)	M (30), F (20)	26.0 (22.7–31.2)	4.4 (3.0–5.5) cm from AV	Yes (43) No (7)	Open (4), LA (14), HA (19), RA (10)
Chouillard et al. [49]	16	57.7 (34–81)	M (6), F (10)	27.9 (21–38)	Mid- or low rectal tumors	NR	SILS, pure
Chen et al. [50]	50	57.3 (29–80)	M (38), F (12)	24.2 (16–37)	5.8 (2–10) cm from AV	Yes (50)	LA, SILS
De'Angelis et al. [54]	32	64.9	M (21), F (11)	25.19	4.0 (2.5–5) cm from AV	Yes (27) No (5)	LA
Perdawood et al. [51]	25	70 (54–76)	M (19), F (6)	28 (18–46)	8.0 (4–10) cm from AV	Yes (7) No (18)	LA
Buchs et al. [52]	20	59.3 (32–87)	M (14), F (6)	27.1 (17.4–38.4)	2.0 (0–7) from anorectal junction	Yes (6) No (14)	LA, RA
Kang et al. [53]	20	58.6 (36–84)	M (12), F (8)	22.2 (16.7–27.5)	6.1 (3–12) cm from AV	Yes (6) No (14)	LA, SILS, pure

(continued)

Table 21.1 (continued)

Transanal platform	Type of resection	Operating time (min)	Final stage (*n*)	Number of lymph nodes collected	TME quality	Positive distal margin	Positive CRM
Transanal platform	Type of resection	Operating time (min)	Final stage (*n*)	Number of lymph nodes collected	TME quality	Positive distal margin	Positive CRM
SILS port (Covidien USA); GelPoint (applied medical)	LAR 65, APR 15	204 (91–447)	ypT0 (6), ypT1 (3), ypT2 (29), ypT3 (42), N0 (44), N1 (21), N2 (15)	14 (6–30)	71 complete, 7 near complete, incomplete 2	0	2
GelPoint (applied medical)	LAR 138, 2 proctocolectomy w IPAA	166 (60–360)	Complete response (15); stage I (34); stage II (43); stage III (39); stage IV (9)	14.7 ± 6.8	Complete 136; nearly complete 3; incomplete 1	N/R	9 (6.4%)
Endorec (aspide) (42), SILS port (Covidien) (11), GelPoint (applied medical) (3)	APR 4, LAR 52	270 (150–495)	NR	12 (7–29)	47 complete, 9 nearly complete, 0 incomplete	N/R	3
SILS port (Covidien)	LAR 25, APR 1	241 (150–360)	pT0 (5), pT1 (7), pT2 (6), pT3 (8), pN+ (7)	10 (median 8)	23 complete, 3 near compete	0	0
TEO (Storz)	LAR 32	240 (165–360)	Stage 0 (2), stage I (7), stage II (10), stage III (12), stage IV (1)	NR	30 complete; 2 near complete	0	0
TEO (Storz)	LAR 30	304 (120–432)	pCR 0, pT1 (1), pT2 (8), pT3 (18), pT4 (3), pN0 (14), pN1 (13), pN2 (3)	13 (8–32)	30 complete	0	4
GelPoint (applied medical)	APR 7 (12%), LAR 43 (86%)	267 (227–331)	pCR (12), pT1 (2), pT2 (11), pT3 (21), pT4 (4); N0 (34), N1 (8), N2 (8)	18 (12–24)	36 complete, 13 near complete, 1 incomplete	1 (2%)	2 (4%)
SILS port (Covidien)	LAR 14, APR 2	265 (155–440)	pTy (1), pT1 (3), pT2 (4), pT3 (7), pT4	17 (12–81)	16 complete	0	0

(continued)

Table 21.1 (continued)

Transanal platform	Type of resection	Operating time (min)	Final stage (*n*)	Number of lymph nodes collected	TME quality	Positive distal margin	Positive CRM
			(1); N0 (11), N1 (4), N2 (1)				
GelPoint (applied medical)	LAR 50	182.1 ± 55.4	ypT1/T2N0 (13); ypT3/T4N0 (12); ypTanyN1-2 (17), pCR (8)	16 (6–42)	NR	0	2 (4%)
GelPoint (applied medical)	LAR 32	195	pT1 (3); ypT2 (12); ypT3 (11); ypT4 (2); N0 (27), N1 (5), N2 (0)	17 (7.14)	27 complete, 3 nearly complete, 2 incomplete	2 (6.2%)	1 (3.1%)
GelPoint (applied medical)	LAR 18, APR 7	NR	T0 (0), T1 (0), T2 (8), T3 (16), T4 (1); N0 (14), N1 (8), N2 (3)	21 (9–42)	20 complete, 5 ncarly complete	0	1 (4%)
Gloveport (4), GelPoint (applied medical) (16)	LAR 16, ELAPE 2, completion proctectomy 1, APR 1	315.3 ± 77.1	T0 (4), T1 (0), T2 (8), T3 (5), T4 (0); N0 (10), N1 (5), N2 (2)	23 (11–45)	16 complete, 1 near complete	0	1 (5.9%)
SILS port (Covidien)	LAR 20	200 (70–420)	Complete response (2), tis (2), stage I (10), stage II (4), stage III (2)	12 (1–20)	18 complete, 2 near complete	0	0

APR abdominoperineal resection; *AV* anal verge; *CRT* chemoradiation therapy, *DL* dentate line; *F* female; *HA* hand-assisted laparoscopy; *LA* laparoscopic-assisted; *LAR* low anterior resection; *M* male; *NR* not reported; *RA* robot-assisted; *TME* total mesorectal excision

injury, one vaginal wall injury, and one prostatic injury. Intraoperative complications typically occurred early during the surgeon's experience. It was noted that laparoscopic assistance, namely performance of these procedures as a 2-team approach, helped identify and avoid critical anatomical structures. The conversion rate to laparotomy was 3%. The average length of hospital stay was 8.1 days (range 4.5–14.0). The rate of postoperative morbidity was 30% and included complications such as transient urinary retention, ileus, obstruction, anastomotic leakage, and pelvic abscess. Follow-up ranged from 5 to 32 months. Regarding functional outcomes, 5 of the 13 studies reported fecal incontinence with an average Wexner score of 6.9 [3–18]. Oncologically, 8 out of the 13 studies report local and distal recurrence with 45 counted local or distant recurrences. The time to recurrence ranged from 5 to 24 months.

Table 21.2 Postoperative outcomes of published clinical series on transanal TME for rectal cancer

Series	Length of stay (*d*)	Intraoperative complications (*n*)	Follow-up period (months)	Morbidity rate (%)	Early postoperative complications (*n*)	Late postoperative complications (*n*)	Functional outcomes	Recurrence
Veltcamp Helbach et al. [41] $N = 80$	8 (3–41)	Laparotomy (4), bleeding (2), perforation (3), abdominal incision for extraction (7)	24	39	Anastomotic leakage, ischemia of proximal limb of colon, small bowel laceration, revision of colostomy, small bowel obstruction, hematoma, full-thickness ischemia of mucosa distal to anastomosis	NR	NR	Local recurrences (2)
Lacy et al. [43] $N = 140$	7.8 (3–39)	None	15.0 ± 9.1	34	Adhesive obstruction (1); anastomotic leak (12); ileostomy obstruction/ileus (11); intra-abdominal collection (4); bleeding (5); anastomotic bleed (3); high ileostomy output (2); acute pancreatitis (1); urinary retention (3); fever (5); blood transfusion (3); ascites (1)	Anastomotic stricture (6); colitis (4); high ileostomy output (3); ileostomy obstruction (2); intestinal obstruction (1); rectovaginal fistula (1)	NR	11 after excluding 9 patients with stage IV lesions (includes 8 with distant mets [6.1], 1 with local recurrence [0.8], and 2 with both distant mets and local recurrence [1.5])
Tuech et al. [44] $N = 56$	10 (6–21)	3 conversion, 6 delayed coloanal anastomosis	29 months (18–52)	26	Anastomotic leak not requiring reoperation (3), pelvic sepsis without evidence of anastomotic leak (3), transient urinary disorders (5), blood transfusion (2), cerebral infarction (1)	NR	Wexner 5 (3–18)	Local recurrence (1), distal recurrence (2)
Muratore et al. [45] $N = 26$	7 (3–25)	0	23 months (16–30)	27	Myocardial infarction (1), asymptomatic anastomotic leak (2), transient urinary retention (1), lymphorrhea (1), intestinal obstruction (2)	NR	NR	Distal recurrence (2)
Serra-Aracil et al. (2015) $N = 32$	8 (4–20)	0	NR	31	Nosocomial infection (3), SSI (3), anastomotic leakage (3), SBO requiring reintervention (1), necrosis of descending colon due to injury of marginal artery (1)	NR	NR	NR

(continued)

Table 21.2 (continued)

Series	Length of stay (*d*)	Intraoperative complications (*n*)	Follow-up period (months)	Morbidity rate (%)	Early postoperative complications (*n*)	Late postoperative complications (*n*)	Functional outcomes	Recurrence
Rouanet et al. [47] *N* = 30	14 (8–25)	2 urethral injury (due to anterior bulky tumor and concurrent prostatic tumor), 1 air embolism	21 (10–41)	30	Sepsis (2), bowel obstruction (1), anastomotic leak (1)	NR	Median Wexner score 11	Local or distal recurrence (14)
Atallah et al. [71] *N* = 50	4.5 (4.0–8.0)	3 (6%), 1 urethral injury, 1 ureteral injury, 1 injury to iliac vessels	15.1 (7.0–23.2)	36	Ileus (9), pelvic abscess (4), anastomotic leak (3), urinary retention (2), pneumonia (1), SSI (1), reoperations (6)	NR	NR	Local recurrence (2), distal recurrence (8)
Chouillard et al. [49] *N* = 16	10.4 (4–29)		9 months (3–29)	19	Intestinal obstruction (2), pelvic abscess (1)	NR		0
Chen et al. (2015) *N* = 50	7.4 (5–18)	2 presacral bleeding, 1 vaginal wall injury		20	UTI (1), pelvic abscess (3), rectovaginal fistula (1), anastomosis defect (3), pseudomembranous colitis (1), bleeding (1)	NR	NR	NR
De'Angelis et al. [54] *N* = 32	7.8	0	32.6 months	25	Urinary disorder (1), urinary infection (1), wound infection (1), anastomotic leak causing pelvic abscess (2), transfusion (1), anastomotic leak medically managed (1), anastomotic leak requiring surgical drainage (1)	NR	Wexner score 9	Local recurrence (1), distal recurrence (1)
Perdawood et al. (2015) *N* = 25	5 (2–43)	2 bleeding	NR	52	Anastomotic leakage requiring readmission (2), high ileostomy output (2), stoma necrosis (1), mechanical obstruction from adhesions (2)	NR	Wexner 4.5 (0–7)	NR
Buchs et al. [52] *N* = 20	7 (3–36)	1 (5%)	10 months (6–21)	30	High ileostomy output, anastomotic leak	Delayed pelvic sepsis secondary to contained anastomotic leak (1)	NR	Distal recurrence (1)
Kang et al. [53] *N* = 20	NR	1 (5%) massive bleeding, 1 (5%) prostate and urethra injury	5 months (1–8)	20	Urethral injury (1), urinary retentions (2), anastomotic hemorrhage (1), mild anastomotic leak (1)	NR	Wexner 5.0 (3–11)	0

The international experience with taTME is still preliminary and based on small to larger single-institutional case series, with no randomized trial comparing taTME with open or laparoscopic TME. However, there have been five retrospective studies that compare outcomes of matched cohorts of patients who underwent taTME versus laparoscopic TME [50, 51, 54–56]. Fernandez-Hevia et al. [55] retrospectively matched 37 cases of laparoscopic-assisted taTME with 37 cases of laparoscopic TME for rectal cancer and demonstrated no significant differences with respect to quality of the mesorectal specimen, lymph node harvest, resection margins, or intraoperative complications. They also demonstrated comparable 30-day postoperative complications, but a statistically significant lower readmission rate in the taTME group (2% vs. 6%) [55]. Velthuis et al. [56] retrospectively matched 25 cases of laparoscopic-assisted taTME with 25 cases of laparoscopic TME and interestingly found that taTME was associated with a significantly higher rate of complete mesorectum than laparoscopic TME (92% vs. 72%). The studies by de'Angelis, Perdawood, and Chen each retrospectively compared laparoscopic-assisted taTME with laparoscopic TME, demonstrating shorter operative times and hospital stays with no differences in intra-/postoperative complications and oncologic outcomes [50, 51, 54]. Currently, the COLOR III trial is in preparation that will compare standard laparoscopic TME versus transanal TME [57].

It is notable that the overall experience for a pure transanal approach to TME without laparoscopic assistance is sparse but growing. Leroy and Zhang described the first two cases of a pure taTME in 2013, demonstrating that it was feasible and safe for mid-to-low-lying rectal cancer [58, 59]. Since then, there have been a total of 21 cases of pure taTME reported [49, 53]. In the study by Chouillard et al., 16 patients underwent taTME, either with or without abdominal assistance. Ten, eight women and two men, out of the 16 were performed in pure fashion, with no ileostomy or conversion to laparoscopy [49]. Kang et al. [53] reported a series of 20 taTME with and without abdominal assistance, 15 of which were performed in pure fashion in nine men and six women. In their experience, pure taTME was easier to perform in women than in men, as demonstrated by the four patients requiring conversion to laparoscopy being all men. Reasons for conversion to laparoscopy included prostatic and urethral injury leading to significant hemorrhage, unsatisfactory exposure accompanied by mild hemorrhage, and having resistance to delivery of the specimen due to bulky mesorectum [53].

Indications for Transanal Total Mesorectal Excision

Although the data with respect to oncologic and functional outcomes have not yet matured, transanal endoscopic proctectomy, with or without TME, has been shown to be feasible and effective in the treatment of benign and malignant disease of the rectum. There is a growing consensus regarding specific indications and contraindications for this approach based on specific pathology, tumor stage, and favorable versus unfavorable anatomical factors.

Benign Indications

Transanal endoscopic completion proctectomy is a particularly attractive approach when seeking to avoid abdominal entry during removal of retained rectal stumps. Indications for a transanal endoscopic approach are the same as for any other approach to completion proctectomy, including inflammatory bowel disease. The transanal approach also lends itself well to intersphincteric proctectomy in cases of refractory radiation proctitis or fecal incontinence, strictures, rectovaginal fistulas, or other complex pelvic fistula, as well as colorectal anastomotic complications. Depending on the length of the residual rectal stump to be removed, a pure transanal endoscopic approach or hybrid approach with laparoscopic or robotic assistance can be performed. Furthermore, depending on the specific pathology warranting proctectomy, rectal dissection can be carried out along the rectal wall with preservation of the

Table 21.3 Published clinical series on taTME for benign indications

Series	Age (year)	Gender	BMI (kg/m²)	Indications	Operative technique	Transanal platform	Type of resection	Operating time (min)	Rectal stump (cm)	Anastomosis	Conversions	Intraoperative complications (*n*)	Morbidity rate	Functional outcomes
De Buck van Overstraeten [60] *N* = 11	34 (22–66)	M (3), F (8)	NR	UC	LA	GelPoint path	Completion proctectomy	160 (133–209)	NR	Stapled (11)	0	0	2 (18%)	NR
Tasende [61] *N* = 18	40.5 (15.7)	M (13), F (5)	26.4 (SD 11.1)	UC	LA	GelPoint path	Restorative proctocolectomy w IPAA	170 (90–300)	NR	Stapled (14), handsewn (2)	0	0	6 (37.5%)	Wexner 1.4 (SD 2.9)
Leo [62] *N* = 16	46 (26–70)	M (10), F (6)	NR	UC	LA	GelPoint path	Restorative proctocolectomy w IPAA	247 (185–470)	NR	Stapled (14), handsewn (2)	3 (18.7%)	0	6 (37.5%)	NR
Wolthuis [63] *N* = 14	65 (38–87)	M (5), F (9)	25 (17–32)	Fistula (1), IBD (2), incontinence (1), circular TVA (2), complication of surgery (3), cancer (5)	LA (11), pure TAMIS (3)	GelPoint path	Coloanal anastomosis (7), intersphincteric proctectomy (7)	55 (35–95)	NR	handsewn (7), end-colostomy (6), end ileostomy (1)	2 (18%)	Maintaining insufflation (2), difficult view due to bleeding (1), fibrosis due to prostate radiotherapy (1), rectal perforation (1),	6 (43%)	NR
Bremers [64] *N* = 9	NR	NR	NR	IBD (6), lynch (1), collagenous colitis (1), anastomotic leak (1)	Transanal	TEM	Proctectomy	161 (107–239)	15 (8–20)	NR	1 (11%)	0	1 (11%)	NR
Liyanage [65] *N* = 12	66 (SD 13)	M (7), F (5)	NR	IBD (9), neoplasia (2), proctitis (1)	Transanal	TEM	Proctectomy	215 (123–345)	17.8 (SD 6.1)	NR	1	0	6 (50%)	NR
McLemore [66] *N* = 6	(22–74)	M (2), F (4)	30.5 (22–51)	Proctitis	LA transanal	GelPoint path	Completion proctectomy (2), APR (1), restorative proctocolectomy with coloanal anastomosis (1), restorative proctocolectomy w IPAA (1)	294 (176–557)	8.5 (8–15)	NR	NR	0	3 (50%)	NR

F female; *IBD* inflammatory bowel disease; *LA* laparoscopic-assisted; *M* male; *NR* not reported; *TAMIS* transanal minimally invasive surgery; *TEM* transanal endoscopic microsurgery; *TVA* tubulovillous adenoma; *UC* ulcerative colitis mesorectum, or in combination with total mesorectal dissection.

There have been seven series published on transanal endoscopic proctectomy for benign indications, describing outcomes in a total of 86 patients [60–66]. These have been outlined in Table 21.3. Procedures performed included completion proctectomy, restorative proctocolectomy with coloanal anastomosis or ileal pouch-anal anastomosis (IPAA), and APR. These were performed primarily in hybrid fashion with transabdominal laparoscopic assistance. Indications were for refractory diversion and radiation proctitis, ulcerative colitis and Crohn's disease, large carpeting villous adenomas of the rectum, fecal incontinence, rectal strictures, and complex fistulas [60–66]. The length of the resected retained rectal stumps ranged from 8 to 30 cm. There were no deaths or major procedural complications, but three patients required conversion to open proctectomy due to intra-abdominal adhesions [62, 63]. The cumulative morbidity across the series was 35% (30/86 cases) and included urinary tract infections, presacral hematoma, several cases of delayed perineal wound healing, a perineal dehiscence requiring reoperation, an incarcerated parastomal hernia, and a colocutaneous fistula to the perineum requiring reoperation. Although these preliminary reports demonstrate the feasibility and procedural safety of a primarily transanal endoscopic approach for distal rectal dissection in ulcerative colitis, data on short-term pouch function are lacking.

Malignant Indications

Unlike benign disease, proctectomy for rectal adenocarcinoma strictly requires TME. Oncologically adequate resection with a complete mesorectum and negative margins is critical to minimize the chance of local recurrence, with the circumferential resection margin being a major determinant of overall survival following curative rectal cancer resection. Of critical importance in the early stages of adoption of taTME was the demonstration of the feasibility of achieving adequate mesorectal dissection and satisfactory short-term oncologic outcomes. The major drive behind increased adoption on this approach has been the suggested improvement in access to the low rectum and mesorectum relative to open and laparoscopic approaches, and an enhanced view of dissection planes achieved through the transanal platforms. This bottom-up approach provides a less obstructed view and manipulation of the perirectal and mesorectal planes, facilitating the mesorectal dissection, especially for low rectal tumors in patients with a narrow pelvis.

Accepted indications and contraindications for taTME are consistent with indications for laparoscopic or robotic TME. Based on standard tumor staging, taTME is warranted for resectable T1 tumors with high-risk histologic features, T2 tumors, and T3 tumors. Although early IRB-approved taTME protocols excluded node-positive disease and metastatic disease, the current indications for taTME have expanded to include these patients if taTME is performed with curative intent, as well as following treatment with neoadjuvant therapy when indicated.

Current indications for taTME also highlight specific tumor and patient characteristics that are well suited for a primarily transanal approach. There is no specified upper BMI limit, but taTME is becoming the preferred approach in morbidly obese patients with resectable rectal tumors. For very low rectal tumors located at or below the dentate line but not invading the external anal sphincter, taTME can be performed in continuity with rectal mucosectomy and partial or total ISR in order to achieve negative distal margins, followed by handsewn anastomosis. For mid-rectal tumors located >5 cm above the anal verge and at least 1 cm above the top of the anorectal ring, full-thickness rectal transection can be performed starting just below a purse-string suture placed to occlude the rectum below the tumor, with preservation of the anal sphincters, and followed by stapled colorectal anastomosis. Transanal TME is not unanimously believed to provide added benefit to a laparoscopic or robotic approach for rectal tumors located >10 cm above the anal verge, with the obvious exception of the obese male. For these tumors, in an effort to preserve rectal function, transanal rectal transection is performed well above the anorectal ring followed by transanal tumor-specific mesorectal excision and stapled colorectal anastomosis.

Currently, taTME is contraindicated for T4 disease and tumors with predicted involved CRM, unless there is evidence of significant downstaging on restaging MRI following neoadjuvant treatment. Transanal TME is also contraindicated for completely or near-completely obstructing rectal tumors. Another relative contraindication, particularly for less experienced operators, includes prior prostatectomy or other complex pelvic resection, prior pelvic radiation for gynecologic or urologic malignancies, and recurrent rectal cancer. This past history in patients can substantially complicate identification of the correct dissection planes from the perineal approach and may increase the risk of organ injury, particularly of the bladder and urethra [67].

Patient Selection

Transanal NOTES is appropriate for patients with benign disease or resectable premalignant and malignant low-to-mid-rectal tumors. These patients should have no history of extensive abdominal or pelvic surgery. Transanal TME is suitable for patients eligible for low anterior resection for low and mid-rectal tumors, but it is most effective in male patients with a narrow pelvis and in patients with a high BMI. Patients with recurrent or T4 disease and those with threatened circumferential resection margins and minimal to no response to neoadjuvant treatment are not usually candidates for taTME with sphincter preservation and most often require APR or extralevator APR and/or exenteration to achieve an R0 resection. Of note, taTME with APR and even extralevator abdominoperineal excision (ELAPE) can be performed using a transanal approach, especially if difficulty with the perineal and abdominal dissection is anticipated, as in obese males with a narrow pelvis.

Preoperative Assessment and Staging

Evaluation of surgical candidates for transanal endoscopic proctectomy follows the same principles as for any other approaches to the rectum. Preoperative workup includes a complete medical and surgical history, colonoscopy with biopsies, and a comprehensive physical examination, including a digital rectal examination (DRE). Preoperative assessment should take into account patients' baseline activity level, defecatory function, as well as urinary and sexual function. For newly diagnosed rectal cancer, laboratory studies including complete blood count, serum chemistries, liver function tests, and baseline serum carcinoembryonic antigen level should be obtained. Staging CT scans of the chest, abdomen and pelvis should be completed in addition to a pelvic MRI for tumor staging and to assess the status of the mesorectal fascia and predict involvement of the CRM. Endorectal ultrasound can be performed in conjunction with pelvic MRI, particularly in cases where differentiating between T2 and T3 disease is equivocal on pelvic MRI. Patients with locally advanced disease should undergo standard long-course neoadjuvant treatment, although in some cases, short-course radiation may be elected, and neoadjuvant treatment may even be avoided altogether in carefully selected T3a rectal tumors [55].

Preoperative DRE should assess baseline anal sphincter function, localize the tumor within the rectum, and determine tumor mobility or fixation, along with distance from the anorectal ring, dentate line, and anal verge. Preoperative evaluation should also include proctoscopy or flexible sigmoidoscopy to localize the rectal tumor and assist surgical planning. DRE, office endoscopy, and/or pelvic MRI may be repeated following completion of neoadjuvant treatment, to assess tumor response, as that may impact the operative plan with respect to sphincter preservation. Transanal proctectomy for rectal cancer is typically performed 8–12 weeks following completion of neoadjuvant treatment, which is the standard of care in the management of locally advanced rectal cancer.

Candidates for sphincter-preserving proctectomy using transanal assistance should be extensively counseled regarding temporary fecal diversion, as well as anticipated functional disturbances and quality of life issues following ileostomy closure. This is particularly important for very low rectal tumors if radiation was administered preoperatively, and where partial or complete ISR might be required to achieve negative resection margins.

Preoperative Preparation

With the exception of completion proctectomy, patients undergoing transanal endoscopic restorative proctectomy usually undergo mechanical bowel preparation the night prior to surgery either with a combination of oral agents and enemas or with enemas alone. Standard perioperative antibiotic and thromboembolic prophylaxis is administered parenterally. General anesthesia with paralytics is recommended to avoid leakage of CO_2 during procedures. However, the surgical team may consider preoperative epidural placement versus patient-controlled analgesia postoperatively or transversus abdominis plane (TAP) block at the end of the procedure.

Operative Setup

Ample time should be reserved for setup on the day of surgery. Regarding intraoperative positioning, most surgeons perform taTME with the patient in lithotomy position, but completion proctectomy can be performed in prone position, which can be helpful in cases where hip flexion is severely limited [66]. Most authors perform on-table rectal irrigation with dilute betadine. A Foley catheter is routinely placed, and the abdomen and perineum are both prepped and draped to allow simultaneous or sequential access during hybrid transanal procedures.

The amount of space in the operating room should be taken into consideration. The majority of taTME procedures are performed using a hybrid rather than a pure transanal endoscopic approach. Therefore, procedures can be performed as either a 1-team approach with a single team performing the abdominal and transanal dissection sequentially or a 2-team approach with a transanal team and an abdominal team working simultaneously (Fig. 21.1). The 2-team approach is preferred for reasons of safety and decreased operative time [43, 53]. If a 1-team approach is used, then it is recommended to have an assistant on standby for transanal delivery of the colon. A 2-team approach at this portion of the case is meant to assist with reach, to ensure correct orientation of bowel and mesentery, confirm adequate blood supply, and reduce tension. There should be one surgical scrub technician with a table for the transanal team, and another surgical technician with a table for the abdominal team.

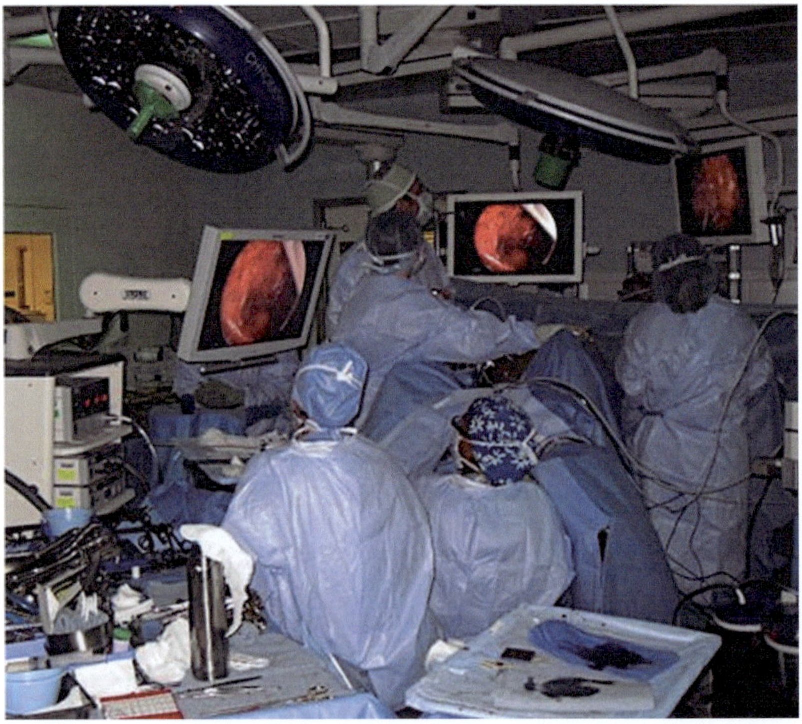

Fig. 21.1 Operative setup demonstrating 2-team approach with a transanal team and an abdominal team working simultaneously

Depending on the transanal platform being used, there must be enough room for one to two surgeons to operate transanally. The TAMIS platform requires a dedicated assistant for camera control, while the TEO/TEM does not. An optimal high-definition video monitor should have a moveable screen on swivel. There is typically one located between the legs facing the transanal surgeon/team at eye level while not obstructing the operative field of the abdominal team. The abdominal team requires a video monitor on the right side of the patient and another on the left.

Instrumentation

The abdominal portion of the case requires instrumentation from a standard laparoscopic or robotic low anterior resection tray, with monopolar hook and scissors, bipolar vessel sealer, trocars, CO_2 insufflator, suction, irrigation, a pelvic drain, and supplies to mature a loop ileostomy.

Instrumentation for the transanal portion of the surgery should include the following:

- Standard anorectal tray with plastic or metal anoscopes. Our preference is to use the graduated plastic disposable anoscope that is part of the procedure for prolapsed hemorrhoid (PPH) stapling kit (Medtronic, Minneapolis, MN);
- Lone Star disposable retractor;
- Head light;
- TES platform that the operator is familiar with (TAMIS, TEO, or TEM);
- Monopolar cautery hook or spatula;
- Bipolar device (although dissection with monopolar cautery is preferred);
- High-flow insufflator and smoke evacuation system (AirSeal®, SurgiQuest, Milford, CT) has become the preferred system worldwide, but other high-flow insufflators are available on the market;
- Suction and irrigation;
- Bariatric length 10-mm camera if a TAMIS platform is used;
- EEA staplers if a stapled anastomosis is to be performed;
- Indocyanine green (ICG) fluorescence imaging may be used to assess the perfusion of colorectal or coloanal anastomoses.

Procedural Steps for taTME

Most surgeons using a 1-team approach will start with the abdominal dissection, with high ligation of the inferior mesenteric artery and division of the inferior mesenteric vein, splenic flexure takedown, and mobilization of the left colon, sigmoid, and proximal rectum. The extent of pelvic dissection is variable, but usually extends to just above the peritoneal reflection anteriorly, and to below the sacral promontory posteriorly, until the deeper mesorectal dissection becomes technically challenging. The team then transitions to transanal dissection. Occasionally, transanal dissection will be initiated first, followed by abdominal access and dissection.

Whether a 1-team or 2-team simultaneous approach is utilized, the steps of transanal dissection depend on the exact tumor level, i.e., distance from the anorectal ring. Following confirmation of the exact location of the tumor by digital and visual inspection with anoscopy, assessment of the required distal margin is made (Fig. 21.2). For tumors above the anorectal ring, a purse-string suture is placed 0.5–1 cm below the rectal tumor. This is completed either directly through a standard anoscope or endoscopically through the TES platform (Fig. 21.3). In the latter case, the transanal platform is inserted first and then followed by purse-string occlusion of the rectum. The purse string usually consists of 2-0 Prolene or 2-0 Vicryl sutures based on the surgeon's preference. Care must be taken to ensure that the purse-string suture is airtight to avoid distention of the proximal colon and spillage of fecal material or tumor cells onto the operative field (Fig. 21.4).

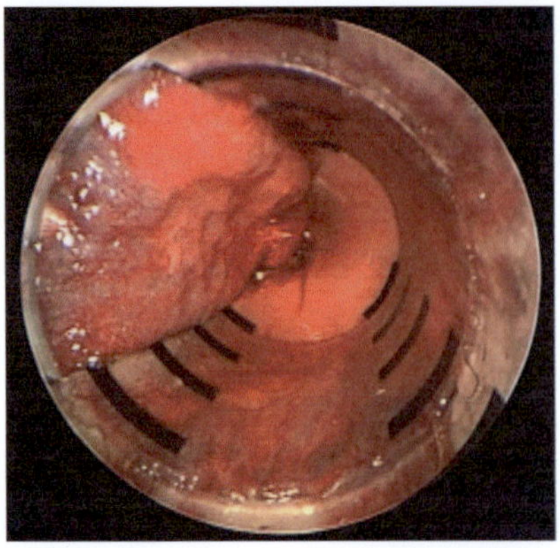

Fig. 21.2 View through a plastic anoscope demonstrating the exact distance between the rectal lesion and the dentate line

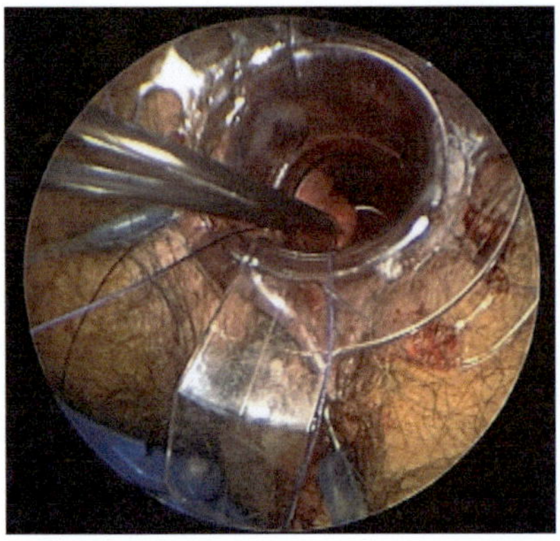

Fig. 21.3 Purse-string suture placement through a plastic anoscope

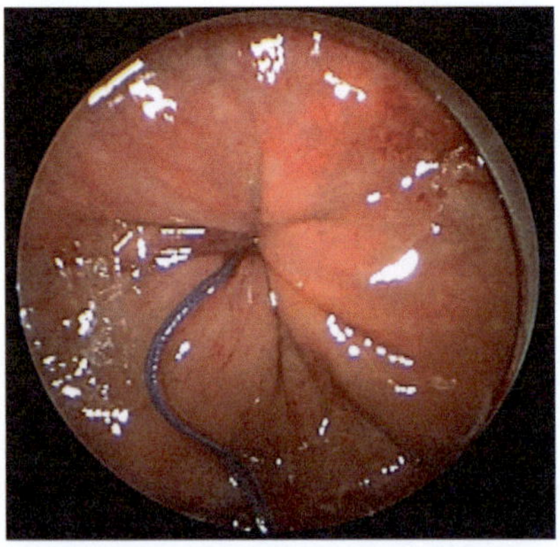

Fig. 21.4 Purse-string occlusion of the rectum below the rectal tumor

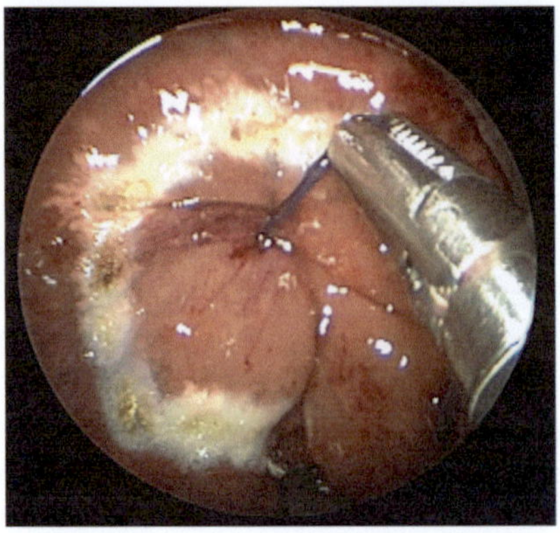

Fig. 21.5 Initiation of circumferential rectal transanal dissection starting just below the purse-string suture

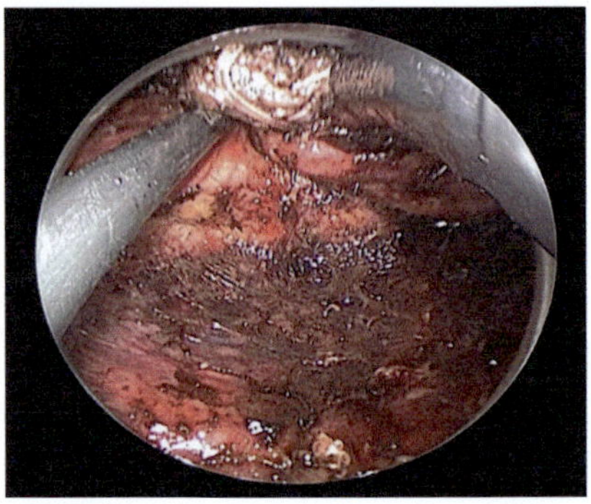

Fig. 21.6 Posterior mesorectal dissection carried out along avascular plane between the mesorectal fascia and the sacrum

After purse-string insertion of the transanal platform and occlusion of the rectum, distention with CO_2 is achieved to a pressure of 10–12 mm Hg. The rectal mucosa is scored circumferentially (Fig. 21.5). Full-thickness rectal and mesorectal mobilization is carried out sequentially using monopolar instruments. Efforts should be made to avoid the use of bipolar energy, which is not needed if dissection carries on along the correct planes. Posterior mesorectal dissection is carried out along the avascular plane between the mesorectal fascia and the sacrum, while anterior dissection is carried between the rectovaginal or rectoprostatic fascia (Figs. 21.6 and 21.7). Laterally, care must be taken to avoid dissection of the pelvic sidewall and damage to

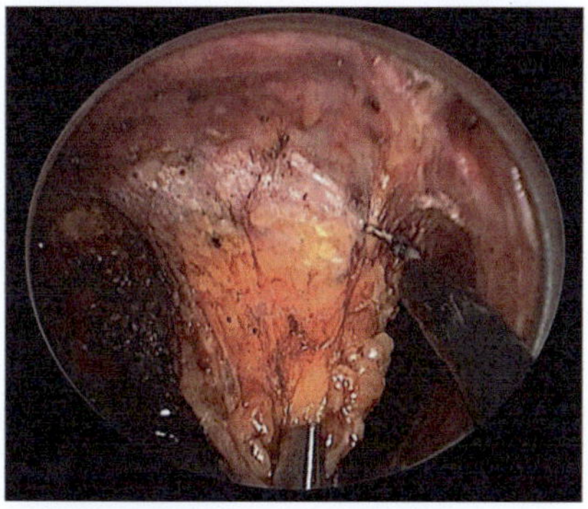

Fig. 21.7 Anterior mesorectal dissection carried out between mesorectum and retroprostatic fascia

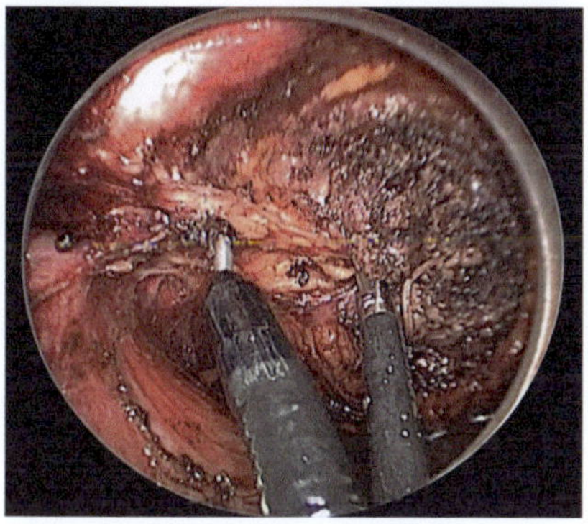

Fig. 21.8 Lateral mesorectal dissection carried out between mesorectum and pelvic sidewall

the pelvic plexus (Fig. 21.8). During the anterolateral dissection of the rectum and mesorectum, care must be taken to avoid injury to the neurovascular bundles bilaterally, which may serve as landmarks for the location of the prostate when difficulties are encountered during anterior mobilization and identification of the posterior aspect of the prostate.

Transanal TME dissection is carried out circumferentially, and in a sequential but symmetric pattern. Every effort should be made to avoid dissecting too far along any given plane to avoid loss of orientation from distorted tissue planes. Posterior mesorectal dissection is technically the easiest because the main landmarks, namely the presacral fascia and the mesorectal fascia, are readily identifiable. Anteriorly, the difficulty is to identify the posterior aspect of the vagina or prostate, which can

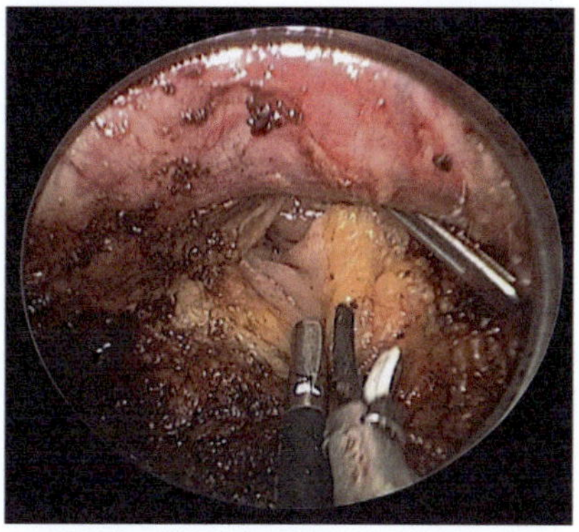

Fig. 21.9 Transanal view of peritoneal entry

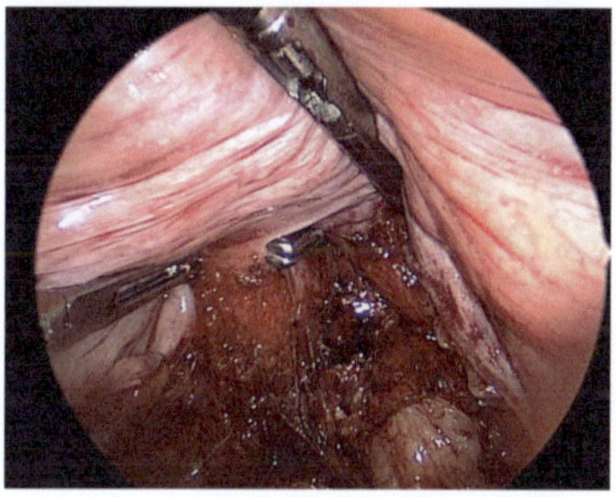

Fig. 21.10 Laparoscopic view of peritoneal entry

be complicated when starting low and having to dissect through the perineal body before identifying the correct anterior mesorectal plane. Ultimately, anterior dissection is carried out cephalad until the peritoneal reflection is reached, which is another landmark that is readily identifiable. Posteriorly, depending on the angulation of the sacral promontory, transanal dissection cannot be extended beyond the top of the sacral promontory and must be assisted by the abdominal team. Even when using a 1-team approach, abdominal assistance during this step is critical, as it allows two teams to work simultaneously to complete mobilization of the rectum and merge the abdominal and transanal planes of dissection. Peritoneal entry is usually performed transanally and under laparoscopic visualization from above (Figs. 21.9 and 21.10).

Following complete mobilization of the TME specimen, the colon is either exteriorized transanally or through an abdominal incision if the specimen is too bulky to permit transanal extraction (Fig. 21.11). After transection of the specimen, a colorectal stapled anastomosis can be performed if the rectum was transected well above the dentate line. A double-purse-string, circular-stapled anastomosis technique is used with either end-to-end, side-to-end, coloanal J-pouch or transverse coloplasty [68]. A protective loop ileostomy is then constructed with placement of closed pelvic drains.

For tumors below the anorectal ring, either partial or complete ISR is performed first to achieve negative distal margins. ISR is performed through a Lone Star retractor with monopolar instruments. Dissection is extended cephalad until the puborectalis muscle and the bottom of the mesorectum are identified, and the rectovaginal or retroprostatic plane is visualized anteriorly. The anorectal stump is then closed with a purse-string suture, and the transanal platform is inserted. Further dissection is needed posteriorly through the anococcygeal raphe to access the presacral space. The inferior aspect of the mesorectum can be identified posteriorly, and the rectovaginal or rectoprostatic plane anteriorly, and taTME may then proceed as described previously. The specimen is extracted and a handsewn coloanal anastomosis is performed using end-to-end, side-to-end, coloanal J-pouch, or transverse coloplasty with a protective ileostomy (Figs. 21.12 and 21.13).

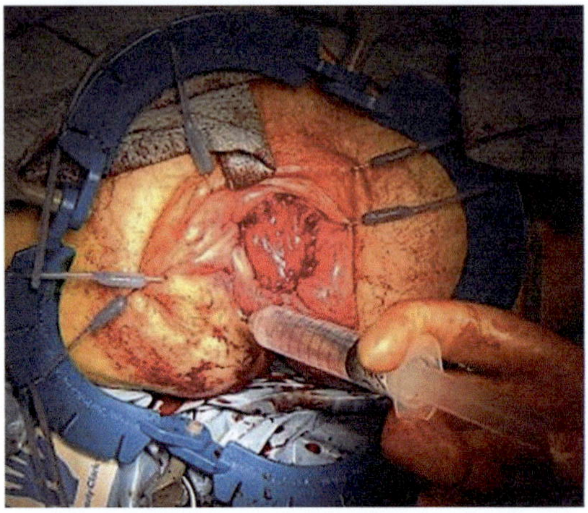

Fig. 21.12 Handsewn coloanal anastomosis

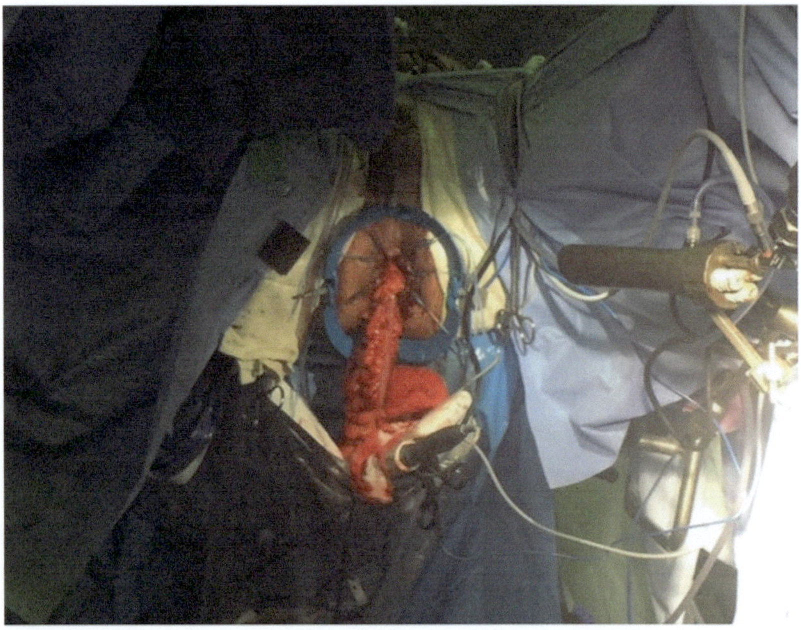

Fig. 21.11 Transanal specimen extraction

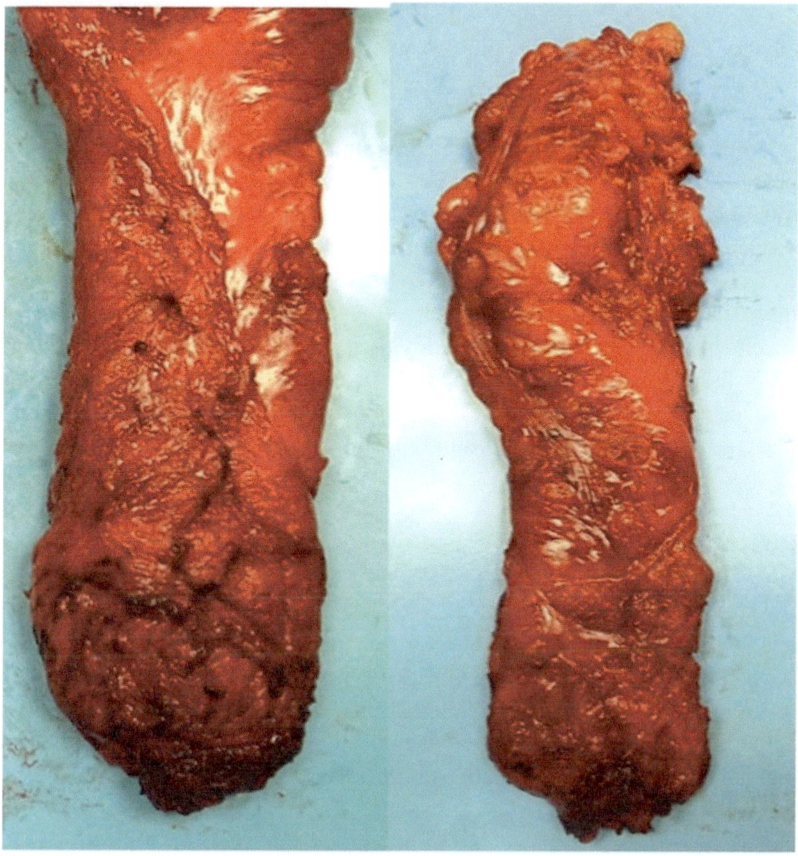

Fig. 21.13 Anterior and posterior views of complete TME specimen

Alternatives

In patients with ulcerative colitis or familial adenomatous polyposis (FAP), where a transanal restorative proctocolectomy or proctectomy with IPAA would be performed, transanal procedures would commence after mobilization of the colon and/or rectum and are initiated with a Lone Star retractor and circumferential rectal mucosectomy starting at the level of the dentate line. Rectal transection is then carried out full-thickness above the anorectal ring with rectal dissection following along the rectal wall and mesorectal plane [66]. Alternatively, one may place a purse-string suture 3 cm above the dentate line followed by circumferential, full-thickness incision of the rectal wall and then close rectal dissection. IPAA is performed with a single-stapled technique following specimen extraction [67].

With transanal endoscopic proctectomy or proctocolectomy with APR, the colon is mobilized followed by ligation of the inferior mesenteric vessels, and TME dissection initiated using an open, laparoscopic- or robotic-assisted transabdominal approach. The anus is sutured closed followed by intersphincteric or standard proctectomy, which may be carried out simultaneously (2-team) or sequentially with the abdominal dissection (1-team). Transanal dissection continues cephalad with division of the perineal body until the rectoprostatic or rectovaginal plane is clearly identified. Posterior dissection is then carried out until the puborectalis is visualized. The transanal platform is then inserted with CO_2 insufflation, and rectal dissection is advanced endoscopically. The posterior dissection can be carried out close to the rectal wall within the mesorectal plane, or along the plane between the mesorectum and presacral fascia depending on the pathology and surgeon's preference. After proctectomy, the specimen is then extracted followed by closure of the perineal wound in layers.

Another alternative to transanal completion proctectomy for benign disease is to initiate transanal, endoscopic, full-thickness, rectal transection through the transanal platform starting well above the dentate line. The rectal dissection, mesorectal dissection, and exteriorization of the specimen are then performed, and intersphincteric dissection of the short anorectal stump is then carried out, followed by extraction of the new specimen and perineal wound closure [64].

Postoperative Care and Follow-Up

A Foley catheter is typically kept in place for at least two days after the procedure given the relatively high incidence of postoperative urinary retention following perineal dissection, especially in males [36, 44, 47]. One to two doses of parenteral antibiotics are administered postoperatively. Patients are often managed using enhanced recovery protocols with immediate initiation of oral intake as tolerated, and pain control with aggressive, non-narcotic regimens. Patients are extensively counseled regarding ostomy management prior to discharge.

Postoperative visits and evaluation following taTME are the same as any rectal cancer resection. In patients with locally advanced rectal cancer undergoing adjuvant treatment, ileostomy closure is usually deferred until completion of adjuvant therapy. Endoscopic and radiographic evaluation of the coloanal anastomosis is performed prior to reversal, and anastomotic complications such as strictures, leaks, and fistulas are managed using standard protocols. Oncologic surveillance following rectal cancer resections typically follows NCCN guidelines. Regarding functional outcomes, patients who have undergone partial or complete ISR are at increased risk for poor functional outcomes and require long-term monitoring of their defecatory function and aggressive management of their fecal incontinence.

Complications

Complication rates reported with taTME performed either in pure or hybrid fashion with abdominal assistance mirror complications rates associated with open or laparoscopic TME and include intraoperative bleeding, organ injury (including rectal perforation, ureteral, and urethral injury), vaginal wall injury, and prostatic injury. Conversion to laparoscopic and/or open techniques is always possible and represents good surgical judgment rather than a complication. Conversion rates can be expected to be higher during a surgeon's early experience.

Maintaining pneumorectum is a technical issue unique to taTME. When encountering loss of pneumorectum, the surgeon should troubleshoot, check for leaks in the platform, and confirm muscle paralysis. One should avoid premature peritoneal entry during the transanal approach and defer this step until complete circumferential TME has been extended as far cephalad as possible.

Urethral injury is not a reported complication of open and laparoscopic TME, and it is a rare complication during difficult APR, with an estimated incidence of 1.5–2% [69, 70]. Although rarely reported in current taTME series, urethral injury has emerged as the most concerning procedure-specific morbidity associated with taTME. Although only four urethral injuries have been described in our review of over 500 published taTME cases to date, the actual incidence of urethral injury is not yet defined. Based on personal communications, there have been more cases of urethral injuries during taTME than have been voluntarily entered in the LOREC international taTME registry, which will soon publish the findings of the first 720 taTME cases entered. The risk of urethral injury seems to be highest during the surgeon's early experience, during difficult anterior dissection, and in patients with bulky anterior rectal tumors or enlarged prostate [47, 48, 53, 71].

To avoid urethral injury, the surgeon must be familiar with the pre-prostatic anatomy from the taTME point of view. The neurovascular bundle of Walsh contains paired arterial vessels that can be recognized during the anterolateral dissection. Dissection must be maintained superficial to these paired vessels to avoid entering into the prostate and risk transecting the prostatic urethra [71].

Commonly reported postoperative complications following taTME are consistent with that from standard TME and include urinary tract infection, surgical site infections, pelvic abscess, anastomotic leaks, ischemic left conduit, and urinary retention. There may be need for readmission and reoperation. Medical complications such as pneumonia, deep venous thrombosis, pulmonary embolism, or other cardiopulmonary complications may occur.

Long-term functional outcomes are largely unknown at this time, and complications likely include functional disturbances that range from urgency, fragmentation, tenesmus, and fecal incontinence, as with any other type of TME. Persistent urinary dysfunction has been reported, but did resolve after 6 months [72]. Overall impact of taTME on defecatory, urinary, and sexual function needs to be further investigated in the setting of large trials. Likewise, long-term oncologic outcomes of these procedures as they relate to surgical technique, tumor stage, quality of TME, and use of neoadjuvant treatment are much needed.

Limitations

Transanal TME does not appear to confer any added benefit to a laparoscopic or robotic approach for upper rectal tumors located >10 cm from the anal verge except in obese male patients. With the available transanal platforms, TAMIS in particular, lesions located in the upper rectum are more difficult to reach for resection. The anastomoses in taTME for lesions at this level are more difficult due to inadequate visual exposure and require endoscopic placement of the purse-string suture rather than by hand [68].

An additional limitation of taTME is the unknown impact of increased use of the transanal platform on anal sphincter function. For TES, anorectal dysfunction ranges from <1 to 4% and is typically transient [73–75]. Patients who undergo TES have been shown to return to their baseline fecal continence within 6–12 weeks [73–75]. However, taTME requires more time in the operating room in comparison with TES. It is suspected that patients undergoing taTME are at greater risk for anal sphincter dysfunction because of the prolonged use of the transanal platform.

Training

Despite the lack of published data on the effect of experience or the impact of inanimate training models on a surgeon's performance during transanal proctectomy, data from prior experimental studies on this technique have highlighted the importance of fresh human cadavers as the best-suited training model for this technique [76]. Total mesorectal dissection is accurately reproducible in human cadavers, as most of the dissection in patients is bloodless, as long as rectal and mesorectal dissection proceeds along the anatomically correct (i.e., avascular) planes. In their series of consecutive transanal endoscopic rectosigmoid resection in 32 human cadavers, based on the significant decrease in operative time in completing the procedures after five cases, the authors concluded that the "learning curve" for taTME was likely around five cadavers with regard to procedural training [76]. To make the most from a cadaver training course, a surgeon aspiring to implement taTME into their practice must have expertise in minimally invasive TME, ISR, as well as TES [77]. Additionally, IRB-approved data collection with publication of outcomes and/or participation in a clinical registry is highly recommended to ensure that taTME is being performed safely as it becomes more widely adopted [57, 77]. Finally, there is strong consensus that surgeons initiating taTME should be proctored during their first few cases in an effort to reduce operative time, help with troubleshooting, and minimize the incidence of intraoperative complications, especially during complicated cases.

Future Directions

The concept of transanal colorectal surgery is undergoing a revolutionary paradigm shift. Transanal rectosigmoid resection has been used in the management of rectal prolapse since the Altemeier procedure, and transanal ISR or the TATA procedure have been well described in the treatment of low rectal cancer. Today, transanal NOTES builds on the concept of transanal rectal dissection by proposing to perform complete rectal, mesorectal, and colon dissection entirely transanally using an endoscopic platform. The techniques for NOTES colorectal procedures derive from TES, and apart from its original use for local resection of rectal tumors, TES platforms have been applied for NOSE and for laparoscopic-assisted transanal rectosigmoidectomy in humans [34, 39, 42]. The experience of pure taTME is growing [49, 53]. Meanwhile, the indications for taTME are expanding from low and mid-rectal tumors to possibly recurrent cancer, reoperative pelvic surgery, and restorative proctocolectomy with IPAA [67]. The current transanal platforms may someday evolve to include robotic platforms. COLOR III, an international, multicenter, superiority, randomized trial designed to compare taTME and conventional laparoscopic TME, will launch in the near future [57]. Though there is potential for even wider adoption and growth of taTME, it must be performed safely in the hands of a surgical team with significant experience in minimally invasive TME, TES, and ISR. Therefore, the development and validation of a taTME training model is critical. With such momentum moving forward, it is no wonder that members of the surgical community are now cautiously optimistic that taTME may become the most commonly performed technique for distal rectal cancer.

References

1. Group COSTS. A comparison of laparoscopically assisted and open colectomy for colon cancer. N Engl J Med. 2004;350(20):2050–59.
2. Guillou P, Quirke P, Thorpe H. Short-term endpoints of conventional versus laparoscopic-assisted surgery in patients with colorectal cancer (MRC CLASICC trial): multicentre, randomised controlled trial. Lancet. 2005;365(9472):1718–26.
3. Fleshman J, Sargent D, Green E. Clinical outcomes of surgical therapy study group. Laparoscopic colectomy for cancer is not inferior to open surgery based on 5-year data from the COST Study Group trial. Ann Surg. 2007;246(4):655–62.
4. Veldkamp R, Kuhry E, Hop W. Colon cancer laparoscopic or open resection study group (COLOR). Laparoscopic surgery versus open surgery for colon cancer: short-term outcomes of a randomised trial. Lancet Oncol. 2005;6(7):477–84.
5. Young M, Pigazzi A. Total mesorectal excision: open, laparoscopic or robotic. Recent Results Cancer Res. 2014;203:47–55.
6. Delmonaco P, Cirocchi R, La Mura F. Trocar site hernia after laparoscopic colectomy: a case report and literature review. ISRN Surg 2011. 2011.
7. Franklin M, Liang S, Russek K. Integration of transanal specimen extraction into laparoscopic anterior resection with total mesorectal excision for rectal cancer: a consecutive series of 179 patients. Surg Endosc. 2013;27(1):127–32.
8. Cheung H, Leung A, Chung C, Ng D, Li M. Endo-laparoscopic colectomy without mini-laparotomy for left-sided colonic tumors. World J Surg 2009. 2009;33(6):1287–91.
9. Leroy J, Constantino F, Cahill R, D'Agostino J, Morales A, Mutter D, et al. Laparoscopic resection with transanal specimen extraction for sigmoid diverticulitis. Br J Surg 2011. 2011;98(9):1327–34.
10. Leroy J, Diana M, Wall J, Marescaux J. NOTES applications in colorectal surgery. 1st ed. In: Kalloo A, Marescaux J, Zorron R, editors. Wiley-Blackwell; 2012.
11. van der Pas M, Haglind E, Cuesta M, Furst A, Lacy A, Hop W, et al. Laparoscopic versus open surgery for rectal cancer (COLOR II): short-term outcomes of a randomised, phase 3 trial. Lancet Oncol. 2013;14(3):210–8.
12. Bonjer J, Deijen C, Abis G, Cuesta M, van der Pas M, de Lange-de Klerk E, et al. A randomized trial of laparoscopic versus open surgery for rectal cancer. N Engl J Med. 2015;372(14):1324–32.
13. Leung K, Kwok S, Lam S, Lee J, Yiu R, Ng S, et al. Laparoscopic resection of rectosigmoid carcinoma prospective randomised trial. Lancet. 2004;363(9416):1187–92.
14. Ng S, Leung K, Lee J, Yiu R, Li J, Hon S. Long-term morbidity and oncologic outcomes of laparoscopic-assisted anterior resection for upper rectal cancer: ten-year results of a prospective, randomized trial. Dis Colon Rectum. 2009;52(4):558–66.
15. Jayne D, Guillou P, Thorpe H, Quirke P, Copeland J, Smith A, et al. Randomized trial of laparoscopic assisted resection of colorectal carcinoma 3 year

results of the UK MRC CLASICC Trial Group. J Clin Oncol. 2007;25(21):3061–8.
16. Kang S, Park J, Jeong S, Nam B, Choi H, Kim D, et al. Open versus laparoscopic surgery for mid or low rectal cancer after neoadjuvant chemoradiotherapy (COREAN trial): short-term outcomes of an open-label randomised controlled trial. Lancet Oncol. 2010;11(7):637–45.
17. Jeong S, Park J, Nam B, Kim S, Kang S, Lim S, et al. Open versus laparoscopic surgery for mid-rectal or low-rectal cancer after neoadjuvant chemoradiotherapy (COREAN trial): survival outcomes of an open-label, non-inferiority, randomised controlled trial. Lancet Oncol. 2014;15(7):767–74.
18. Fleshman J, Branda M, Sargent D, Boller A, George V, Abbas M, et al. Effect of laparoscopic-assisted resection vs open resection of stage II or III rectal cancer on pathologic outcomes: the ACOSOG Z6051 randomized clinical trial. JAMA. 2015;314(13):1356–64.
19. Stevenson A, Solomon M, Lumley J, Hewett P, Clouston A, Gebski V, et al. Effect of laparoscopic-assisted resection vs open resection on pathological outcomes in rectal cancer: the ALaCaRT randomized clinical trial. JAMA. 2015;314 (13):1356–63.
20. Lee G, Sylla P. Shifting paradigms in minimally invasive surgery: applications of transanal natural orifice transluminal endoscopic surgery in colorectal surgery. Clin Colon Rectal Surg. 2015;28(3):181–93.
21. Jayne D, Brown J, Thorpe H, Walker J, Quirke P, Guillou P. Bladder and sexual function following resection for rectal cancer in a randomized clinical trial of laparoscopic versus open technique. Br J Surg. 2005;92(9):1124–32.
22. Breukink S, van der Zaag-Loonen H, Bouma E, Pierie J, Hoff C, Wiggers T, et al. Prospective evaluation of quality of life and sexual functioning after laparoscopic total mesorectal excision. Dis Colon Rectum. 2007;50(2):147–55.
23. Jayne D, Thorpe H, Copeland J, Quirke P, Brown J, Guillou P. Five-year follow-up of the Medical Research Council CLASICC trial of laparoscopically assisted versus open surgery for colorectal cancer. Br J Surg. 2010;97(11):1638–45.
24. Xiong B, Ma L, Zhang C, Cheng Y. Robotic versus laparoscopic total mesorectal excision for rectal cancer: a meta-analysis. J Surg Res. 2014;188 (2):404–14.
25. Quirke P, Steele R, Monson J, Grieve R, Khanna S, Couture J, et al. Effect of the plane of surgery achieved on local recurrence in patients with operable rectal cancer: a prospective study using data from the MRC CR07 and NCIC-CTG CO16 randomised clinical trial. Lancet. 2009;373(9666):821–8.
26. Leite J, Martins S, Oliveria J, Cunha M, Castro-Sousa F. Clinical significance of macroscopic completeness of mesorectal resection in rectal cancer. Colorectal Dis. 2011;13(4):381–6.
27. Maslekar S, Sharma A, Macdonald A, Gunn J, Monson J, Hartley J. Mesorectal grades predict recurrences after curative resection for rectal cancer. Dis Colon Rectum. 2007;50(2):168–75.
28. Rickles A, Dietz D, Chang G, Wexner S, Berho M, Remzi F, et al. High rate of positive circumferential resection margins following rectal cancer surgery: a call to action. Ann Surg. 2015;262(6):891–8.
29. Wexner S, Berho M. Transanal total mesorectal excision of rectal carcinoma: evidence to learn and adopt the technique. Ann Surg. 2015;261(2):234–6.
30. Marks J, Frenkel J, D'Andrea A, Greenleaf C. Maximizing rectal cancer results: TEM and TATA techniques to expand sphincter preservation. Surg Oncol Clin N Am. 2011;20(3):501–20.
31. Atallah S. Transanal total mesorectal excision: full steam ahead. Tech Coloproctol. 2015;19(2):57–61.
32. Buess G, Theiss R, Gunther M, Hutterer F, Pichlmaier H. Endoscopic surgery in the rectum. Endoscopy. 1985;17(1):31–5.
33. Atallah S, Albert M, Larach S. Transanal minimally invasive surgery: a giant leap forward. Surg Endosc. 2010;24(9):2200–5.
34. Bonin E, Gostout C. Anal route: transrectal/transcolonic access. In: Kalloo A, Marescaux J, Zorron R, editors. Natural orifice translumenal endoscopic surgery (NOTES): textbook and video atlas. Oxford, UK: Wiley-Blackwell; 2012. p. 53–5.
35. Singh R, Omiccioli A, Hegge S, McKinley C. Does the extraction-site location in laparoscopic colorectal surgery have an impact on incisional hernia rates? Surg Endosc. 2008;22(12):2596–600.
36. Sylla P, Bordeianou L, Berger D, Han K, Lauwers G, Sahani D, et al. A pilot study of natural orifice transanal endoscopic total mesorectal excision with laparoscopic assistance for rectal cancer. Surg Endosc. 2013;27(9):3396–405.
37. Whiteford M, Denk P, Swanstrom L. Feasibility of radical sigmoid colectomy performed as natural orifice translumenal endoscopic surgery (NOTES) using transanal endoscopic microsurgery. Surg Endosc. 2007;21(10):1870–4.
38. Lacy A, Saavedra-Perez D, Bravo R, Adelsdorfer C, Aceituno M, Balust J. Minilaparoscopy-assisted natural orifice total colectomy: technical report of a minilaparoscopy-assisted transrectal resection. Surg Endosc. 2012;26(7):2080–5.
39. Fuchs K, Breithaupt W, Varga G, Schulz T, Reinisch A, Josipovic N. Transanal hybrid colon resection: from laparoscopy to NOTES. Surg Endosc. 2013;27(3):746–52.
40. Vahdad M, Cernaianu G, Semaan A, Klein T, Faran S, Zemon H, et al. An experimental study in six fresh human cadavers using a novel approach to avoid abdominal wall incisions in total colectomy: totally transanal laparoendoscopic single-site pull-through colectomy with J-pouch creation. Surg Endosc. 2015. Epub 20 Oct 2015.

41. Veltcamp Helbach M, Deijen C, Velthuis S, Bonjer J, Tuynman J, Sietses C. Transanal total mesorectal excision for rectal adenocarcinoma: short-term outcomes and experience after 80 cases. Surg Endosc. 2014;30(2):464–70.
42. Sylla P, Rattner D, Delgado S, Lacy A. NOTES transanal rectal cancer resection using transanal endoscopic microsurgery and laparoscopic assistance. Surg Endosc. 2010;24(5):1205–10.
43. Lacy A, Tasende M, Delgado S, Fernandez-Hevia M, Jimenez M, De Lacy B, et al. Transanal total mesorectal excision for rectal cancer: outcomes after 140 patients. J Am Coll Surg. 2015;221(2):415–23.
44. Tuech J, Karoui M, Lelong B, De Chaisemartin C, Bridoux V, Manceau G, et al. A step toward NOTES total mesorectal excision for rectal cancer: endoscopic transanal proctectomy. Ann Surg. 2015;261 (2):228–33.
45. Muratore A, Mellano A, Marsanic P, De Simone M. Transanal total mesorectal excision (taTME) for cancer located in the lower rectum: short- and mid-term results. Eur J Surg Oncol. 2015;41 (4):478–83.
46. Serra-Aracil X, Mora-Lopez L, Casalots A, Pericay C, Guerrero R, Navarro-Soto S. Hybrid NOTES: TEO for transanal total mesorectal excision: intracorporeal resection and anastomosis. Surg Endosc. 2016;30(1):346–54.
47. Rouanet P, Mourregot A, Azar C, Carrere S, Gutowski M, Quenet F, et al. Transanal endoscopic proctectomy: an innovative procedure for difficult resection of rectal tumors in men with narrow pelvis. Dis Colon Rectum. 2013;56(4):408–15.
48. Burke J, Martin-Perez B, Khan A, Nassif G, deBeche-Adams T, Larach S, et al. Transanal total mesorectal excision for rectal cancer: early outcomes in 50 consecutive patients. Colorectal Dis. 2016. Epub 8 Jan 2016.
49. Chouillard E, Chahine E, Khoury G, Vinson-Bonnet B, Gumbs A, Azoulay D, et al. NOTES total mesorectal excision (TME) for patients with rectal neoplasia: a preliminary experience. Surg Endosc. 2014;28(11):3150–7.
50. Chen C, Lai Y, Jiang J, Chu C, Huang I, Chen W, et al. Transanal total mesorectal excision versus laparoscopic surgery for rectal cancer receiving neoadjuvant chemoradiation: a matched case-control study. Ann Surg Oncol. 2016;23 (4):1169–76.
51. Perdawood S, Al Khefagie G. Transanal vs laparoscopic total mesorectal excision for rectal cancer: initial experience from Denmark. Colorectal Dis. 2016;18(1):51–8.
52. Buchs N, Nicholson G, Yeung T, Mortensen N, Cunningham C, Jones O, et al. Transanal rectal resection: an initial experience of 20 cases. Colorectal Dis. 2016;18(1):45–50.
53. Kang L, Chen W, Luo S, Luo Y, Liu Z, Huang M, et al. Transanal total mesorectal excision for rectal cancer: a preliminary report. Surg Endosc. 2015. Epub 27 Aug 2015.
54. de'Angelis N, Portigliotti L, Azoulay D, Brunetti F. Transanal total mesorectal excision for rectal cancer: a single center experience and systematic review of the literature. Langenbecks Arch Surg. 2015;400 (8):945–59.
55. Fernandez-Hevia M, Delgado S, Castellis A, Tasende M, Momblan D, Diaz del Gobbo G, et al. Transanal total mesorectal excision in rectal cancer: short-term outcomes in comparison with laparoscopic surgery. Ann Surg. 2015;261(2):221–7.
56. Velthuis S, Nieuwenhuis D, Ruijter T, Cuesta M, Bonjer H, Sietses C. Transanal versus traditional laparoscopic total mesorectal excision for rectal carcinoma. Surg Endosc. 2014;28(12):3494–9.
57. Diejen C, Velthuis S, Tsai A, Mavroveli S, de Lang-de Klerk E, Sietses C, et al. COLOR III: a multicentre randomised clinical trial comparing transanal TME versus laparoscopic TME for mid and low rectal cancer. Surg Endosc. 2015. Epub 4 Nov 2015.
58. Leroy J, Barry B, Melani A, Mutter D, Marescaux J. No-scar transanal total mesorectal excision: the last step to pure NOTES for colorectal surgery. JAMA Surg. 2013;148(3):226–30.
59. Zhang H, Zhang Y, Jin X, Li M, Fan J, Yang Z. Transanal single-port laparoscopic total mesorectal excision in the treatment of rectal cancer. Tech Coloproctol. 2013;17(1):117–23.
60. de Buck van Overstraeten A, Wolthuis A, D'Hoore A. Transanal completion proctectomy after total colectomy and ileal pouch-anal anastomosis for ulcerative colitis: a modified single stapled technique. Colorectal Dis. 2016;18(4):141–4.
61. Tasende M, Delgado S, Jimenez M, del Gobbo G, Fernandez-Hevia M, DeLacy B. Minimal invasive surgery: NOSE and NOTES in ulcerative colitis. Surg Endosc. 2015;29(11):3313–8.
62. Leo C, Samaranayake S, Perry-Wood Z, Vitone L, Faiz O, Hodgkinson J, et al. Initial experience of restorative proctocolectomy for ulcerative colitis by transanal total mesorectal excision and single incision abdominal laparoscopic surgery. Colorectal Dis. 2016.
63. Wolthuis A, de Buck van Overstraeten A, D'Hoore A. Dynamic article: transanal rectal excision: a pilot study. Dis Colon Rectum. 2014;57(1):105–9.
64. Bremers A, van Laarhoven K, van der Kolk B, de Wilt J, van Goor H. Transanal endoscopic microsurgery approach for rectal stump resection as an alternative to transperitoneal stump resection. Br J Surg. 2013;100(4):568–71.
65. Liyanage C, Ramwell A, Harris G, Levy B, Simson J. Transanal endoscopic microsurgery: a new technique for completion proctectomy. Colorectal Dis. 2013;15(9):542–7.
66. McLemore E, Leland H, Devaraj B, Pola S, Docherty M, Patel D, et al. Transanal endoscopic surgical proctectomy for proctitis case series report:

diversion, radiation, ulcerative colitis, and Crohn's disease. Glob J Gastroenterol Hepatol. 2013;1:51–7.
67. Borstlap W, Harran N, Tanis P, Bemelman W. Feasibility of the TAMIS technique for redo pelvic surgery. Surg Endosc. 2016. Epub 11 Apr 2016.
68. Penna M, Knol J, Tuynman J, Tekkis P, Mortensen N, Hompes R. Four anastomotic techniques following transanal total mesorectal excision (TaTME). Tech Coloproctol. 2016;20(3):185–91.
69. Ng K, Ng D, Cheung H, Wong J, Yau K, Chung C, et al. Laparoscopic resection for rectal cancers: lessons learned from 579 cases. Ann Surg 2009. 2016;249(1):82–6.
70. Andersson A, Bergdahl L. Urologic complications following abdominoperineal resection of the rectum. Arch Surg 1976. 1976;111(9):969–71.
71. Atallah S, Albert M, Monson J. Critical concepts and important anatomic landmarks encountered during transanal total mesorectal excisions (taTME): toward the mastery of a new operation for rectal cancer surgery. Tech Coloproctol. 2016;20(7):483–94.
72. Kim JY, Kim NK, Lee KY, Hur H, Min BS, Kim JH. A comparative study of voiding and sexual function after total mesorectal excision with autonomic nerve preservation for rectal cancer: laparoscopic versus robotic surgery. Ann Surg Oncol. 2012;19(8):2485–93.
73. Tsai B, Finne C, Nordenstam J, Christoforidis D, Madoff R, Mellgren A. Transanal endoscopic microsurgery resection of rectal tumors: outcomes and recommendations. Dis Colon Rectum. 2010;53(1):16–23.
74. Cataldo P, O'Brien S, Osler T. Transanal endoscopic microsurgery: a prospective evaluation of functional results. Dis Colon Rectum. 2005;48(7):1366–71.
75. Hompes R, Ashraf S, Gosselink M, van Dongen K, Mortensen N, Lindsey I, et al. Evaluation of quality of life and function at 1 year after transanal endoscopic microsurgery. Colorectal Dis. 2015;17(2):54–61.
76. Telem D, Han K, Kim M, Ajari I, Sohn D, Woods K, et al. Transanal rectosigmoid resection via natural orifice translumenal endoscopic surgery (NOTES) with total mesorectal excision in a large human cadaver series. Surg Endosc. 2013;27(1):74–80.
77. McLemore E, Harnsberger C, Broderick R, Leland H, Sylla P, Coker A, et al. Transanal total mesorectal excision (taTME) for rectal cancer: a training pathway. Surg Endosc. 2015. Epub 10 Dec 2015.

Transanal Endoscopic Microsurgery 22

Jean Salem and John H. Marks

Abstract

Transanal endoscopic microsurgery (TEM) represents the embodiment of natural orifice translumenal endoscopic surgery (NOTES). Its indications range from excision of benign lesions of the rectum to select cancers after neoadjuvant therapy. It has the advantage of resecting the lesion without entering the abdominal cavity which translates into less morbidity and mortality. TEM also offers chances for sphincter preservation in very low rectal lesions. We describe herein the indications of TEM and the workup of patients presenting with rectal tumors, and then, we explain the technical aspects of this procedure.

Keywords

TEM · NOTES · TAMIS · taTME · Sphincter preserving surgery · Rectal cancer · Rectal adenoma

Introduction

Since its introduction in 1983, transanal endoscopic microsurgery (TEM) has emerged as a safe and effective method to treat rectal lesions. Its indications have expanded from the treatment of benign lesions to excision of early rectal cancers to more advanced cancers after the treatment with neoadjuvant therapy. There has been ongoing interest in TEM due to its increase in sphincter preservation, better functional outcomes, and reduced short-term morbidity and mortality [1, 2].

This minimally invasive technique represents the embodiment of natural orifice translumenal endoscopic surgery (NOTES) and offers superior visualization of the lesion, lower margin positivity, and lower recurrence rates compared with the traditional transanal excision [3].

J. Salem · J.H. Marks (✉)
Department of Colorectal Surgery, Lankenau Medical Center, 100 Lancaster Avenue, Wynnewood, PA 19096, USA
e-mail: MarksJ@mlhs.org

J. Salem
e-mail: jean.salem@lycos.com

J.R. Romanelli et al. (eds.), *NOTES and Endoluminal Surgery*, Clinical Gastroenterology, DOI 10.1007/978-3-319-50610-4_22

Indications

TEM was initially used exclusively for benign lesions and for invasive cancers in patients with multiple comorbidities who were considered to be at high risk of radical surgery. However, as experience with TEM has grown, its indications have been expanded. It has been selectively used in the treatment of fistulous disease, anastomotic strictures, and invasive cancers [4, 5].

The current indications for invasive rectal cancers are selected T1 lesions, as well as T2 or T3 lesions, after chemoradiation that has regressed into the bowel wall [6, 7]. The cancer should be less than 3 cm in size and mobile.

Workup

- **Full history and physical examination**: Evaluate both the general health condition of the patient and the extent of the disease. It is important to inquire about bowel habits, anal sphincter function, bladder and sexual function, past medical history, and past surgical history. Digital rectal examination is the single most important component of the preoperative evaluation for lesions in the distal half of the rectum. The status of sphincter tone must always be checked as it impacts significantly on treatment decisions.
- **Flexible sigmoidoscopy and rigid proctoscopy**: Flexible sigmoidoscopy provides a clear image of the lesion and its characteristics: level in the rectum, mobility/fixation, size of the tumor, circumferential involvement, obstruction, ulceration, and estimation of the clinical stage of disease. Rigid proctoscopy offers a more accurate localization of the tumor's position (anterior/posterior or right/left). While stated separately, the digital rectal examination and the endoscopic evaluation are carried out together and provide a fuller characterization of the rectal lesion.
- **Full colonoscopy**: This should always be performed to assess the entire colon for potential synchronous lesions.
- **Preoperative laboratory studies**: In addition to normal preoperative blood work prior to general anesthesia, serum testing for carcinoembryonic antigen (CEA) should be obtained in case of malignancy.
- **Preoperative imaging**: Computed tomography (**CT**) of the chest, abdomen, and pelvis should be obtained to rule out metastatic disease. Magnetic resonance imaging (MRI) with rectal protocol should also be considered to assess T and N stages and potential adjacent organ involvement.
- **Endoscopic rectal ultrasound**: to view the depth of invasion of the tumor and to evaluate for lymph node involvement.
- Either rectal endoscopic ultrasound or MRI is an excellent source of information regarding the T stage of the lesion. The choice of modality used should be based on your local radiologic expertise.
- If the patient has a malignant lesion that is unfavorable (≥T3 or N+) at any level in the rectum, or a favorable cancer in the distal one-third of the rectum, neoadjuvant chemoradiation is recommended. Surgical decision making is based on the evaluation of the tumor at 8–12 weeks after the completion of the neoadjuvant treatment in order to maximize the effect of tumor downstaging.

Our treatment algorithm is shown in Fig. 22.1. Full-thickness local excision via a TEM approach is offered in these categories of patients:

1. Medically compromised patients who can not undergo a major surgery.
2. Staged: patients who would tolerate a radical total mesorectal excision (TME) operation, but in whom, because of comorbidities, the morbidity/mortality rate would be significantly increased.
3. Elective: good operative candidates who have had impressive downstaging or refuse radical surgery.

For the staged/elective groups, if the pathology is ≥ypT3 or N+, radical surgery is recommended.

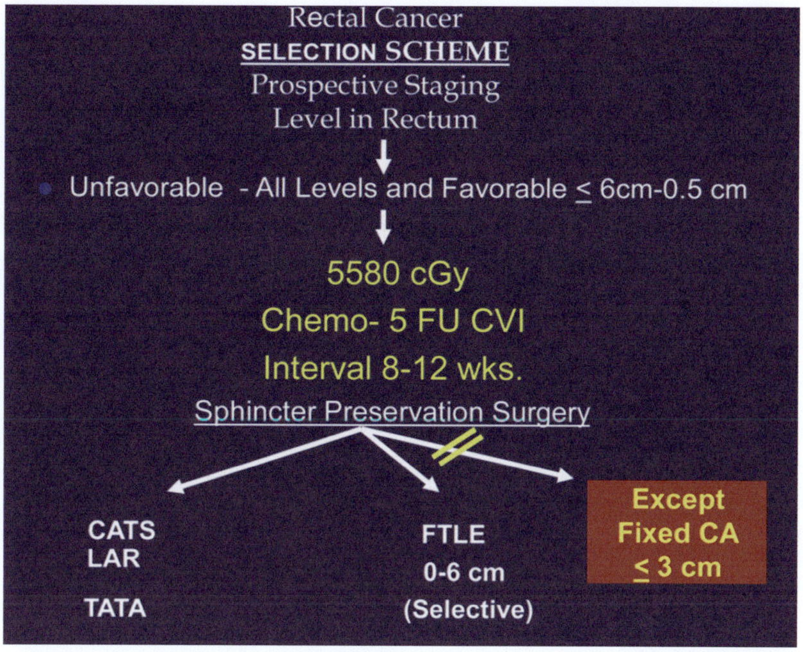

Fig. 22.1 Treatment algorithm

Equipment

- **Operating rectoscope**: It is 4 cm in diameter and either 12 or 20 cm in length, with a beveled or straight-faced end. The surgeon's end has an airtight faceplate with four ports sealed by capped rubber sleeves through which the optical stereoscope, suction, and two long-shafted instruments are inserted. The rectoscope and its attachments are secured to the operating room table using a Martin arm. The straight-faced rectoscope is utilized for low tumors to avoid loss of the pneumorectum, and it allows the surgeon the benefit of the improved optics for this low level (Fig. 22.2).
- **Stereoscope**: The surgeon can visualize the field through the binocular stereoscopic eyepiece, which provides a precise three-dimensional view of the operative field with up to sixfold magnification. The stereoscopic eyepiece itself includes dual lenses, an insufflation channel, and lens irrigator. An accessory monocular scope is connected to a video screen (Fig. 22.3).
- **Long-handled instruments**: All operating instruments are 5 mm in diameter and include graspers, scissors, monopolar cautery hook, needle driver, and clip applier. The graspers are either straight or more commonly angled at the tip. This allows an increased range of grasp by rotating the handle of the instrument (Fig. 22.4).
- **Endosurgical unit**: This unit provides a light source, carbon dioxide (CO_2) insufflation, suction, irrigation, and continuous monitoring of intrarectal pressure. Simultaneously, an integrated roller pump provides constant low-volume suction at the same rate as the gas insufflation. This permits adjustable effective suction that does not collapse the lumen. The insufflation allows for stable gas pressure in order to maintain visualization of the distended rectum without insufflation of the more proximal colon. Most importantly, this avoids the ballooning effect of using a standard laparoscopic insufflation that turns on and off every few seconds.

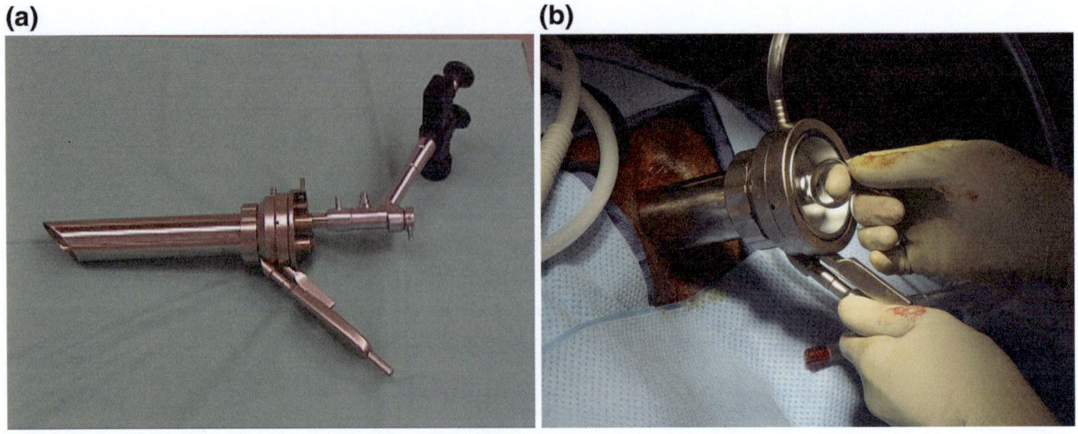

Fig. 22.2 **a** TEM rectoscope. **b** Insertion of TEM rectoscope. After gentle dilation of the anus, the rectoscope is inserted with an obturator in place for an atraumatic entry

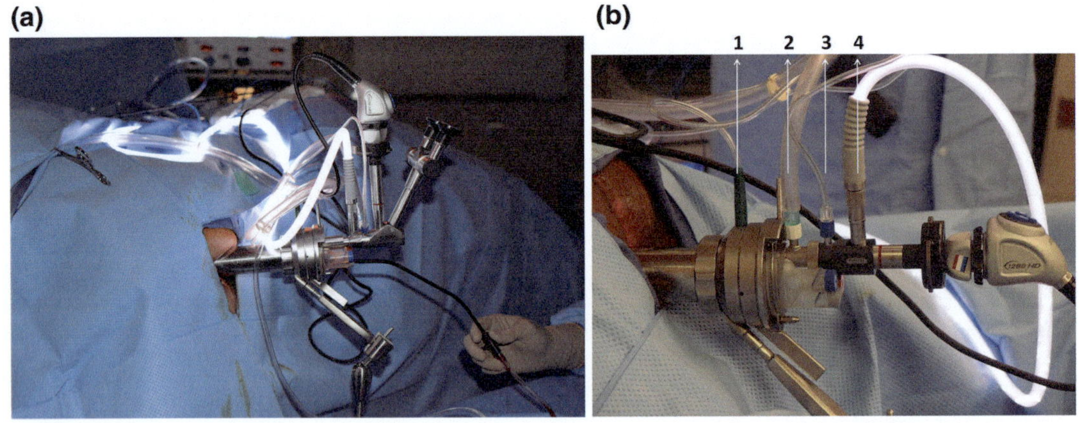

Fig. 22.3 **a** Finalized assembly of the TEM rectoscope. **b** The four pieces of tubing are connected into their respective ports in the apparatus. The four ports are used for suction *1*, continuous insufflation *2*, irrigation *3*, and the light source *4*. The connectors are all different to avoid attaching the tubes to the wrong location

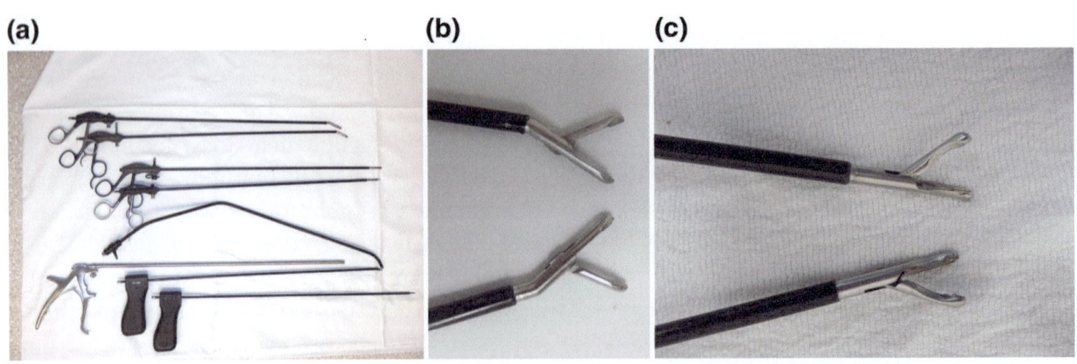

Fig. 22.4 **a** Important TEM instruments. From *top* to *bottom*: curved monopolar grasping forceps for *left* and *right* hands, straight monopolar grasping forceps for *left* and *right* hands, suction tube, suture clip forceps, articulated monopolar knife, and straight monopolar knife. **b** Close-up of curved forceps. **c** Close-up of straight forceps

Operative Technique

It is essential that the position of the patient is known before surgery. This is because the TEM equipment reach is limited to the bottom 180° of the field of vision. The preoperative rigid sigmoidoscopy is used to localize the tumor and determine the quadrant location of the tumor in order to plan the operative positioning of the patient to allow the lesion of interest to lie at the 6 o'clock position. Patients with an anterior-based lesion are positioned in the prone jackknife position, while those with a posterior lesion are positioned in lithotomy (Fig. 22.5). Laterally located lesions are best approached with patients in the appropriate lateral decubitus position.

All patients receive a mechanical bowel preparation the day before surgery, as well as preoperative antibiotic prophylaxis. TEM is performed under general anesthesia, and a Foley catheter is inserted in all patients.

The procedure is started by gentle dilatation of the anus and insertion of the rectoscope. The position of the mass is confirmed with the glass faceplate, functioning as a large rigid sigmoidoscope at this point. Once this is confirmed, the rectoscope is fixed to the operating table using a Martin arm. The stereoscope is then introduced and attached to the endosurgical unit to provide insufflation, suction, and irrigation (Fig. 22.6). After adjusting the rectoscope to get the optimal view, the tumor is well delineated. Using the

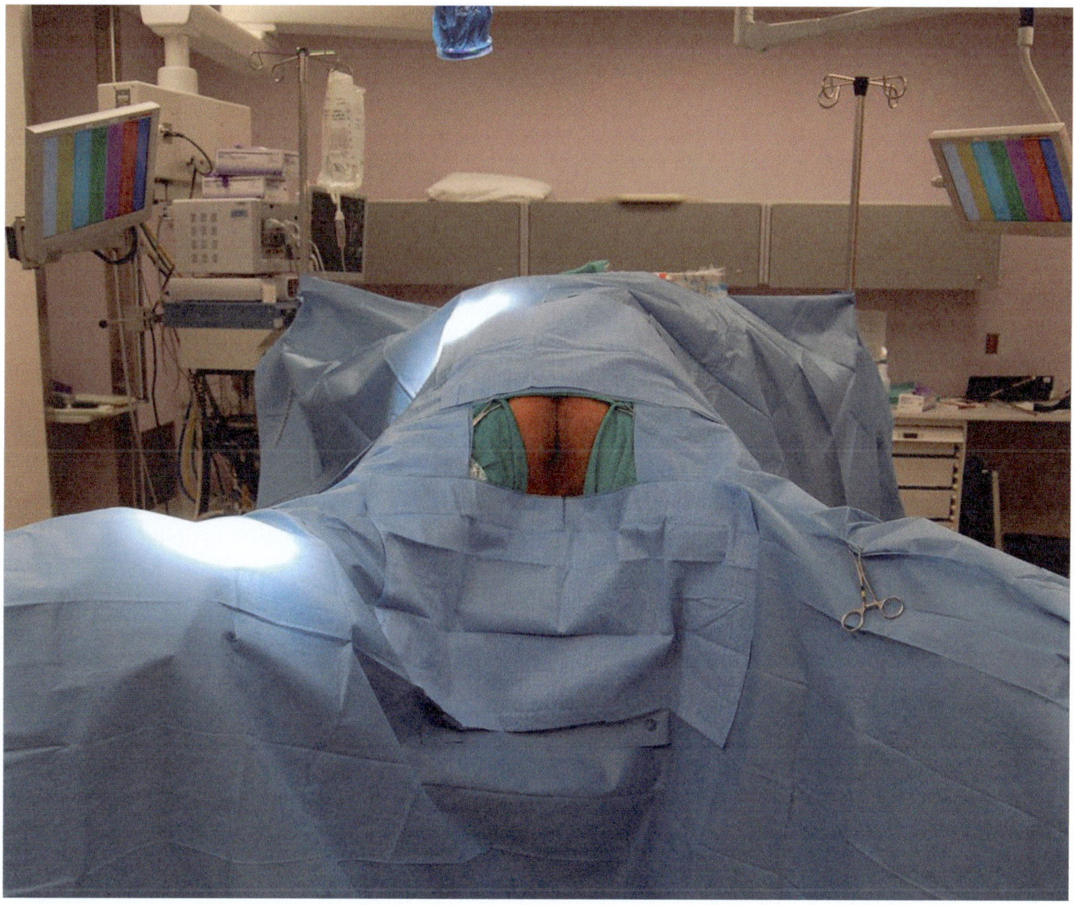

Fig. 22.5 Prone position: ideal for patients with anteriorly located lesions. The arms are resting without straining on arm boards

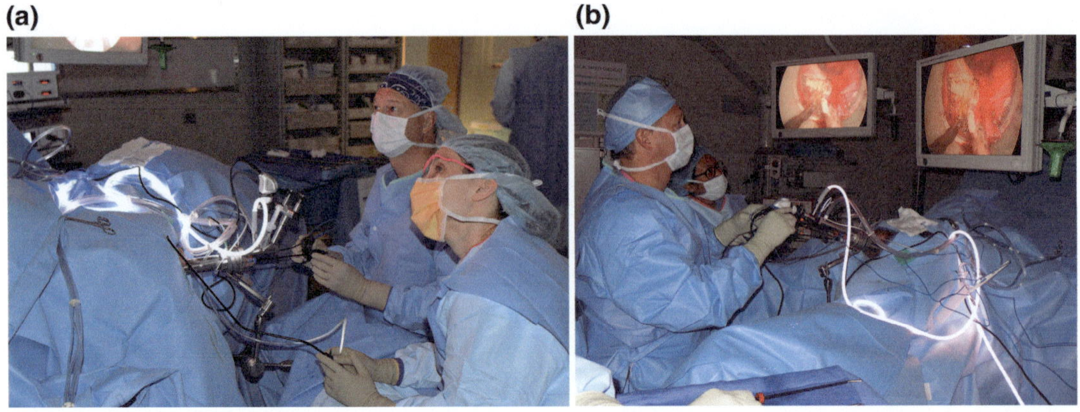

Fig. 22.6 a, b Surgical team setup. The surgeon is in a seated position in between the patient's legs, with the assistant positioned to his or her *left* side. The monitors are placed in front of the surgeon. The operating rectoscope is fixed to the operating table with a Martin arm for stability

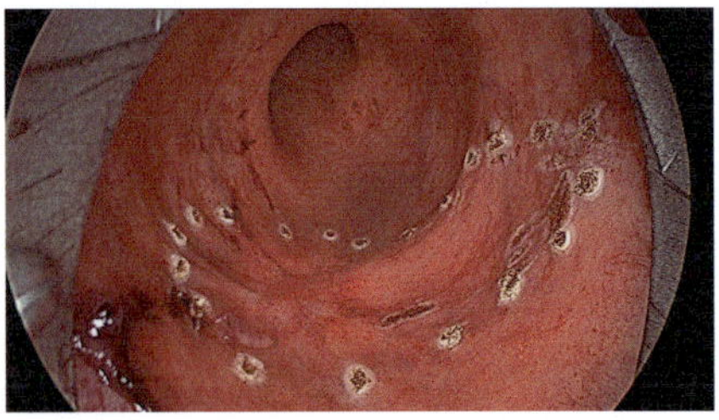

Fig. 22.7 Marking of the lesion. The margin of resection is marked circumferentially using electrocautery

monopolar cautery, the mucosa is scored circumferentially, marking the resection margins (Fig. 22.7). For benign lesions, a 5-mm margin is adequate. For invasive cancers, a 1-cm margin is required. Using a grasper with the left hand, the mucosa is lifted and a full-thickness excision is performed using electrocautery. One should make sure to reach the perirectal fat. Often, a layer of adipose tissue is found below the submucosa before entering the muscularis propria. This should not be mistaken with the perirectal fat.

Five layers of transection are possible:

1. submucosal,
2. intramuscular,
3. full thickness through the muscularis propria,
4. partial-thickness mesorectum, and
5. TME-level mesorectal excision.

A marking suture is placed at the inferior border of the specimen prior to removal to ensure the maintenance of proper orientation of the specimen (Fig. 22.8).

Unlike in laparoscopy, there is no ability to move the instrument in a left or right fashion as the shafts are passing through a 20-cm tube. Movement of the instrument is in a piston-like in/out fashion. Constant repositioning of the TEM scope using the Martin arm allows for the surgery to be performed using only these maneuvers.

After the lesion is dissected and ready to be removed (Fig. 22.9), the insufflation is turned off and the tumor is grasped and pulled into the operating proctoscope. The faceplate is removed, and the specimen is delivered. The faceplate, the defect, and the instruments are washed and irrigated with dilute Betadine to reduce the risk of tumor implantation.

The closure of the rectal wall defect is performed in a running, full-thickness fashion with a 2-0 PDS suture (Fig. 22.10). Knot tying using TEM equipment is very difficult and is instead achieved using silver clips which are secured onto the suture. Once the closure is complete, any slack in the suture line can be fixed by gently pulling up on one end of the suture and applying another clip to tighten it.

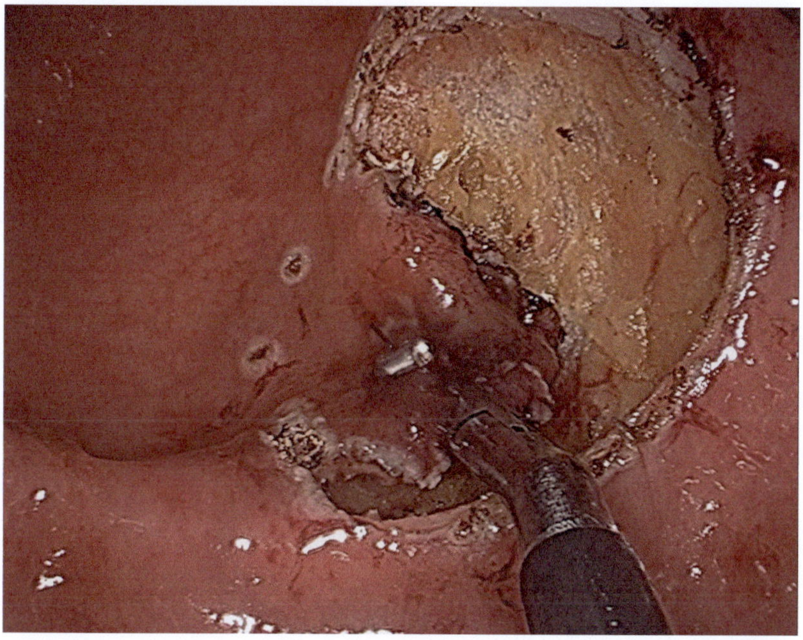

Fig. 22.8 Placement of a marking suture. Prior to complete excision, a marking suture is placed in the distal margin of the target lesion for orientation

(a) (b)

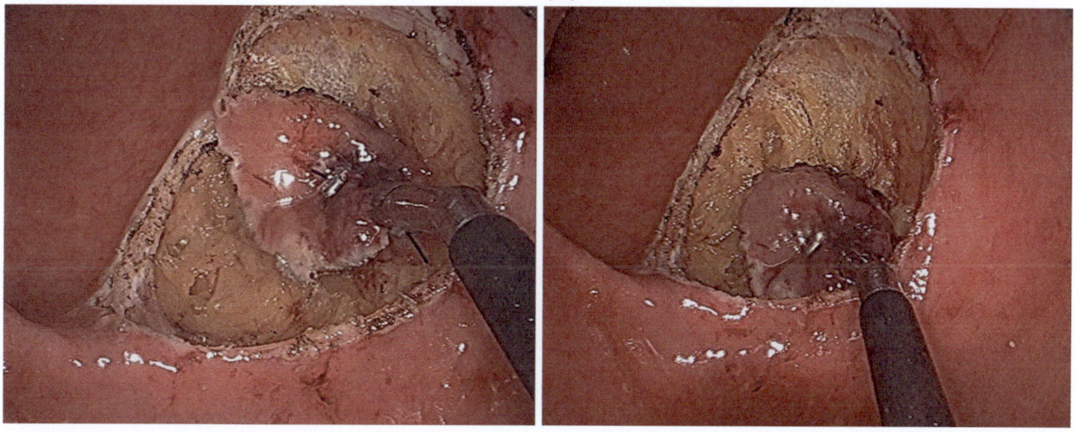

Fig. 22.9 **a**, **b** Operative pictures show the full-thickness circumferential dissection of a malignant lesion. Notice that the dissection is carried through the entire bowel wall until the *yellow* fat of the perirectal tissues is reached

Technical Variations

- Submucosal excision: For benign lesions, a full-thickness excision is not required. One can dissect in the submucosal plane circumferentially to excise the lesion.
- High anterior lesions should not be approached via TEM due to the risk of inadvertent entry into the peritoneal cavity. These patients

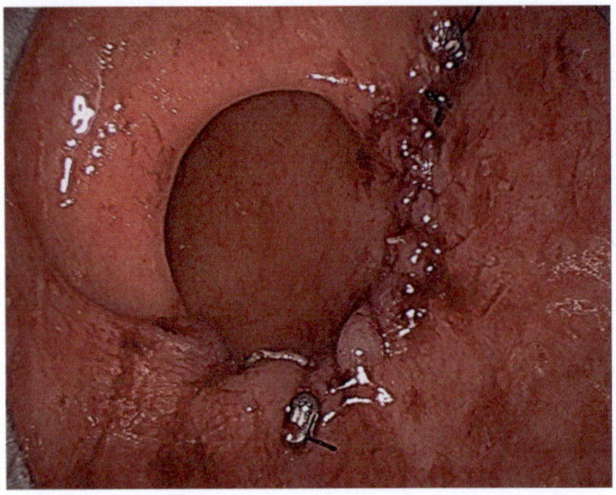

Fig. 22.10 Closure of the defect

are best served by a low anterior resection. However, in very experienced hands, entry into the peritoneal cavity is permissible. Closure is preferably performed in two layers. Entry into the peritoneal cavity is safe in experienced hands and does not increase the risk of carcinomatosis or sepsis [8].

Outcomes

For rectal cancers, when indicated, TEM is much safer than TME with lower rates of morbidity and mortality [2].

From a functional standpoint, satisfaction with fecal continence is generally high with TEM. For very low early rectal cancers, TEM can spare the patients from having a permanent colostomy while preserving an appropriate sphincter function [9].

From an oncological standpoint, TEM and radical surgery for T1 cancers have similar rates of recurrence and survival [6]. For T2 rectal cancers, after neoadjuvant therapy, a prospective randomized study comparing TEM and TME showed a local recurrence rate of 5.7% (2 of 35) in the TEM group and 2.8% (1 of 35) in the TME group [7]. Although not stated by the authors, this difference is not statistically significant, and both groups had a 94% disease-free survival at the end of the 84-month follow-up period.

Conclusion

TEM offers both the patient and the surgeon a unique opportunity to perform endoluminal surgery and avoid the need for any abdominal operation. This is an exciting technology that represents a true NOTES experience. The ability to definitively treat benign lesions as well as select cancers with or without neoadjuvant therapy is an exciting option that TEM surgery provides. The increased visualization, reach, and ability to handle the tissue endoluminally, as well as the excellent outcomes, have led to the increase in the utilization of the TEM approach.

References

1. Allaix ME, Arezzo A, Giraudo G, Morino M. Transanal endoscopic microsurgery vs. laparoscopic total mesorectal excision for T2N0 rectal cancer. J Gastrointest Surg. 2012;16:2280–7.
2. De Graaf EJ, Doornebosch PG, Tollenaar RA, et al. Transanal endoscopic microsurgery versus total mesorectal excision of T1 rectal adenocarcinomas with curative intention. Eur J Surg Oncol. 2009;35:1280–5.
3. Clancy C, Burke JP, Albert MR, et al. Transanal endoscopic microsurgery versus standard transanal excision for the removal of rectal neoplasms: a systematic review and meta-analysis. Dis Colon Rectum. 2015;58(2):254–61.
4. Bochove-Overgaauw DM, Beerlage HP, Bosscha K, Gelderman WA. Transanal endoscopic microsurgery for correction of rectourethral fistulae. J Endourol. 2006;20(12):1087–90.
5. Kato K, Saito T, Matsuda M, Imai M, Kasai S, Mito M. Successful treatment of a rectal anastomotic stenosis by transanal endoscopic microsurgery (TEM) using the contact Nd:YAG laser. Surg Endosc. 1997;11(5):485–7.
6. Winde G, Nottberg H, Keller R, Schmid KW, Bünte H. Surgical cure for early rectal carcinomas (T1). Transanal endoscopic microsurgery vs. anterior resection. Dis Colon Rectum. 1996;39(9):969–76.

7. Lezoche G, Baldarelli M, Guerrieri M, et al. A prospective randomized study with a 5-year minimum follow-up evaluation of transanal endoscopic microsurgery versus laparoscopic total mesorectal excision after neoadjuvant therapy. Surg Endosc. 2008;22(2):352–8.
8. Marks JH, Frenkel JL, Greenleaf CE, D'Andrea AP. Transanal endoscopic microsurgery with entrance into the peritoneal cavity: is it safe? Dis Colon Rectum. 2014;57:1176–82.
9. Valsdottir EB, Yarandi SS, Marks JH, Marks GJ. Quality of life and fecal incontinence after transanal endoscopic microsurgery for benign and malignant rectal lesions. Surg Endosc. 2014;28(1):193–202.

Transvaginal NOTES Nephrectomy 23

Xiaofeng Zou, Yijun Xue and Guoxi Zhang

Abstract

Natural orifice translumenal endoscopic surgery (NOTES) nephrectomy has been reported by several centers. Between May 2010 and January 2015, we have performed 178 transvaginal NOTES nephrectomies. Eighteen of these underwent pure transvaginal NOTES nephrectomies. At first, two umbilical trocars and one transvaginal trocar were used during the procedure. Then, one umbilical trocar and a transvaginal multi-instrument access port were used. At last, there was no umbilical trocar. Dissection was performed according to the method of a standard laparoscopic transabdominal nephrectomy. The specimen was placed inside a homemade bag and removed through an extended incision at the posterior vaginal fornix. Transvaginal NOTES nephrectomy was successfully completed in 172 patients. Five patients were converted to open surgery, and 1 patient was converted to suprapubic-assisted laparoendoscopic single-site surgery. At a mean range follow-up of 51.8 (10–69) months, the posterior colpotomy incision healed well, and the scars were nearly invisible on the abdominal wall. The female sexual function index (FSFI) questionnaire showed that transvaginal NOTES nephrectomy did not affect the female sexual function. Therefore, NOTES nephrectomy using the vagina as an entry point to the peritoneal cavity is very promising.

X. Zou (✉) · Y. Xue · G. Zhang
Department of Urology, First Affiliated Hospital of Gannan Medical University, No. 23, Qing Nian Road, Ganzhou 341000, Jiangxi Province, China
e-mail: gyfyurology@126.com

Y. Xue
e-mail: sudaxyj@163.com

G. Zhang
e-mail: zgx8778@163.com

J.R. Romanelli et al. (eds.), *NOTES and Endoluminal Surgery*, Clinical Gastroenterology, DOI 10.1007/978-3-319-50610-4_23

Keywords
Natural orifice translumenal endoscopic surgery (NOTES) · Transvaginal approach · Transperitoneal approach · Laparoscopy · Nephrectomy · Cosmetic result

Introduction

The first open nephrectomy procedure described in 1861 by Wolcott remained unchanged for nearly 130 years [1]. However, the introduction of minimally invasive surgery, namely laparoscopic surgery, revolutionized the approach to nephrectomy. Currently, laparoscopic nephrectomy has assumed a central role in the surgical treatment of benign and malignant kidney diseases [2]. Although laparoscopy is well recognized in decreasing surgical morbidity, it still requires three to five incisions each, at least 0.5–1 cm in length. Each incision carries risks of bleeding, visceral organ damage, pain, and incisional hernia.

Technologic advancements have challenged minimally invasive surgery to reduce patient morbidity further, and to improve convalescence. One such development is natural orifice translumenal endoscopic surgery (NOTES), whereby abdominal access is gained through a single transvisceral incision [3]. The potential benefits of this method include reducing the incidence of vascular and visceral injuries owing to the reduced number of incisions required, reduced risk of incisional hernia, and reduced postoperative pain with earlier return to normal function. Furthermore, NOTES is intuitively attractive for patients regarding body image and cosmetic issues, and it may result in diminished psychological opposition to the prospect of surgical intervention.

In urology, the concept of NOTES was initiated with the use of natural orifices to extract surgical specimens. Vaginal extraction of an intact kidney following laparoscopic nephrectomy was first reported by Breda [4], with a larger series reported by Gill et al. [5]. While many routes of access have been used for transvisceral surgery [6–10], the transvaginal route is most commonly used in the field of human urology. In this chapter, we will discuss our institutional experience with hybrid transvaginal NOTES nephrectomy, and a step-wise transition toward pure transvaginal NOTES nephrectomy.

Preclinical Development of NOTES Nephrectomy

Prior to the introduction of NOTES nephrectomy into the clinical setting, this surgical technique underwent several iterations in animal models. Gettman et al. [7] published a seminal NOTES study in 2002, which actually predated the coining of the 'NOTES' acronym, after performing 6 transvaginal laparoscopic nephrectomies in a pig model; a hybrid NOTES technique involving a concurrent transabdominal laparoscopic port was used in 5 of these nephrectomies, with one pure NOTES nephrectomy, in which no external incision was performed. The operative time in the pure NOTES nephrectomy was 360 min, compared with a mean operative time of 210 min in the five hybrid procedures. One of the main limitations in performing NOTES nephrectomy highlighted by Gettman et al. [7] was the cumbersome nature of the standard laparoscopic instruments. The available instruments did not enable robust retraction of the retroperitoneal tissue, or the ability to perform controlled blunt dissection that is vital to the dissection of the renal unit. This is especially true in humans, who have substantially more perinephric fat than pigs. Furthermore, the available instruments were inserted parallel to the endoscope, which limited effective traction, counter traction, and visibility. After these initial reports, a series of proof-of-principle animal and cadaveric studies continued to refine the surgical techniques for NOTES nephrectomy [11–22].

To address some of the technical challenges facing NOTES nephrectomy, several methodological adaptations were explored. Multitasking platforms, such as the TransPort™ multilumen operating platform (USGI Medical, San Clemente, CA), were identified as tools that could facilitate NOTES [12, 13]. The novelty of the TransPort™ multilumen device, in particular, was that it remained flexible during insertion but could be locked in place to create a rigid working platform for visualization, and up to four instruments. In addition, Zeltser et al. [23] developed a magnetically anchored guidance system, which they used to perform a laparoscopic nephrectomy with instruments inserted via a single transabdominal port in a pig model. They concluded that this guidance system enabled unhindered intracorporeal manipulation of instruments and might be amenable to pure NOTES.

Robotic platforms represent another logical avenue of exploration in NOTES, especially given its widespread adoption in urology. Robots hold additional promise in improving visualization and in articulating laparoscopic instruments that are particularly well suited to suturing and knot tying. However, initial attempts to incorporate conventional robotic platforms into NOTES procedures performed in pigs were affected by substantial extracorporeal clashing of the robotic arms, owing to the extreme proximity of the robotic ports during such procedures [13].

Entry of Hybrid NOTES in the Clinical Setting

The vagina gained acceptance as a viable extraction portal in women after laparoscopic nephrectomy over two decades ago [4, 5], but the concept of a transvaginal nephrectomy did not materialize until 2008 when Branco et al. [24] first demonstrated that the vagina could also be used as a working port in a 23-year-old woman with recurrent UTIs and a nonfunctioning kidney. They used a hybrid NOTES technique with two 5-mm laparoscopic ports, a double-channel flexible endoscope, and a polypectomy snare to complete the procedure. Operative time was 170 min, estimated blood loss was 350 ml, no operative complications occurred, and the patient recovered uneventfully within a 12-h hospitalization.

Subsequent to this report, hybrid NOTES nephrectomy underwent further technical modifications, and the indications in which this approach was used were expanded. Alcaraz [25] demonstrated the feasibility of hybrid NOTES nephrectomy in the treatment of patients with kidney cancer. Kaouk [26] reduced the number of laparoscopic ports necessary for retraction of the mobilized kidney from two to one. Porpiglia [27] reduced the size of the laparoscopic ports to 3.5 mm. Sotelo [28] utilized the transvaginal port to perform the majority of the intraoperative dissection. Finally, Alcaraz [29] and Kaouk [30] demonstrated the safety of NOTES-assisted living-donor nephrectomy. Indeed, transvaginal hybrid NOTES living-donor nephrectomy was reported to have no adverse effects on graft functioning in the recipient or the sexual activity of the donor. However, these reports highlighted some important perioperative challenges, including rectal injury caused during vaginal entry of the trocar, failure to progress with the dissection, intraoperative hemorrhage, and postoperative pelvic abscess [25–30]. Although these refinements in technique represented important developments, the holy grail of a pure NOTES approach had not yet been realized.

Pure NOTES Nephrectomy in the Clinic

In 2010, Kaouk et al. [31] at the Cleveland Clinic in Ohio reported the first pure transvaginal NOTES nephrectomy in a 58-year-old woman with an atrophic right kidney. Pneumoperitoneum was obtained via introduction of a blunt tip trocar into the peritoneal cavity through the vagina. Two standard 10-mm trocars and a 5-mm trocar were placed through a GelPort® (Applied Medical, Rancho Santa Margarita, CA) placed within a 30-mm posterior colpotomy. A 5-mm deflecting laparoscope was used, along with a standard endovascular stapler for ligation of the hilar structures. The remaining upper pole and posterior attachments of the kidney were dissected using a monopolar J-hook. Although no perioperative complications were noted, the authors concluded that the procedure was tedious, time-consuming (taking 420 min), and technically demanding. For these reasons, hybrid NOTES is often performed in lieu of pure NOTES, and so several additional modifications to the hybrid NOTES technique have been developed as will be described below.

Robot-Assisted NOTES Nephrectomy

The incorporation of robotic technology has allowed surgeons to overcome some of the limitations in NOTES nephrectomy, especially regarding issues of triangulation, maintaining orientation, and overly flexible endoscopic instruments. Hagen et al. [32] attempted transvaginal pure NOTES in a cadaver model using the lithotomy position, and intersecting robotic instruments. However, the lithotomy position was found to be incompatible with the da Vinci® (Intuitive Surgical, Sunnyvale, CA, USA) robotic platform due to the clashing of the robotic arms. In response, Laydner et al. [33], also using a cadaver model, reported the feasibility of a robot-assisted transvaginal pure NOTES technique using a novel prone jackknife position and retroperitoneal approach, which avoided clashing of the robotic arms. Although many of these techniques are starting to be established in the field of urology, many challenges persist and continue to limit widespread clinical integration of NOTES.

Transvaginal NOTES Nephrectomy at Our Institution

Between May 2010 and January 2015, at the Department of Urology, First Affiliated Hospital of Gannan Medical University, Ganzhou, China, we have performed 178 transvaginal NOTES nephrectomies (simple 149, radical 29). Eighteen of these underwent pure transvaginal NOTES nephrectomies (simple 17, radical 1).

Indications

The indications continue to expand as surgeons' expertise grows, and we feel that all female patients who are a candidate for laparoscopic nephrectomy for benign or malignant disease should be considered for a transvaginal NOTES approach.

Contraindications

The transvaginal NOTES nephrectomy cannot be applied to all female patients. There is no work showing what would constitute relative and absolute contraindications to the procedure, but based on our experience, we cite the following situations as contraindications:

- Lacking visibility of the cervix,
- Ongoing pregnancy,
- Genital infections,
- Known endometriosis,
- Neoplasms of the vulva, vagina, or cervix, and
- Intact hymen.
- Prior hysterectomy
- Vaginal narrowing identified as the inability to insert two fingers into the vagina [34].

Consent

Transvaginal NOTES nephrectomy demands special skills, and it is important to discuss with your patients that there are specific risks that they must be aware of before consenting to this approach:

- Possible risks of unrecognized injury to nearby structures during the placement of a vaginal trocar, particularly the rectum and sigmoid colon
- The possibility of postoperative dyspareunia
- Possible risks of inadvertent injury to another organ during the dissection of the kidney
- Possible risks access of bleeding from the artery and vein
- The potential need to convert to the traditional open or laparoscopic surgery if difficulties arise.

Preoperative Evaluation

- A meticulous past history and physical examination is the initial step in patient evaluation. Emphasis is placed on pulmonary, cardiac and renal status, sexual history, obstetric history, and past medical history along with a careful history of prior abdominal surgery. It is highly recommended that all patients undergo routine gynecological exam. The exam should include a complete pelvic exam, bimanual exam, and breast exam.
- Basic laboratory blood work,
- Pregnancy test to rule out unexpected early gestation,
- Sonography, nephrogram, intravenous urogram, and computerized tomography,
- Further cardiac/pulmonary workup when indicated.

Preoperative Preparation

Vaginal irrigation with iodophor is performed, and oral metronidazole and norfloxacin are given for 3 days before surgery. Each patient undergoes a mechanical bowel preparation with the use of enema the morning of surgery, and has a clear liquid diet 1 day prior to surgery.

Surgical Technique

Patient Positioning

We begin by placing a soft beanbag on the surgical table. The beanbag is primarily placed under the torso. A nasogastric tube and transurethral catheter are placed to decompress the stomach and bladder. The patients are placed in lithotomy position with the affected side elevated at 30–60°; the kidney rest is minimally raised, and the table is slightly flexed. The patient is secured with adhesive tape, ensuring adequate padding on the bony prominences. The surgical field was prepared with povidone iodine.

Port Placement

Hybrid Transvaginal NOTES (Two Umbilical Trocars and One Transvaginal Trocar)

5- and 10-mm trocars were placed at the right and left medial margins of the umbilicus through two separate umbilical incisions. A lengthened 10-mm or 5-mm trocar was placed through the posterior vaginal fornix into the abdominal cavity under direct vision using a 10-mm 30° or flexible-tip 5.4-mm 0° laparoscopes (Olympus Optical, Tokyo, Japan). Dissection was performed transumbilically using standard

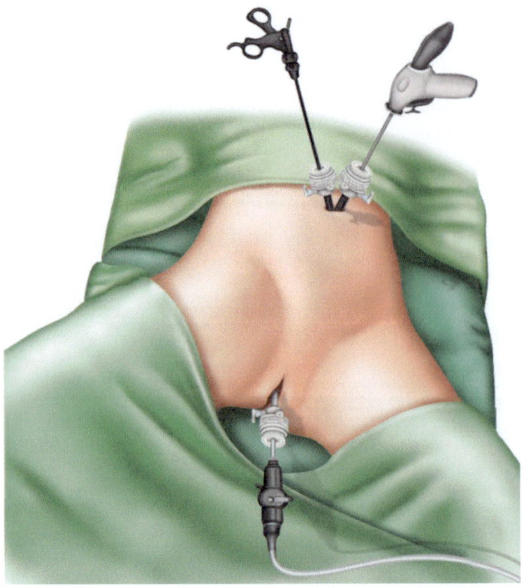

Fig. 23.1 Patient and trocar placement for hybrid transvaginal NOTES nephrectomy (two umbilical trocars and one transvaginal trocar). Reprinted with permission from Elsevier. Yijun Xue, Xiaofeng Zou, Guoxi Zhang, Yuanhu Yuan, Rihai Xiao, Yunfeng Liao, Xin Zhong, Bo Jiang, Ruiquan Xu, Yuhua Zou, Gang Xu, Kunlin Xie, Xu Zhang. Transvaginal Natural Orifice Translumenal Endoscopic Nephrectomy in a Series of 63 Cases: Stepwise Transition From Hybrid to Pure NOTES, *European Urology* 2015;68(2):302–310

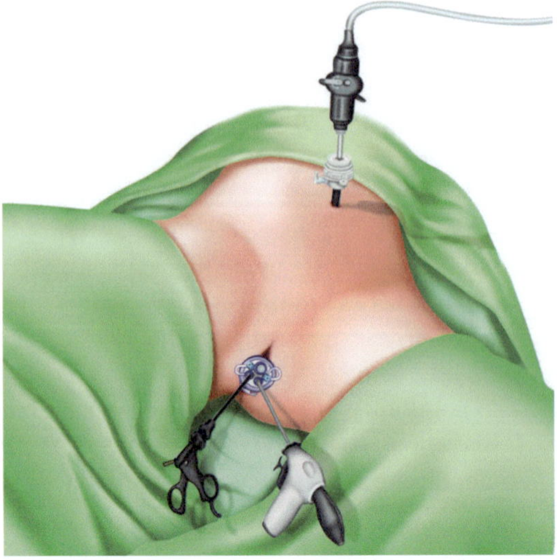

Fig. 23.2 Patient and trocar placement for hybrid transvaginal NOTES nephrectomy (one umbilical trocar and a transvaginal multi-instrument access port). Reprinted with permission from Elsevier. Yijun Xue, Xiaofeng Zou, Guoxi Zhang, Yuanhu Yuan, Rihai Xiao, Yunfeng Liao, Xin Zhong, Bo Jiang, Ruiquan Xu, Yuhua Zou, Gang Xu, Kunlin Xie, Xu Zhang. Transvaginal Natural Orifice Translumenal Endoscopic Nephrectomy in a Series of 63 Cases: Stepwise Transition From Hybrid to Pure NOTES, *European Urology* 2015;68(2):302–310

laparoscopic instruments and a 5-mm ultrasonic shears (Harmonic scalpel; Ethicon Endosurgery, Cincinnati, OH, USA) (Fig. 23.1).

Hybrid Transvaginal NOTES(One Umbilical Trocar and a Transvaginal Multi-instrument Access Port)

A 10-mm umbilical trocar was introduced into abdominal cavity, and a flexible-tip 5.4-mm 0° laparoscope was used. A multi-instrument access port (TriPort; Olympus Medical System Corp, Tokyo, Japan) was deployed across the vaginal incision under direct vision (Fig. 23.2, and used for a 5-mm ultrasonic dissector and a 5-mm flexible forceps.

Pure Transvaginal NOTES (No Umbilical Trocar)

A 5-mm trocar was introduced into the pelvic cavity through the vaginal incision, guided by a 5-mm blunt-tipped forceps, and a flexible-tip 5.4-mm 0° laparoscope was used to confirm no rectal injury. Then, a self-developed three-channel Zou-port (Zhouji Medical Instruments Co Ltd., Zhejiang, China) was deployed across the vaginal incision, into which the flexible-tip laparoscope and instruments were all introduced (Fig. 23.3).

Technical Details of the Procedure

Dissection was performed according to the method of a standard laparoscopic transabdominal nephrectomy. Using the ultrasonic dissector,

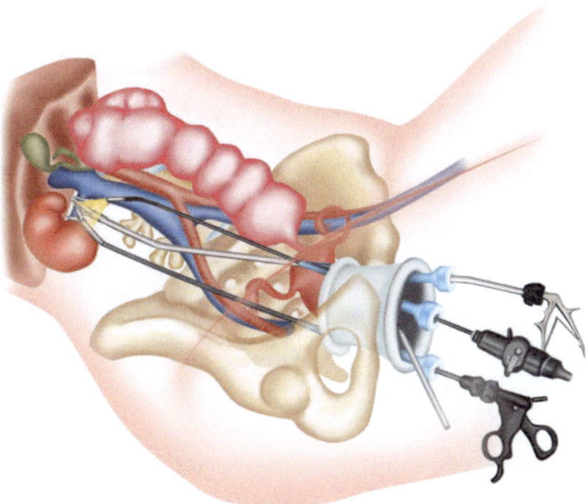

Fig. 23.3 Diagrammatic representation of the use of extra-long pre-bent instruments during pure transvaginal NOTES nephrectomy. Reprinted with permission from Elsevier. Yijun Xue, Xiaofeng Zou, Guoxi Zhang, Yuanhu Yuan, Rihai Xiao, Yunfeng Liao, Xin Zhong, Bo Jiang, Ruiquan Xu, Yuhua Zou, Gang Xu, Kunlin Xie, Xu Zhang. Transvaginal Natural Orifice Translumenal Endoscopic Nephrectomy in a Series of 63 Cases: Stepwise Transition From Hybrid to Pure NOTES, *European Urology* 2015;68(2):302–310

the peritoneum was incised along the line of Toldt, and the colon was mobilized and retracted medially. The ureter was identified proximal to the iliac vessels and ligated using 5- or 10-mm Hem-o-lok clips (Teleflex Medical China, Shanghai, China). Proximal mobilization of the ureter up to level of the ureteropelvic junction was performed. The mobilized ureter was used for the retraction of the kidney and the lower pole of the kidney was mobilized, followed by posterior dissection. The lower pole was lifted laterally to define the renal hilum. After the hilum was identified, it was dissected using the ultrasonic dissector or pre-bent instruments and flexible forceps. The Hem-o-lok applier was used to control the artery, and then the vein. In cases of severe hydronephrosis, the collecting system was drained, as needed, to achieve better exposure to the renal pedicle. If dense adhesions around the renal artery precluded skeletonizing it, the renal artery was doubly clipped with its surrounding fibrous tissues, and the kidney was mobilized outside Gerota's fascia. Remaining attachments of the upper pole of the kidney medially, superiorly, posteriorly, and laterally were progressively freed using straight, flexible, or pre-bent instruments to retract the dissected kidney, and the kidney was released. A homemade bag was introduced into the abdominal cavity through the 10-mm working channel of the transvaginal Zou-port. The specimen was placed inside the bag and removed through an extended incision at the posterior vaginal fornix (Fig. 23.4a, b). For hybrid transvaginal NOTES nephrectomy, one or no drain was placed at the renal bed, and one was placed at pelvic cavity through the vagina. We placed the intra-abdominal drain through the umbilical incision in order to remove the abdominal fluid, which can also help us early find postoperative problems. However, in the first 10 cases, we found that the postoperative drainage from intra-abdominal drains was little (less than 20 ml each day). Furthermore, the fluid may flow out of the pelvic drain when the patient is in the semi-recumbent position. Therefore, we consider that it is not necessary to place an intra-abdominal drain. There was no intra-abdominal drain in later patients. For pure transvaginal NOTES nephrectomy, the drain tube was placed at pelvic cavity through the vagina. The vaginal wound and the 10-mm umbilical fascial defect were closed using a 2-0 absorbable suture. Finally, a vaginal tamponade with a sterile vaginal pack dressing was applied in all the patients. Complete sexual abstinence lasting 3 months was advised for all cases.

Postoperative Care

- Patients received intravenous fluid until recovery of bowel sounds.
- Intravenous broad-spectrum antibiotic (ceftriaxone) and injection tramadol on patient demand were administered.
- The drainage tube output, if less than 30 ml in 24 h, was removed.
- Patients can resume their normal daily activities as soon as they are comfortable doing them.

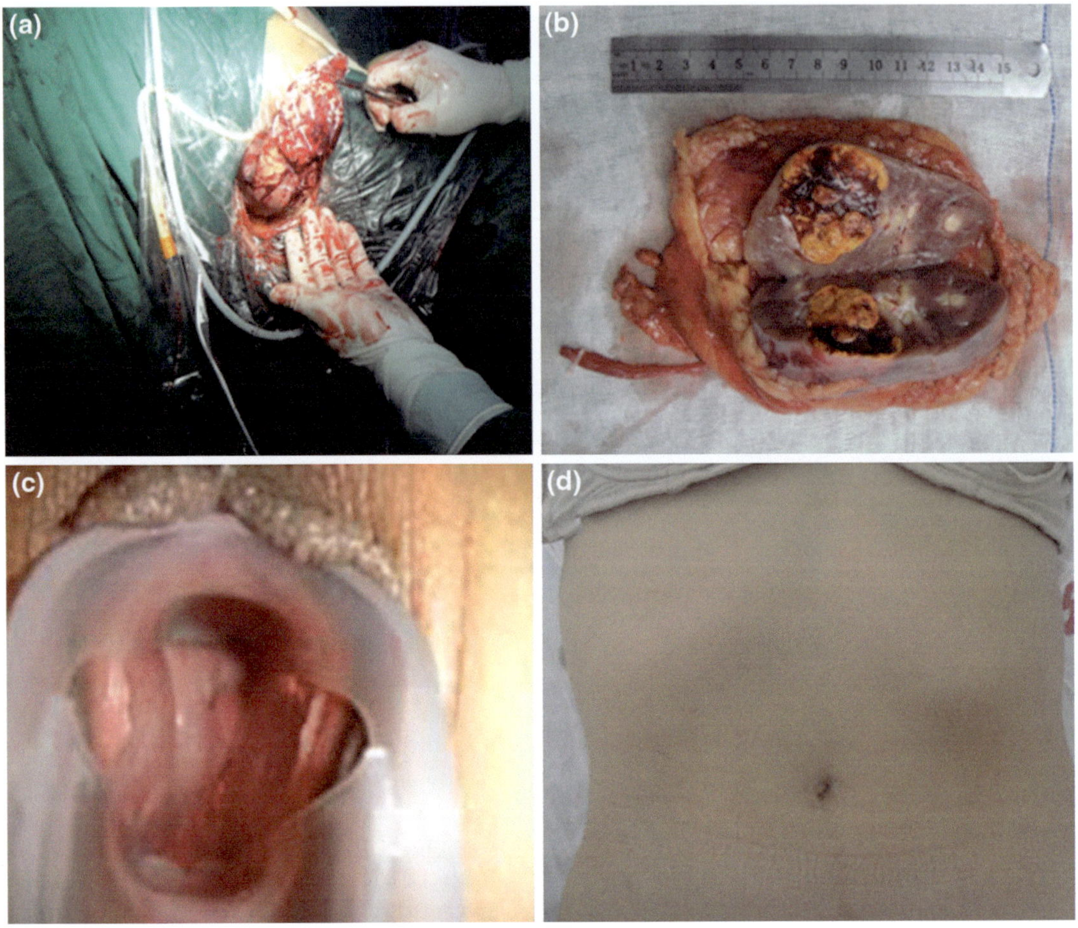

Fig. 23.4 **a** Specimen extraction through the vagina. **b** Intact excised specimen shows the lower-pole tumor. **c** Three-month postoperative appearance of posterior colpotomy incision. **d** Three-month postoperative appearance of umbilical incision. Reprinted with permission from Elsevier. Yijun Xue, Xiaofeng Zou, Guoxi Zhang, Yuanhu Yuan, Rihai Xiao, Yunfeng Liao, Xin Zhong, Bo Jiang, Ruiquan Xu, Yuhua Zou, Gang Xu, Kunlin Xie, Xu Zhang. Transvaginal Natural Orifice Translumenal Endoscopic Nephrectomy in a Series of 63 Cases: Stepwise Transition From Hybrid to Pure NOTES, *European Urology* 2015;68(2):302–310

- Fluid intake was encouraged to prevent constipation.
- Some light vaginal bleeding is expected and may continue for several days following the procedure. Occasionally (during the first week), patients may have an episode of heavy bleeding when the patients stand up or after urinating. If the bleeding is excessive (more than a menstrual period or completing soaks a large pad in 1 h), the patient should contact the physician. To promote healing and reduce the risk of infection, patients should not put anything in their vagina for the first 8–12 weeks until the tissues have had time to completely heal. This includes tampons and douches that involve the vagina. Complete sexual abstinence lasting 3 months was advised for all patients.
- Showers are permitted, but tub baths and swimming should be avoided until the incisions are healed.
- Patients are instructed to notify the doctor or go to the emergency department if any of the following happens: abdominal distention or pain;increased or bright red bleeding from the vagina;foul smelling vaginal flow;redness,

pus-like (yellow or green) discharge or swelling from the cuts;fever/chills with temperature over 38.5 °C.

Results

For hybrid transvaginal NOTES nephrectomy, the mean operative time was 105 min (range: 70–280 min), and the mean estimated blood loss was 80 ml (range: 30–800 ml). There were 19 intraoperative complications. Five patients were converted to open surgery. There were 15 postoperative complications:14 minor complications (Clavien 1–2) and 1 major complication (Clavien 3b, postoperative bleeding). The patient subsequently underwent exploratory laparotomy revealing a clip dislodgment from the gonadal vein. For pure transvaginal NOTES nephrectomy, the procedures were successfully performed in all patients without additional trocars except for one patient who experienced a rectal injury caused by a forceps during the placement of the Zou-Port, and immediate repair was performed. The patient was converted to suprapubic-assisted laparoendoscopic single-site surgery (SA-LESS) nephrectomy in which 5- and 10-mm trocars were inserted at the medial margin of the umbilicus through two separate incisions and a 10-mm trocar was inserted into the abdominal cavity below the pubic hairline. The technique for the SA-LESS is similar to that of the standard laparoscopy, with conventional instruments placed in the abdominal trocars, under direct vision achieved by a 5.4-mm flexible-tip laparoscope placed through the trocar below the pubic hairline [35]. The kidney specimen was removed after the incision below the pubic hairline was enlarged. Postoperative major complications included a right external iliac artery thrombosis on postoperative day 2, which was successfully treated by thrombus removal. This complication may be related to the patient's poor vascular condition, and the long-time compression and repeated friction injury of the vascular intima. There was no other intraoperative abdominal and pelvic organs injury. The mean operative time was 190 min (range: 160–320 min), and the mean estimated blood loss was 170 ml (range: 100–500 ml).

At a mean range follow-up of 51.8 (10–69) months, all the patients were in good condition. The posterior colpotomy incision healed well (Fig. 23.4c). The scars were nearly invisible on the abdominal wall (Fig. 23.4d). There were no infections, umbilical hernias, or uterine prolapse. All patients who underwent nephrectomy for malignant suspicion were alive without evidence of tumor recurrence or metastasis. One hundred and sixty eight patients completed the female sexual function index (FSFI) questionnaire, and analysis did not show any difference in FSFI scores before and after surgery.

Stepwise Transition from Hybrid to Pure Transvaginal NOTES Nephrectomy

Our transvaginal NOTES nephrectomy schedule has evolved as a stepwise process [36]. Prior to proceeding with NOTES in humans, we underwent extensive training in the animal laboratory to investigate operative safety and to prepare for transition to human clinical application. Different methods of peritoneal access were evaluated, and the transvaginal route was finally determined to be an ideal approach for nephrectomy. For our initial human experience, we performed five cases of transumbilical, multiport laparoscopic nephrectomy with intact specimen extraction through the vagina [37]. We think that this method is an effective technique by itself and an ideal way to train for the hybrid transvaginal NOTES technique. In our hybrid NOTES series, vaginal access was used to insert a laparoscope, and two umbilical trocars were used as main working ports. We then transitioned to a single umbilical trocar used for the laparoscope, with the transvaginal approach used for the majority of the dissection. Working toward pure transvaginal NOTES nephrectomy, we firstly performed pure transvaginal NOTES renal cyst decortication in 5 patients using extra-long pre-bent instruments [38]. Finally, we moved to a pure transvaginal NOTES nephrectomy. Based on our experience, we offer the following recommendations:

- This relatively slow and graded introduction of pure transvaginal NOTES nephrectomy into clinical practice is pragmatic, so this procedure can be explored safely.
- Highly judicious patient selection (thinner patients [BMI < 30] with limited prior abdominal surgery and favorable disease processes) is of utmost importance in the early phase of NOTES skill acquisition, to minimize complications and optimize surgical outcomes.
- In situations where there is lack of progression or other concerns about patient safety, the transition to at least standard laparoscopy is advisable.
- Triangulation is one of the fundamental concepts of laparoscopic surgery. NOTES seeks to decrease morbidity and improve cosmesis by placing all surgical instruments through a single transvisceral incision. This "in-line" placement of instruments invariably results in clashing, imprecise tissue handling, and retraction. We strongly recommend starting NOTES with regular and extensive practice in standard laparoscopy.

Conditions Necessary for Progression to Pure Transvaginal NOTES Nephrectomy

- Placement of a transvaginal port is a crucial first step.
- Gradually increasing the use of the transvaginal port for actual intraoperative steps, including mobilize/dissect colon and ureter, individually dissect/control renal artery and vein with clips, respectively, and mobilize kidney completely, must be performed.
- Preoperative mechanical bowel preparation is recommended for intestinal repair in case of an intestinal injury.
- The dissection of the cephalad aspect of the hilum and the upper pole is very challenging, because it is difficult to obtain the correct working angles. An additional problem is the considerable distance between the introitus and the upper pole of the kidney; the use of extra-long pre-bent or flexible instruments is required. Pre-shaped, rigid instruments with different profiles were introduced with the aim of minimizing instrument clashing outside the port, providing triangulation in the operative field and better force application at instrument tip during dissection. They are also cost-effective, because they are reusable compared to the single-use disposable flexible instruments.

Instrumentation

The flexible-tip laparoscope provided excellent visualization, even considering the atypical transvaginal perspective. This scope has a distally mounted image capture chip and a built-in light cable which gives the handle a streamlined profile compared to a typical rod-lens scope with a light cable connected at a 90° angle and a bulky image capture coupler which can interfere with the instrument handles being used in close proximity to the scope (Fig. 23.5a). The flexible forceps help with intracorporeal instrument triangulation and proper tissue retraction. The introduction of extra-long pre-bent instruments has the advantage of minimizing instrument clashing, providing triangulation in the operative field and better force distribution during dissection (Fig. 23.5b). Although these instruments have facilitated our pure transvaginal NOTES approach, they are still relatively laborious, with suboptimal ergonomics. Continuing refinement of instrumentation and, most importantly, development of purpose-specific robotic platforms may overcome current limitations of NOTES.

We developed a three-channel port for pure transvaginal NOTES nephrectomy procedures (Fig. 23.6a, b). Several aspects of the port

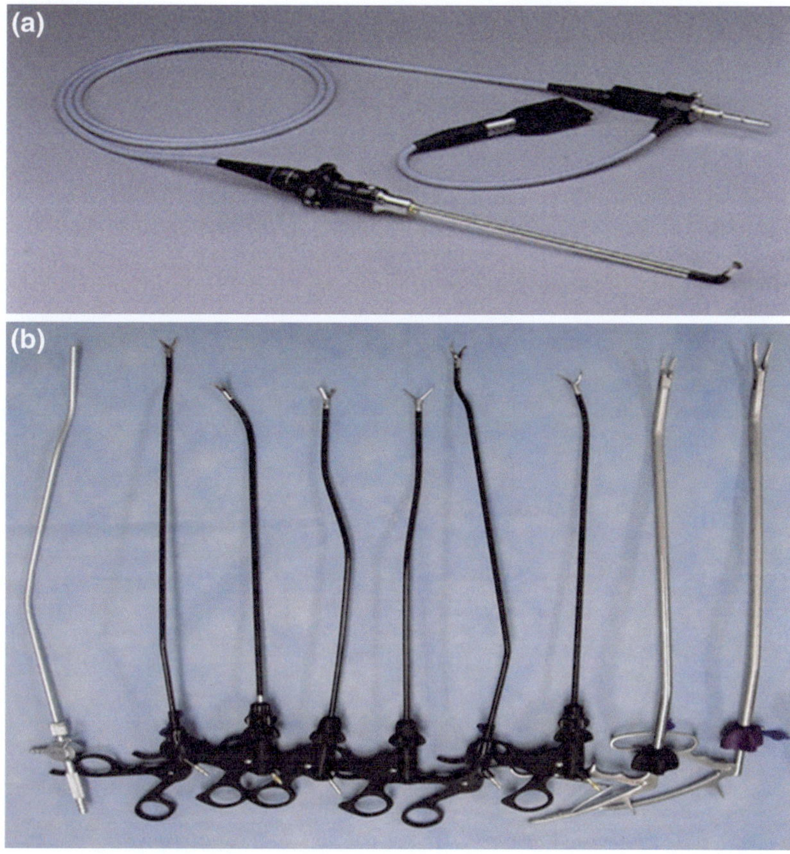

Fig. 23.5 **a** A flexible-tip 5.4-mm 0° laparoscope. **b** Extra-long flexible and pre-bent instruments for pure transvaginal NOTES nephrectomy. Reprinted with permission from Elsevier. Yijun Xue, Xiaofeng Zou, Guoxi Zhang, Yuanhu Yuan, Rihai Xiao, Yunfeng Liao, Xin Zhong, Bo Jiang, Ruiquan Xu, Yuhua Zou, Gang Xu, Kunlin Xie, Xu Zhang. Transvaginal Natural Orifice Translumenal Endoscopic Nephrectomy in a Series of 63 Cases: Stepwise Transition From Hybrid to Pure NOTES, *European Urology* 2015;68(2):302–310

deserve a special mention. It was long enough to bypass the pelvic organs once it was inserted transvaginally. This characteristic precluded the chance of pelvic organ injury during passage of the instruments toward the target organ. Moreover, the port material is elastomeric, and the original length is 25 cm, which can be trimmed with a knife depending on the individual anatomy.

Complications

Although the vagina seems to be an ideal portal of entry for NOTES nephrectomy, several reports have indicated that considerable morbidity can accompany this approach. In one case series of 102 transvaginal NOTES procedures [39], three major complications occurred, specifically rectal injury, omental bleeding, and abscess formation. In an international multicenter trial on NOTES (IMTN) registry [40], an overall complication rate of 6.9% (grade I–II: 5.33%; grade III–IV: 1.57%) was reported for 319 transvaginal NOTES patients. There were 40 complications (22.47%) in our NOTES nephrectomy, including 13 major complications (7.3%), which was similar to that of reported standard laparoscopic nephrectomy [41].

Postoperative Sexual Function

The effect of transvaginal NOTES on postoperative sexual function is a major concern. However, current literature suggests that sexual dysfunction is a rare event after vaginal surgery [39, 40]. Our experience confirmed this, because the satisfaction of the patients with the result of the operation was high, and no patient reported

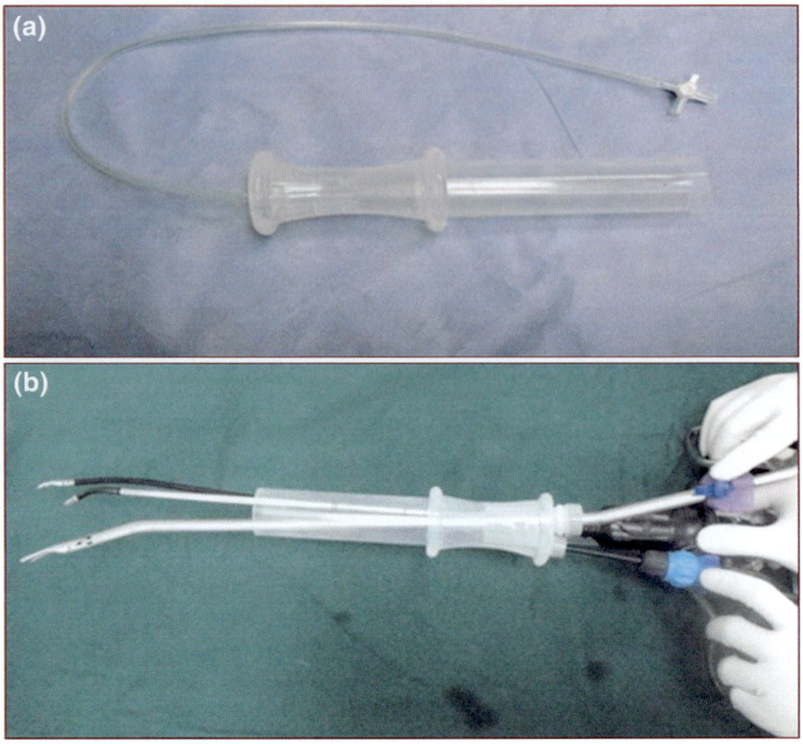

Fig. 23.6 **a** The self-developed three-channel Zou-port. **b** Mock intraoperative view of the three-channel Zou-port. Reprinted with permission from Elsevier. Yijun Xue, Xiaofeng Zou, Guoxi Zhang, Yuanhu Yuan, Rihai Xiao, Yunfeng Liao, Xin Zhong, Bo Jiang, Ruiquan Xu, Yuhua Zou, Gang Xu, Kunlin Xie, Xu Zhang. Transvaginal Natural Orifice Translumenal Endoscopic Nephrectomy in a Series of 63 Cases: Stepwise Transition From Hybrid to Pure NOTES, *European Urology* 2015;68(2):302–310

dyspareunia by a standardized questionnaire. This finding is consistent with a recently published study evaluating the short-term sexual function with the same FSFI questionnaire after transvaginal NOTES nephrectomy [42]. A previous study by Solomon et al. [43] may explain why female sexual function is not affected by a transvaginal procedure. These investigators showed that somatic vaginal innervation is concentrated distally and anteriorly along the vaginal walls, leaving the posterior fornix with sparse sensory innervations.

Recommendations and Conclusions

NOTES nephrectomy using the vagina as an entry point to the peritoneal cavity is very promising. With the development of new instruments and platforms that facilitate handling and stabilization of flexible endoscopes, the surgical approach has the potential to have broad clinical applications in the future.

References

1. Barker AE. Nephrectomy by abdominal section. Med Chir Trans. 1880;63:181–215.
2. Kerbl DC, McDougall EM, Clayman RV, et al. A history and evolution of laparoscopic nephrectomy: perspectives from the past and future directions in the surgical management of renal tumors. J Urol. 2011;185:1150–4.
3. Kobiela J, Stefaniak T, Mackowiak M, et al. NOTES-third generation surgery. Vain hopes or the reality of tomorrow? Langenbecks Arch Surg. 2008;393:405–11.
4. Breda G, Silvestre P, Giunta A, Xaus D, Tamai A, Gherardi L. Laparoscopic nephrectomy with vaginal delivery of the intact kidney. Eur Urol. 1993;24:116–7.
5. Gill IS, Cherullo EE, Meraney AM, et al. Vaginal extraction of the intact specimen following laproscopic radical nephrectomy. J Urol. 2002;167:238–41.
6. Matthes D, Menke P, Koheler M, Nieman W, Brugge J, Hochberg. Feasibility of endoscopic transgastric (ETGN) and transvaginal (ETVN) nephrectomy. Gastrointest Endosc. 2007;65:AB290.
7. Gettman MT, Lotan T, Nappa CA, et al. Transvaginal laparoscopic nephrectomy: development and feasibility in the porcine model. Urology. 2002;59:446–50.

8. Bazzi WM, Wagner O, Stroup SP, et al. Transrectal hybrid natural orifice transluminal endoscopic surgery (NOTES) nephrectomy in a porcine model. Urology. 2011;77:518–23.
9. Baldwin DD, Tenggardjaja C, Bowman R, et al. Hybrid transureteral natural orifice translumenal endoscopic nephrectomy: a feasibility study in the porcine model. J Endourol. 2011;25:245–50.
10. Lima E, Rolanda C, Pego JM, et al. Transvesical endoscopic peritoneoscopy: a novel 5 mm port for intra-abdominal scarless surgery. J Urol. 2006;176:802–5.
11. Lima E, Rolanda C, Pego JM, et al. Third-generation nephrectomy by natural orifice transluminal endoscopic surgery. J Urol. 2007;178:2648–54.
12. Clayman RV, Box GN, Abraham JB, et al. Rapid communication: transvaginal single-port NOTES nephrectomy: initial laboratory experience. J Endourol. 2007;6:640–4.
13. Box GN, Lee HJ, Santos RJ, et al. Rapid communication: robot-assisted NOTES nephrectomy: initial report. J Endourol. 2008;22:503–6.
14. Isariyawongse JP, McGee MF, Rosen MJ, et al. Pure natural orifice transluminal endoscopic surgery (NOTES) nephrectomy using standard laparoscopic instruments in the porcine model. J Endourol. 2008;22:1087–91.
15. Haber GP, Brethauer S, Crouzet S, et al. Pure natural orifice transluminal endoscopic surgery for transvaginal nephrectomy in the porcine model. BJU Int. 2009;104:1260–4.
16. Raman JD, Bergs RA, Fernandez R, et al. Complete transvaginal NOTES nephrectomy using magnetically anchored instrumentation. J Endourol. 2009;23:367–71.
17. Perretta S, Allemann P, Asakuma M, et al. Feasibility of right and left transvaginal retroperitoneal nephrectomy: from the porcine to the cadaver model. J Endourol. 2009;23:1887–92.
18. Aron M, Berger AK, Stein RJ, et al. Transvaginal nephrectomy with a multichannel laparoscopic port: a cadaver study. BJU Int. 2009;103:1537–41.
19. Sánchez-Margallo FM, Pérez FJ, Sánchez MA, et al. Transvaginal NOTES-assisted laparoscopic nephrectomy: a survival study in a sheep model. Surg Endosc. 2012;26:926–32.
20. Lima E, Branco F, Parente J, et al. Transvesical natural orifice transluminal endoscopic surgery (NOTES) nephrectomy with kidney morcellation: a proof of concept study. BJU Int. 2012;109:1533–7.
21. Bazzi WM, Stroup SP, Cohen SA, et al. Feasibility of transrectal hybrid natural orifice transluminal endoscopic surgery (NOTES) nephrectomy in the cadaveric model. Urology. 2012;80:590–5.
22. Eyraud R, Laydner H, Autorino R, et al. Robot-assisted transrectal hybrid natural orifice translumenal endoscopic surgery nephrectomy and adrenalectomy: initial investigation in a cadaver model. Urology. 2013;81:1090–4.
23. Zeltser IS, Bergs R, Fernandez R, et al. Single trocar laparoscopic nephrectomy using magnetic anchoring and guidance system in the porcine model. J Urol. 2007;178:288–91.
24. Branco AW, Branco Filho AJ, Kondo W, et al. Hybrid transvaginal nephrectomy. Eur Urol. 2008;53:1290–4.
25. Alcaraz A, Peri L, Molina A, et al. Feasibility of transvaginal NOTES-assisted laparoscopic nephrectomy. Eur Urol. 2010;57:233–7.
26. Kaouk JH, White WM, Goel RK, et al. NOTES transvaginal nephrectomy: first human experience. Urology. 2009;74:5–8.
27. Porpiglia F, Fiori C, Morra I, et al. Transvaginal natural orifice transluminal endoscopic surgery-assisted minilaparoscopic nephrectomy: a step towards scarless surgery. Eur Urol. 2011;60:862–6.
28. Sotelo R, de Andrade R, Fernandez G, et al. NOTES hybrid transvaginal radical nephrectomy for tumor: stepwise progression toward a first successful clinical case. Eur Urol. 2010;57:138–44.
29. Alcaraz A, Musquera M, Peri L, et al. Feasibility of transvaginal natural orifice transluminal endoscopic surgery-assisted living donor nephrectomy: is kidney vaginal delivery the approach of the future? Eur Urol. 2011;59:1019–25.
30. Kaouk JH, Khalifeh A, Laydner H, et al. Transvaginal hybrid natural orifice transluminal surgery robotic donor nephrectomy: first clinical application. Urology. 2012;80:1171–5.
31. Kaouk JH, Haber GP, Goel RK, et al. Pure natural orifice translumenal endoscopic surgery (NOTES) transvaginal nephrectomy. Eur Urol. 2010;57: 723–6.
32. Hagen ME, Wagner OJ, Inan I, et al. Robotic single-incision transabdominal and transvaginal surgery: initial experience with intersecting robotic arms. Int J Med Robot. 2010;6:251–5.
33. Laydner H, Autorino R, Isac W, et al. Robotic retroperitoneal transvaginal natural orifice translumenal endoscopic surgery (NOTES) nephrectomy: feasibility study in a cadaver model. Urology. 2013;81:1232–7.
34. Nunns D, Williamson K, Swaney L, et al. The morbidity of surgery and adjuvant radiotherapy in the management of endometrial carcinoma. Int J Gynecol Cancer. 2000;10:233–8.
35. Zou X, Zhang G, Xue Y, et al. Suprapubic-assisted laparoendoscopic single-site surgery (LESS) in urology: our experience. BJU Int. 2013;112:92–8.
36. Xue Y, Zou X, Zhang G, et al. Transvaginal natural orifice transluminal endoscopic nephrectomy in a series of 63 cases: stepwise transition from hybrid to pure NOTES. Eur Urol. 2015;68:302–10.
37. Zou X, Zhang G, Xue Y, et al. Transumbilical multiport laparoscopic nephrectomy with specimen extraction through the vagina. Urol Int. 2014;92:407–13.

38. Zou X, Zhang G, Yuan Y, et al. Pure transvaginal natural orifice translumenal endoscopic surgery for renal cyst decortication: report of initial five cases. Int J Urol. 2014;21:64–8.
39. Wood SG, Panait L, Duffy AJ, et al. Complications of transvaginal natural orifice transluminal endoscopic surgery: a series of 102 patients. Ann Surg. 2013;259:744–9.
40. Zorron R, Palanivelu C, Galvão Neto MP, et al. International multicenter trial on clinical natural orifice surgery-NOTES IMTN study: preliminary results of 362 patients. Surg Innov. 2010;17:142–58.
41. Xu H, Ding Q, Jiang HW, et al. Fewer complications after laparoscopic nephrectomy as compared to the open procedure with the modified Clavien classification system-a retrospective analysis from southern China. World J Surg Oncol. 2014;12:4097–106.
42. Peri L, Musquera M, Vilaseca A, et al. Perioperative outcome and female sexual function after laparoscopic transvaginal NOTES-assisted nephrectomy. World J Urol. 2015. Doi:10.1007/s00345-015-1573-9.
43. Solomon D, Lentz R, Duffy AJ, et al. Female sexual function after pure transvaginal appendectomy: a cohort study. J Gastrointest Surg. 2012;16:183–7.

Index

Note: Page numbers followed by *f* and *t* indicate figures and tables respectively

J.R. Romanelli et al. (eds.), *NOTES and Endoluminal Surgery*, Clinical Gastroenterology, DOI 10.1007/978-3-319-50610-4

O

P

MIX
Papier aus verantwortungsvollen Quellen
Paper from responsible sources
FSC® C105338

If you have any concerns about our products,
you can contact us on
ProductSafety@springernature.com

In case Publisher is established outside the EU,
the EU authorized representative is:
Springer Nature Customer Service Center GmbH
Europaplatz 3, 69115 Heidelberg, Germany

Printed by Libri Plureos GmbH
in Hamburg, Germany